Experimenting in the Hearing and Speech Sciences

Experimenting in the Hearing and Speech Sciences

Barry Voroba, Ph.D.
Director of Auditory Research & Education
Starkey Laboratories, Inc.

 Starkey Laboratories Inc., Eden Prairie, Minnesota

Library of Congress
Catalog Card Number 78-63106

ISBN 0-9601970-0-1 (3-ring binder)
ISBN 0-9601970-1-X (Soft cover edition)
ISBN 0-9601970-2-8 (Hard cover edition)

©1978 by Starkey Laboratories Inc.
  6700 Washington Avenue
  Eden Prairie, Minnesota 55344

All rights reserved. This book is protected by copyright. No part of this book may be reproduced in any translation, form or by any means, including photocopying, or utilized by any information storage and retrieval system without written permission from the copyright owner.

Printed in the United States of America

Table of Contents

CONTENTS v
PREFACE viii
ACKNOWLEDGMENTS ix
**PART I — LABORATORY INSTRUMENTATION:
PRINCIPLES AND FUNCTIONS** 1
  SIMPLE HARMONIC MOTION 3
    Sine Wave Generators 5
  THE CONCEPT OF PHASE 5
    Phase Controls 5
    Phase Test Monitor 6
  INTRODUCTION TO THE DECIBEL 6
  WORKING WITH DECIBELS 8
  THE CONCEPT OF ZERO DECIBELS 9
  DECIBELS OF GAIN 9
    Attenuators 10
    Monitor Level Meter 11
  COMBINING SIGNALS TO FORM COMPLEX SOUNDS 11
    Mixer-Amplifiers 12
  PERIODIC COMPLEX SOUNDS 12
    "Buzz" Generator 13
  APERIODIC COMPLEX SOUNDS (NOISE) 13
    Noise Generator 14
  BASIC CONCEPTS OF FILTERING 15
    Filter Operation 17
  SWITCHING OF SIGNALS 18
    Programmable Electronic Gates 19
    Digital Event Programmer 19
    Entering Commands 20
    Special Programmer Functions 20
    Probability Gating 22
  STIMULI AMPLIFICATION AND TRANSDUCTION 22
    Input Preamplifiers 22
    Output Amplifiers 23
    Bone Vibrator Amplifier 24
  OUTPUT LIMITATION 24
    Adjustable Peak Clipper 25
    Automatic Gain Control 25

PART II—DEMONSTRATIONS AND EXPERIMENTS.................27
  I. FUNDAMENTAL CONCEPTS............................29
    I-1: Law of Superposition (Interference)..............30
    I-2: Fourier's Theorem...............................32
    I-3: Quality of Synthesized Complex Waves............34
    I-4: Peak, Average, and RMS Amplitude of Signals.....36
    I-5: Reduction of Acoustic Feedback..................38
  II. THRESHOLD OF AUDIBILITY..........................41
    II-1: Psychometric Function for Human Hearing........42
    II-2: Yes-No Procedure...............................44
    II-3: Receiver Operating Characteristic...............46
    II-4: Adaptive Test Procedures.......................48
    II-5: Two Interval Forced Choice Procedure...........50
    II-6: Hearing Threshold Levels and the Audiometer....52
    II-7: The Occlusion Effect...........................54
    II-8: Cancellation of Bone Conducted Sound...........56
  III. INTENSITY AND LOUDNESS..........................59
    III-1: The Differential Threshold for Intensity......60
    III-2: Pedestal Experiments (The SISI Test)..........62
    III-3: Equal Loudness Contours.......................64
    III-4: The Sone Scale................................66
    III-5: The Psychophysical Power Law..................68
    III-6: Alternate Binaural Loudness Balancing.........70
    III-7: "Recruitment" in Normal Ears..................72
    III-8: The Relationship Between Intensity and Pitch..74
  IV. FREQUENCY AND PITCH..............................77
    IV-1: Ohm's Acoustic Law.............................78
    IV-2: Objective Beats................................80
    IV-3: Consonance, Dissonance, and Musical Intervals..82
    IV-4: Combination Tones..............................84
    IV-5: Pitch of Complex Tones
        ("The Case of the Missing Fundamental")..........86
    IV-6: The Relationship Between Frequency and Pitch...88
    IV-7: The JND for Frequency..........................90
    IV-8: The Effects of Phase on the Pitch of a Complex Sound........92
  V. AUDITORY TEMPORALITY..............................95
    V-1: Waveform Duration and Perceived Tonality........96
    V-2: The Rise and Fall of Waveforms..................98
    V-3: Temporal Integration...........................100
    V-4: Flutter Fusion.................................102
    V-5: Acoustic Temporal Order........................104
    V-6: Auditory Numerosity............................106
    V-7: Differential Sensitivity for Duration..........108
  VI. MASKING PHENOMENA...............................111
    VI-1: Tone-on-Tone Masking..........................112
    VI-2: The Critical Band.............................114

VI-3: The Relationship Between Masking Level and Threshold Shift..116
VI-4: Central Masking..118
VI-5: Forward and Backward Masking..........................120
VI-6: Pulsation Threshold (The "Continuity Effect")..........122
VI-7: Two-Tone Suppression..................................124

VII. BINAURAL HEARING..127
VII-1: Binaural Summation...................................128
VII-2: Binaural Fusion of Pulsed Stimuli....................130
VII-3: Time-Intensity Tradeoff in Lateralization............132
VII-4: The Stereophonic Effect..............................134
VII-5: The Precedence Effect................................136
VII-6: Binaural Beats.......................................138
VII-7: Masking Level Differences............................140
VII-8: The JND for Dichotic Phase...........................142
VII-9: Interaural Attenuation of Air Conduction Signals.....144

VIII. SPEECH PERCEPTION..147
VIII- 1: Synthetic Vowels...................................148
VIII- 2: The Electrolarynx..................................150
VIII- 3: The Performance-Intensity Function.................152
VIII- 4: The Perception of Low Pass and High Pass Filtered Speech...154
VIII- 5: Binaural Alternation of Speech.....................156
VIII- 6: Symmetrical Peak Clipping of Speech and Pure Tones...158
VIII- 7: Minimizing Peak Clipping Distortion................160
VIII- 8: Asymmetric Peak Clipping...........................162
VIII- 9: "Center Clipping" of Speech (Crossover Distortion)...164
VIII-10: Intelligibility of Dichotically Filtered Speech....166
VIII-11: The Intelligibility of Interrupted Speech..........168
VIII-12: The Transfer Functions for Input and Output Compression Systems...170
VIII-13: AGC and Dynamic Signals............................172
VIII-14: Oscilloscopic Speech Displays......................174

APPENDIX..177
INDEX...191

Preface

Sophisticated laboratory instrumentation and techniques have become an indispensible part of professional activities in the Hearing, Speech, and Psychological Sciences. The study of auditory and acoustic phenomena is another ongoing and common concern to the diverse areas of specialization within these three broad disciplines.

This text and the Hearing Science Laboratory system were developed by the author to meet the growing needs of researchers, educators, clinical practitioners, and their students for new literature and equipment to pursue their respective endeavors.

Part one of this book deals with introductory concepts in physical acoustics as well as the electronic generation and processing of sound stimuli. The function and operation of each module in the Hearing Science Laboratory system is also described in this section.

The balance and bulk of this text takes the form of a compendium of 66 experiments and demonstrations that can be performed with the Hearing Science Laboratory or, in many instances, with familiar laboratory electronic devices that may be available to the reader. Each experiment includes: a general statement of purpose; background principles and information regarding the phenomena under investigation; procedures, block diagrams, and wiring guides necessary for implementing the listening tasks; questions and exercises for student consideration; and a selected bibliography of historical and current references.

As indicated in the Table of Contents, the diverse experimental topics have been organized into eight general areas of study that can provide the educator with the syllabus and supporting textual material suitable for coursework in the auditory and instrumentation sciences. It was the author's intention that this text would provide the reader with an introduction and overview to a wide range of classical and contemporary research issues and serve as a reference source and "springboard" for further investigation and experimentation by the interested student and professional. The supplementary blank experiment format sheets which are included in the appendix to the book should prove useful for recording student ideas and experimental designs for research studies.

Acknowledgments

I am indebted to many people for their enthusiastic support and technical contributions to this ambitious project. I wish to acknowledge the engineering and graphics department of Starkey Laboratories for their help in making the Hearing Science Laboratory system and this text a reality. In particular I wish to thank Messrs. W. C. Ausman, A. A. Beex, W. A. Johnson, K. G. Nybakke, D. A. Preves, and C. W. Reynolds for their talented assistance. My appreciation is also extended to Mrs. R. D. Nemitz and Mrs. E. B. Shapiro for their help in the typing and organization of the manuscript. I am most grateful to Patrick W. Moore and Vergal J. Buescher for their excellent renderings of the many illustrations and graphics that were chosen for this text. My thanks also go to the authors and publishers who graciously gave permission for the use of those illustrations cited in this book.

I would like to pay special tribute to my close friend and colleague, Dr. Mitchell B. Kramer, whose editorial expertise and counsel I so treasure. The innumerable comments and criticisms that arose from his most diligent and painstaking review of the evolving manuscript have surely enhanced the accuracy and value of this book.

Finally, I wish to express my deepest gratitude to my wife Sue Ann for her unflagging patience and loving support during the long and arduous development period of this entire enterprise. She has always encouraged and shared my dreams.

Barry Voroba

Laboratory Instrumentation: Principles and Functions

Part I

Laboratory Instrumentation: Principles and Functions

SIMPLE HARMONIC MOTION

Sound is one form of physical energy which bombards us every moment of our lives. *Physical Acoustics* is that branch of science which deals with the nature and behavior of sound in different environments. The hearing sciences of *Psychoacoustics* and *Audiology* are concerned with the human response to sound. The subjective perceptions of listeners to a wide variety of sound stimuli have revealed much about the fundamental nature of the normal and impaired human hearing process.

All sounds are produced by vibrating objects which create physical disturbances in the surrounding environment or *sound medium.* Consider, for example, the sequence of events which occurs when a tuning fork in air is struck and its tines are set into motion. Because solid substances possess a natural tendency to retain their original shapes, the tuning fork tines will spring back and forth, or *oscillate,* from their resting positions in a manner known as *simple harmonic motion.* These vibrations will continue so long as the energy imparted to the tuning fork is sufficient to do the work of

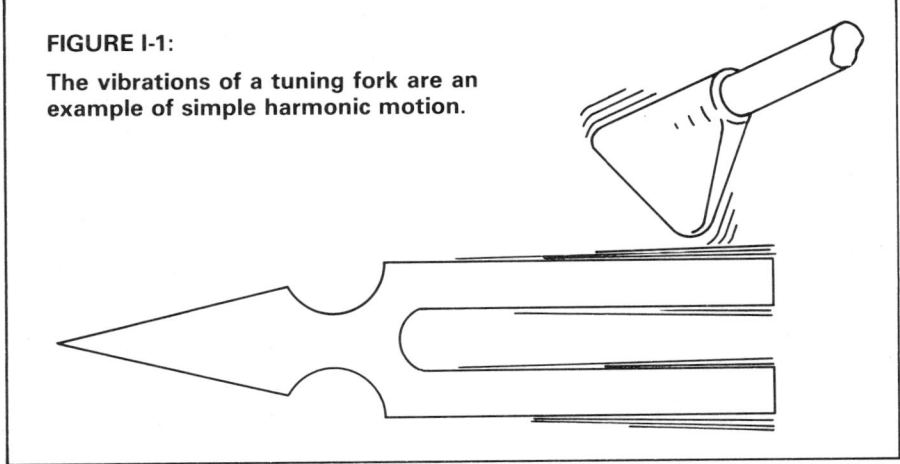

FIGURE I-1:

The vibrations of a tuning fork are an example of simple harmonic motion.

displacing the tines (see Figure I-1). The air molecules which surround the tuning fork are normally in a state of incessant and random motion prior to the physical disturbance caused by the vibrating tuning fork. These molecules are constantly colliding with the surfaces of any containers

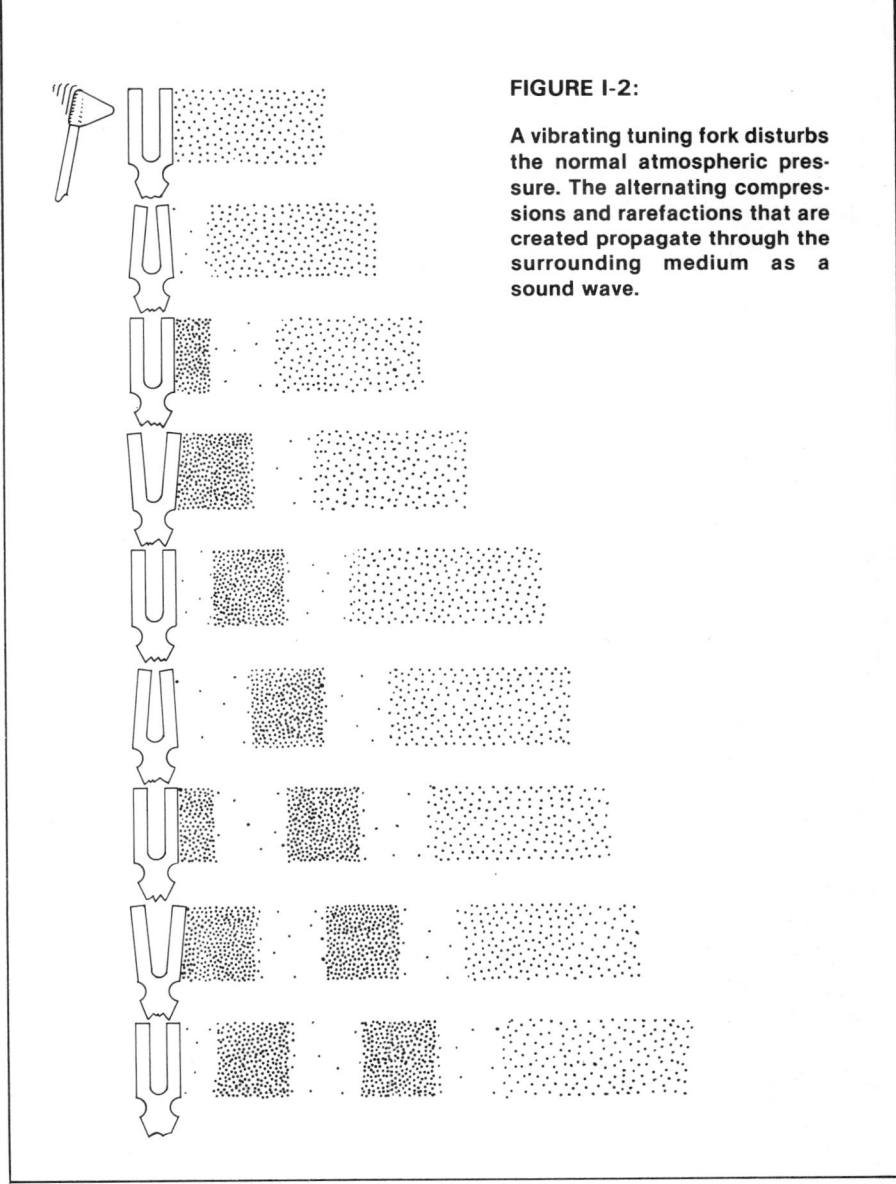

FIGURE I-2:

A vibrating tuning fork disturbs the normal atmospheric pressure. The alternating compressions and rarefactions that are created propagate through the surrounding medium as a sound wave.

which may enclose them and with every other material object they encounter, including each other. It is this bombardment and interaction between molecules and their surrounding surfaces that produce the *ambient*, or normal, background air pressure. Each outward movement of a tuning fork tine will crowd a greater than normal amount of air molecules into the adjacent volume of space, creating a *compression*, or higher than ambient pressure zone. When the tines move inward, the adjacent volume of space will contain less than the normal number of air molecules and form a relatively low-pressure condition called a *rarefaction*. Individual molecules will, in turn, imitate the behavior of the tuning fork tines and disturb their neighboring particles. This results in a kind of chain reaction that conveys or *propagates* the alternating compressions and rarefactions through the medium. We call this traveling disturbance a sound wave. Several stages in this process are illustrated in Figure I-2. A number of fundamental properties or *measures* of sound waves may be revealed by tracing the tuning fork vibrations over time onto graph paper. The back and forth vibrations of the fork produce a line whose vertical dimension or *amplitude* reveals the displacement of a tine from its original resting position (see Figure I-3A). The *peak amplitude*, or maximum displacement in either direction, as well as the total *peak-to-peak amplitude* are two common examples of the measures used to describe the magnitude of the wave (see the upcoming section dealing with attenuators and Laboratory Experiment I-4 for more details about these and other sound magnitude measurements).

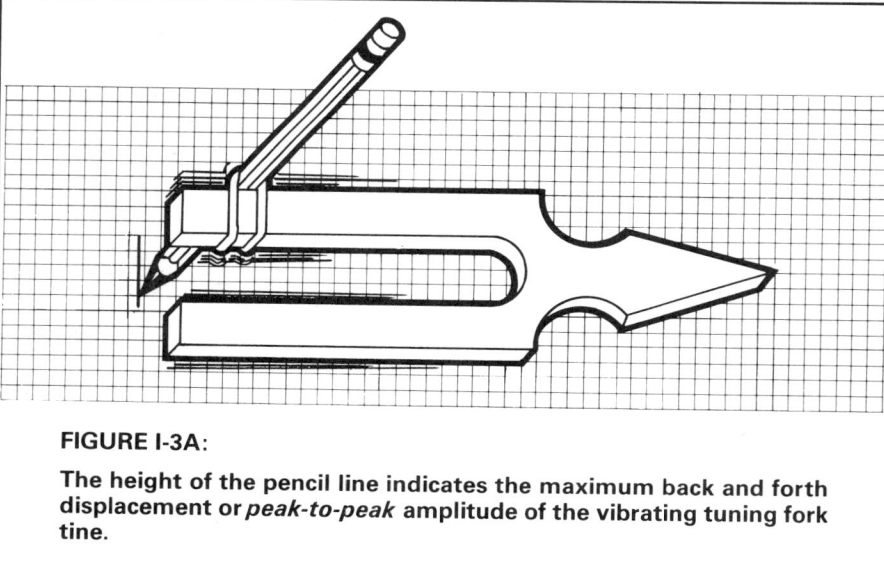

FIGURE I-3A:
The height of the pencil line indicates the maximum back and forth displacement or *peak-to-peak* amplitude of the vibrating tuning fork tine.

It takes a certain amount of time for the tuning fork to execute one complete repetition, or *cycle*, of its motion. This duration is known as the *period* of the wave and may be described by the term *seconds per cycle*. Conversely, the number of cycles that occur per second is called the repetition rate or *frequency* of the sound wave. The term *cycles per second* is now more commonly replaced by an equivalent unit called the *hertz (Hz)*. Because the period and frequency of a wave share such an *inverse* or *reciprocal* relationship with each other, we can easily determine the value of one measure from its counterpart. A sound of 1000 cycles per second, or 1000 hertz, would, for example, have a period of 1/1000th of a second (1 millisecond) per cycle.

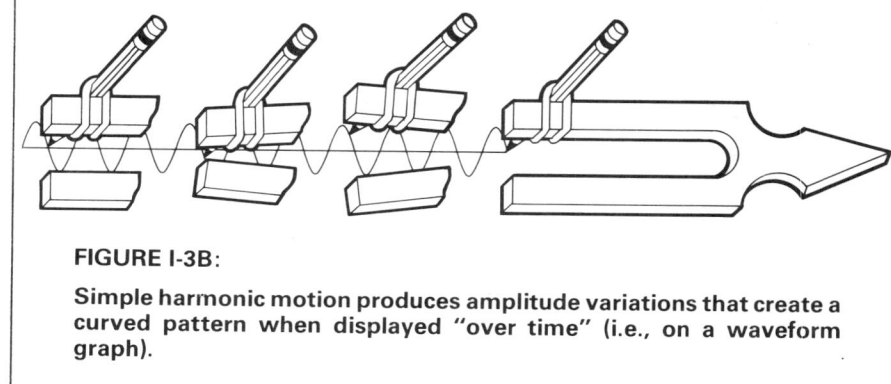

$$\text{Frequency} = \frac{1}{\text{Period}}; \text{ expressed in hertz or cycles per second}$$

$$\text{Period} = \frac{1}{\text{Frequency}}; \text{ expressed in seconds per cycle}$$

Note in Figure I-3B that sliding the tuning fork across the paper creates a curved pattern whose amplitude changes from moment to moment. A display which shows changes in the magnitude of an event as time passes is called a *waveform graph*. Consider a circle uniformly rotating, as shown in Figure I-3C. Changes in amplitude, identical to those of the tuning fork

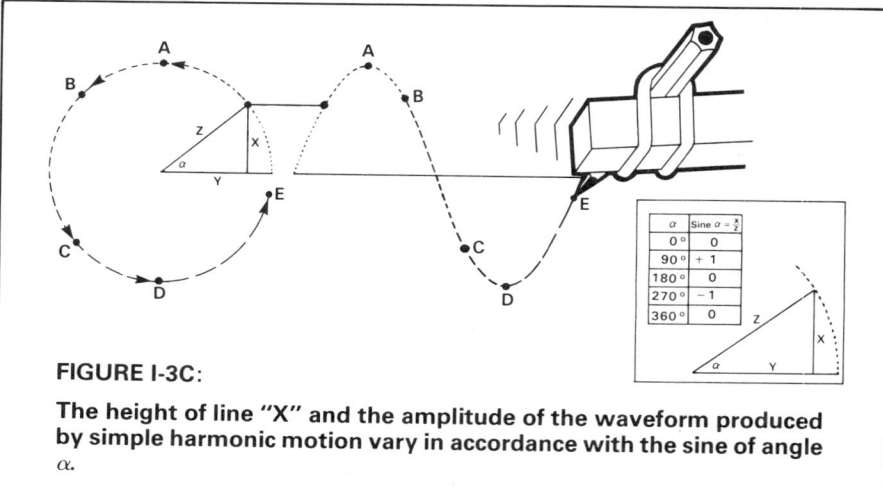

FIGURE I-3B:
Simple harmonic motion produces amplitude variations that create a curved pattern when displayed "over time" (i.e., on a waveform graph).

tine, occur in the vertical height of a line dropped to the horizontal axis from a point on the circumference of this circle. Note that at each instant in time, a different triangle will be formed by the changing vertical line, the rotating radius of the circle, and the horizontal axis. The numerical value of the *sine* of angle (α) varies from +1 to −1 as the radius of the circle rotates

FIGURE I-3C:
The height of line "X" and the amplitude of the waveform produced by simple harmonic motion vary in accordance with the sine of angle α.

from zero through 360 degrees. Because of this link to the mathematical sine function, the graphic patterns that can be produced by simple harmonic motion are called *sinusoids*, or *sine waves*. The sounds produced by objects vibrating with simple harmonic motion are often called *pure tones* and comprise some of the most commonly used sound stimuli in hearing science.

LABORATORY INSTRUMENTATION: PRINCIPLES AND FUNCTIONS

FIGURE I-4:

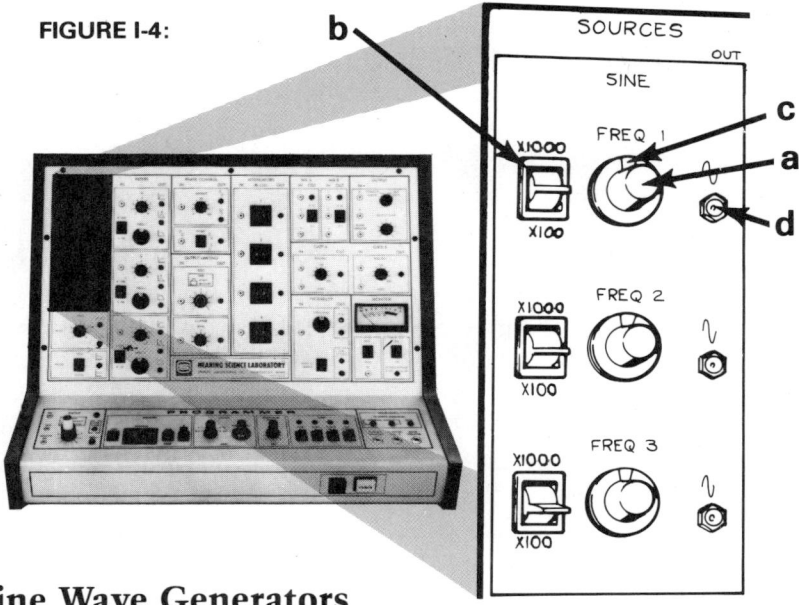

Sine Wave Generators

The three Sine Wave Generators on the Hearing Science Laboratory are shown in Figure I-4. Each module produces a sinusoidal signal having a uniform magnitude at all operating frequencies. Stimulus frequencies from 100 to 10,000 hertz may be selected by adjusting the Frequency Control Knob (I-4a) and Range Switch (I-4b). Multiplying the number which appears in the Control Dial Window (I-4c) by the Range Switch setting value will provide a guide to the test tone frequency. When more precise calibration is called for, an external frequency counter or calibrated oscilloscope should be employed. The output from each Sine Wave Generator emerges from the black Output Jack (I-4d) to the right of the Frequency Control Knob and may be routed to the input of any other laboratory module by means of a single patch cord.

THE CONCEPT OF PHASE

The various points in time or place on a sine wave are often described in terms of the angles associated with circular or simple harmonic motion. Figure I-5, for example, shows that the quarter, half, three-quarter, and full-period landmarks on the sine wave correspond, respectively, to the 90, 180, 270, and 360 (or zero) degree angles formed by a radius at various positions within the circle. These so called *phase angles* may also be used to compare and relate corresponding points on different waves. Consider, for example, the two sine waves shown in Figure I-6A, which possess identical frequencies and amplitudes. If both signals start at the same instant in time, each point on one wave will remain exactly in step with corresponding points on the second wave. The two sinusoids are said to be *in phase* with each other (i.e., they share a zero-degrees phase relationship). If, however, one wave is allowed to complete half a cycle before the start of the second stimulus, corresponding points on the two waves will always be one half period, or 180 degrees, *out of phase* with each other (see Figure I-6B). Intermediate phase relationships ranging between zero and 360 degrees are also possible (see examples shown in Figure I-6C). In the up-

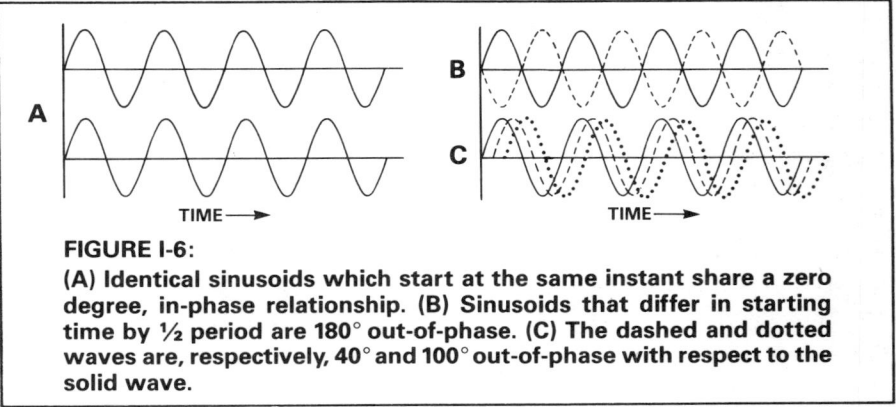

FIGURE I-6:
(A) Identical sinusoids which start at the same instant share a zero degree, in-phase relationship. (B) Sinusoids that differ in starting time by ½ period are 180° out-of-phase. (C) The dashed and dotted waves are, respectively, 40° and 100° out-of-phase with respect to the solid wave.

coming section on mixers, we shall consider how the particular phase relationship that exists between test signals affects the total sound magnitude produced by the waves. The effects of phase upon a listener's ability to detect sound and perceive changes in its quality and location in space are considered in several experiments in this text.

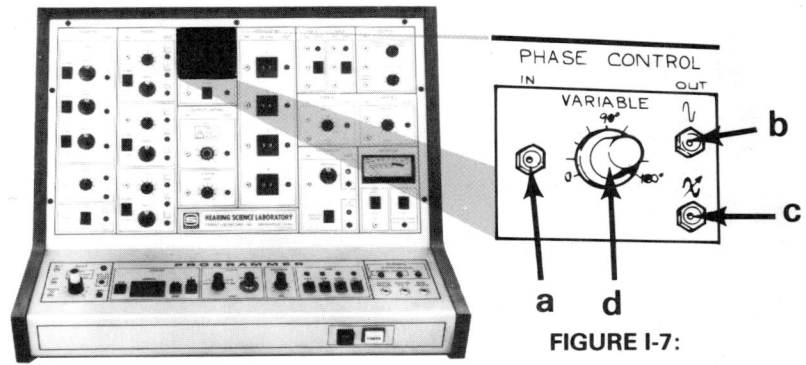

FIGURE I-7:

Phase Controls

Two types of phase control are possible with the Hearing Science Laboratory. A pure tone signal that is routed to the Input Jack of the Variable Phase Shifter (Figure I-7a) will produce two signals at the black Output Jacks of the device (Figure I-7b, c). The upper, Reference Phase Output Jack (I-7b), will provide the same frequency and magnitude tone as the original input signal. The lower, Variable Phase Output Jack (I-7c), will contain a phase shifted version of the signal at the reference jack. By adjusting the Phase Shift Control Knob (Figure I-7d), it is possible to continuously vary the phase relationship between the reference and phase shift output signals between zero and 180 degrees. (Note: When any complex input signal is used, such as speech or noise, the same number of degrees of phase shift will be applied to those component frequencies which lie between 100 and

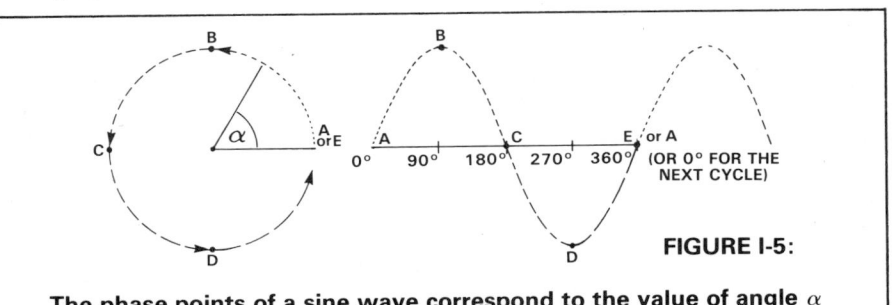

FIGURE I-5:

The phase points of a sine wave correspond to the value of angle α which changes during uniform circular motion.

6 EXPERIMENTING IN THE HEARING AND SPEECH SCIENCES

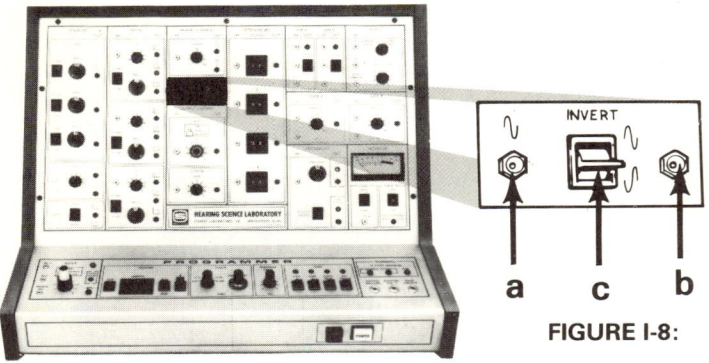

FIGURE I-8:

6000 hertz.) A second type of phase control is provided by the Phase Inverter module (Figure I-8). Any signal delivered to the white Input Jack (I-8a) of this device will appear at the Output Jack (I-8b) as either an exact replica of the input or a phase inverted, "mirror image" signal which has had each component frequency phase shifted by 180 degrees. The position of the Phase Reversal Switch (I-8c) determines whether or not the signal will be inverted at the Output Jack. Specifically, the upper switch position is for the non-inverting mode; the lower switch setting is for the inverting condition.

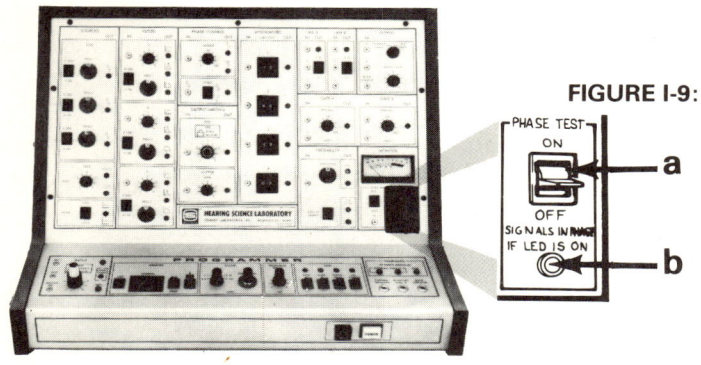

FIGURE I-9:

Phase Test Monitor

The Phase Test Monitor (Figure I-9), located at the lower right hand corner of the front panel, provides confirmation of whether the electrical signals delivered to either two headphones or loudspeakers are zero degrees in phase or 180 degrees out of phase. When the Phase Test Switch (I-9a) is in the "on" position, the red *light-emitting diode (LED)* (I-9b) will flash briefly and then remain on if the signals are in phase or flash and stay off if the signals are out of phase. If the two signals share a phase relationship other than zero or 180 degrees, the phase test light will pulsate on and off continually. Random light flashes can be prevented by setting the Phase Test Switch to the "off" position, which disengages the circuit.

INTRODUCTION TO THE DECIBEL

The exact nature of any sinusoid can be totally defined by specifying its magnitude plus its frequency and phase relationship to other signals. The most common measures of sound magnitude are *power*, *intensity*, and *pressure*. While people tend to use these terms interchangeably in everyday parlance, their scientific definitions and units are quite different.

Consider, for example, the softest 1000 hertz tone that a normal human listener can typically detect. It may be described as having either an intensity of 0.0000000000000001 *watt per square centimeter (W/cm²)* or a sound pressure of 20 *micropascals (μPa)*. At the opposite end of the scale of human sensitivity to sound, we find that signals having intensities near 0.01 watt per square centimeter, equivalent to pressures of 200,000,000 micropascals, can cause considerable pain to a listener. The range of sound magnitudes lying between the limits of detectability and pain is called the *dynamic range* of hearing. Our senses are remarkable in that this range encompasses a physical ratio of 100 trillion to one for sound intensities and 10 million to one for sound pressures! It would be extremely awkward to represent such a wide range of numbers on a graph scale having equidistant lines representing equal increments in sound magnitude (i.e., on so called *arithmetic* or *linear* ruled graph paper). Indeed, a very large piece of paper would have to be used in order to accommodate the many millions of line markings needed to display the entire dynamic range of hearing. When dealing with such large ranges of numerical values, scientists employ scales upon which each division represents a ratio between two numbers, rather than a simple fixed difference. The entire dynamic range can neatly fit within the ratio or *geometric scale* shown in Figure I-10A where each

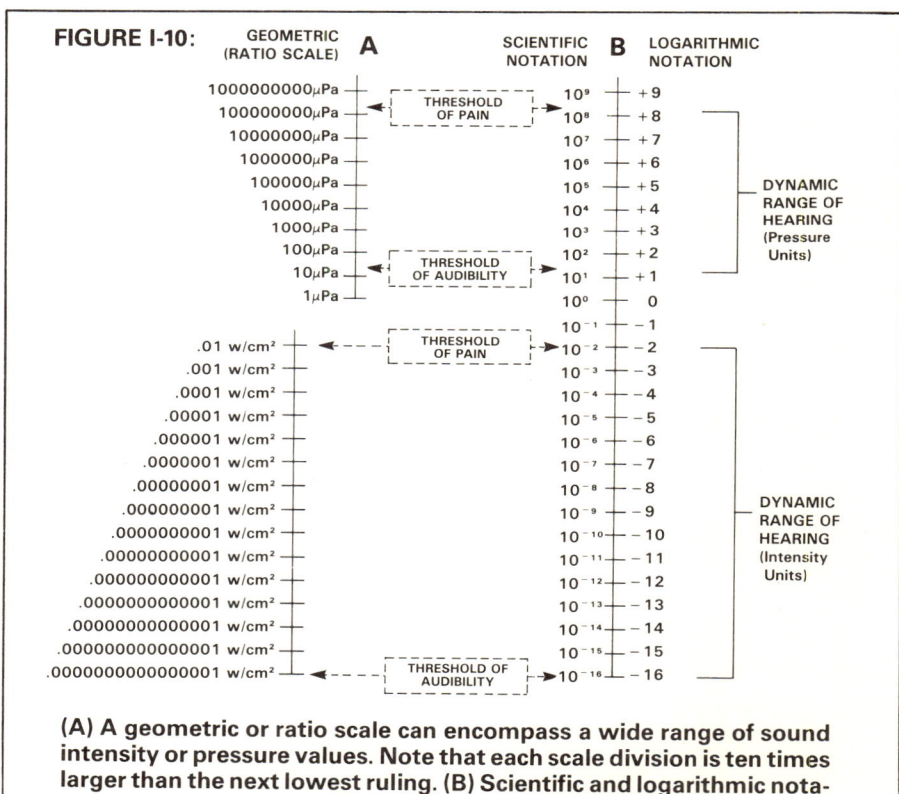

(A) A geometric or ratio scale can encompass a wide range of sound intensity or pressure values. Note that each scale division is ten times larger than the next lowest ruling. (B) Scientific and logarithmic notations express cumbersome numbers in a convenient mathematical "short hand."

scale division is 10 times greater in numerical value than the line below. By using such a multiplication factor, far fewer increments are needed on the graph to encompass the entire dynamic range of hearing.

Engineers and scientists have developed a convenient mathematical shorthand called *scientific notation* which keeps track of the correct location of the decimal point and replaces the cumbersome zeros that typically accompany scales and computations that involve large numerical ranges and values. The number one million, for example, is transformed below into a much simpler format by scientific notation. Note that a multiplication factor, or *base number*, of 10 is shown to be "self multiplied" six times to yield a value of one million. The small superscript numeral placed to the upper right of the base number indicates how many self-multiplications are occurring. This symbol is variously called the *exponent, power,* or *logarithm* of the number. To the left of the base is the *coefficient* which serves as a multiplication factor for the logarithmic portion of the number. Although any number may serve as a base, 10 is commonly used in hearing science, with base 2 and base 2.71 also finding wide usage in the computer and mathematical sciences.

$$1{,}000{,}000 = 10 \times 10 \times 10 \times 10 \times 10 \times 10$$
$$= 1 \times 10^6 \leftarrow \text{exponent or logarithm}$$
$$\uparrow \qquad \nwarrow$$
$$\text{coefficient} \quad \text{base}$$

Thus, the logarithm of one million in the base 10 system is 6. The ranges of sound intensities and pressures associated with the dynamic range of hearing are expressed in scientific and logarithmic notation in Figure I-10B. A table of logarithms or a calculator must be employed to determine the logarithms of numbers other than the simple multiples of ten which have been discussed so far (e.g., log 2 = 0.3; log 200 = 2.3; log 1776 = 3.25). The examples shown below highlight some basic rules for the use of this scientific notation:

Multiplication: $\log A \cdot B = \log A + \log B$
$\log 200 = \log (2 \cdot 100) = \log 2 + \log 100$
$= 0.3 + 2 = 2.3$

Division: $\log \frac{A}{B} = \log A - \log B$
$\log 2 = \log \frac{200}{100} = \log 200 - \log 100$
$= 2.3 - 2 = 0.3$

Exponentiation: $\log (A^n) = n \log A$
$\log (200)^2 = 2 \log 200$
$= (2)(2.3) = 4.6$

The ability of logarithms to compress a wide range of numbers into a smaller scale has prompted engineers and scientists to define units of sound magnitudes themselves in logarithmic, rather than absolute physical terms. Research has shown that this practice is also convenient because of the way in which our senses respond over such a great range of physical stimulus amplitudes.

The unit called the *bel*, in honor of telephone inventor and deaf educator Alexander Graham Bell (1847-1922), has been arbitrarily defined as the logarithm of the ratio of two acoustic intensities or powers.

Specifically:
$$1 \text{ bel} = \log \frac{I_2}{I_1}; \text{ where Intensity}_2 \text{ is tenfold greater than Intensity}_1$$

The measured stimulus (i.e., the numerator) has thus been compared to some *reference level* (i.e., the denominator of the fraction). The normal "dynamic range" of human hearing, which spans an intensity ratio of 100 trillion or 10^{14} to 1, can be seen from the example shown below to encompass 14 bels (i.e., one bel for each multiple of ten contained in the intensity ratio).

Number of bels in dynamic range $= \log \dfrac{\text{Intensity}_2}{\text{Intensity}_1}$

$= \log \dfrac{10^{-2} \text{ watt/cm}^2}{10^{-16} \text{ watt/cm}^2}; \dfrac{\text{greatest intensity in dynamic range}}{\text{least intensity (1kHz threshold)}}$

$= \log 10^{14}$

$= 14 \text{ bels}$

The bel turns out to be a fairly large unit for acoustical purposes and has for convenience been divided into ten, more commonly used *decibels (dB)*. The calculation of the total number of decibels in the dynamic range of hearing is illustrated below:

Number of decibels in dynamic range $= 10 \log \dfrac{I_2}{I_1}$

$= 10 \log \dfrac{10^{-2} \text{ watt/cm}^2}{10^{-16} \text{ watt/cm}^2}$

$= 10 \log 10^{14}$

$= (10)(14) = 140 \text{ dB}$

Because decibels are dimensionless numbers derived from the ratio between two intensity values, the unit itself would be meaningless unless there were common conventions as to how each part of the ratio has been defined and specified. The denominator of the ratio in the decibel equation shown above represents the *reference level* for the particular dB system in use and is an important landmark to which the observed or measured sound value, represented by the numerator, is compared. Although the choice of a reference level is essentially arbitrary, several values have been adopted as standards within various scientific disciplines. One such value is the sound intensity associated with the one thousand hertz pure tone threshold of audibility for normal hearing human listeners mentioned above. Decibels that are calculated with respect to this reference level of

10^{-16} watts per square centimeter are called *decibels Intensity Level (dB IL)*. The names of most decibel systems are adopted by convention and reflect the particular reference that is employed.

The term *decibels Sound Pressure Level (dB SPL)* indicates that a sound pressure, rather than an intensity, is being compared to a reference sound pressure value of 20 micropascals or 0.0002 dynes/cm² (i.e., the approximate sound pressure equivalent of the 10^{-16} w/cm² reference for dB IL). Due to a special relationship that exists between the measures of intensity and pressure, however, and in order to remain consistent with physical events, the coefficient in our original decibel equation must be changed from 10 to 20 when calculating dB SPL. This alteration comes about in the following manner:

The basic dB equation:	$dB = 10 \log \dfrac{\text{Intensity}_2 \text{ (measured)}}{\text{Intensity}_1 \text{ (reference)}}$
The relationship between intensity and pressure:	Intensity varies in direct proportion with the **square** of the pressure (i.e. $I \propto P^2$)
Substituting $(P)^2$ for I, in the dB SPL equation:	$dB\ SPL = 10 \log \dfrac{(\text{Pressure})^2 \text{ measured}}{(\text{Pressure})^2 \text{ reference}}$
The squaring of a number is the same as doubling its logarithm:	$dB\ SPL = (10)(2) \log \dfrac{(P) \text{ measured}}{(P) \text{ reference}}$
	$= 20 \log \dfrac{\text{Pressure measured}}{\text{Pressure reference}}$

It is important to realize that the difference in the dB equations, seen when measuring pressure and intensity, reflects the fact that the two formulas are structured such that dB calculations remain consistent with events in the real world. A doubling of pressure, for example, results in a 6 dB increase in a sound. This is a 6 dB increase in both dB SPL *and* dB IL (although physical intensity has more than doubled; in fact, it has quadrupled). Similarly, doubling intensity results in a 3 dB increase in sound pressure level (although pressure has less than doubled — in fact, it has increased by a factor of 1.41). Calculated examples of this follow below.

WORKING WITH DECIBELS

Assume that a sound having an intensity of roughly 10^{-8} w/cm², equivalent to a pressure of 2×10^5 micropascals, is produced three feet away from a crying baby. It should be clear that these sound magnitudes are enormously greater than the 10^{-16} watt/cm², 20 μ Pa, lower limit of human audibility! In the examples shown below, the dB IL and dB SPL equivalents for these observed intensity and pressure values have been calculated and are shown to be **identical.**

$$dB\ IL = (10) \log \frac{10^{-8} \text{ watt/cm}^2}{10^{-16} \text{ watt/cm}^2}$$
$$= (10) \log 10^8$$
$$= (10)(8)$$
$$= 80\ dB\ IL$$

$$dB\ SPL = (20) \log \frac{2 \times 10^5\ \mu Pa}{2 \times 10^1\ \mu Pa}$$
$$= (20) \log (1 \times 10^4)$$
$$= (20)(4)$$
$$= 80\ dB\ SPL$$

How is it possible for the number of dB IL to equal the number of dB SPL, in light of the fact that intensity and pressure do not share the same units, nor are related to each other in a simple one to one fashion? The reasons which underlie the equivalence between dB IL and dB SPL values have already been introduced. Recall that both decibel systems employ the same 1000 Hz threshold of audibility as a reference level (20 micropascals $\simeq 10^{-16}$ watt/cm²) while the fundamental difference between the measures of pressure and intensity is reconciled and compensated by the use of two different coefficients for the two decibel equations.

Because decibels are logarithmic in nature, it is not meaningful, under most circumstances, simply to add or subtract them like ordinary arithmetic numbers. Consider, for example, the decibel level that is developed by two crying babies, each of whom generates the identical 80 dB IL sound. Is the total sound produced, 160 dB IL, equivalent to that of a rocket blastoff!? Fortunately, for the well being of all, the answer is no. In each of the two examples which follow, the actual dB IL value created by the two children has been calculated by a different method.

Example I

In this first method, both 80 dB IL values have been converted back to their original physical sound intensities of 10^{-8} watt/cm² each. It is permissible to add the two physical sound intensities and use the combined intensity to recompute the total number of dB IL.

One baby: $\quad 80\ dB\ IL = 10^{-8}$ watt/cm²
Two babies: $\quad 10^{-8} + 10^{-8} = 2 \times 10^{-8}$ watt/cm²

$\text{Total dB IL} = (10) \log \dfrac{2 \times 10^{-8}\ \text{watt/cm}^2}{1 \times 10^{-16}\ \text{watt/cm}^2};$ simplifying the fraction....

$= (10) \log (2 \times 10^8)$

$= (10)(\log 2 + \log 10^8);$ Note: $\log 2 = 0.3$

$= (10)(0.3 + 8)$

$= 83\ dB\ IL$

Example II

We have just seen that doubling the number of identical sound sources usually also increases the resulting physical intensity by 2 to 1. The number of additional decibels that arise from a doubled intensity ratio is easily determined from the general form of the decibel equation:

$$\text{\# of dB increase} = 10 \log \frac{\text{Intensity produced by two sound sources}}{\substack{\text{Intensity produced by one sound source} \\ \text{(i.e., the reference condition)}}}$$

$$= (10) \log \frac{2}{1}$$
$$= (10)(0.3)$$
$$= 3 \text{ dB increase}$$

Now simply add the 3 dB increment to the original reference level value for the final answer:

$$80 \text{ dB IL} + 3 \text{ dB increase} = 83 \text{ dB IL}$$

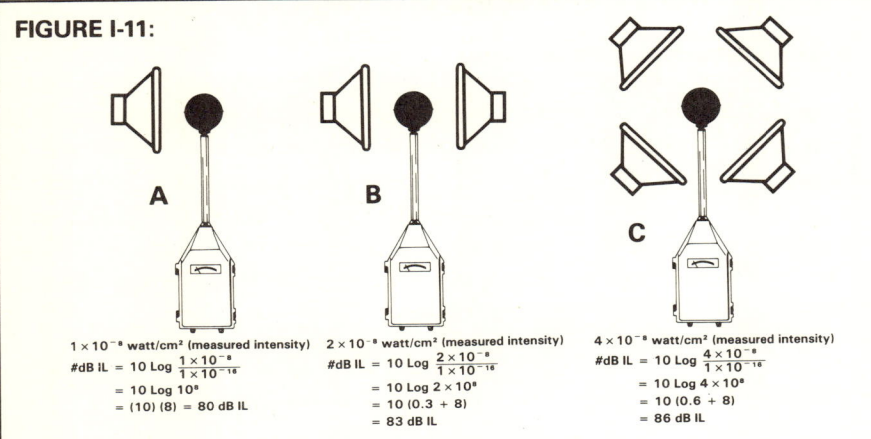

FIGURE I-11:

(A) A sound intensity of 1×10^{-8} watt/cm^2 = 80 dB IL. **(B)** Two identical sound sources produce twice the intensity and an increment of 3 dB. **(C)** Four identical sound sources quadruple the intensity but only double the sound pressure which creates a 6 dB increase over the single loudspeaker condition.

Since dB IL and dB SPL have been shown for practical purposes to be numerically equivalent, doubling the number of identical sound sources will typically yield the same 3 dB increment in either system. Take care, however, **not** to conclude from this corresponding 3 dB increase in dB SPL that a doubling in the **Sound Pressure** has also occurred. The special relationship between pressure and intensity, mentioned earlier, indicates that sound pressure would double only after the number of identical sound sources (and their respective intensities) have quadrupled. Under the exceptional circumstances where the identical sound waves from two sound sources were precisely *correlated*, or coincided at each moment in time and point in space, a doubling in sound pressure equal to a 6 dB increment actually would take place (see Figure I-15A). For practical purposes, however, we may assume that the signals reaching the *sound level meter* shown in Figure I-11 are uncorrelated.

Is the sound magnitude difference between 20 and 40 dB SPL the same as a change from 100 to 120 dB SPL? Although both sets of values certainly reflect a twenty decibel difference in **Sound Pressure Level,** these identical decibel increments do not represent the same change in the actual physical **pressure** of the stimulus. Since decibels are derived from the ratio formed by comparing two sound magnitudes, any 10-fold sound pressure increase always results in a 20 dB increase. Thus, 2000 μPa (40 dB SPL) is ten times the pressure of 200 μPa (20 dB SPL), and 2×10^7 μPa (120 dB SPL) is ten times the pressure of 2×10^6 μPa (100 dB SPL); however, the absolute difference between these physical magnitudes are unequal.

It is important to recognize that the physical pressure (or intensity) value of each decibel increment grows progressively larger as one proceeds toward the top of the logarithmically based decibel scale.

THE CONCEPT OF ZERO DECIBELS

What would be the resulting decibel level for a measured sound pressure or intensity that happens to be equal to the reference value of the dB system itself? It is important to recognize that the reference level, or *zero point* on a decibel scale, or any other logarithmic scale, does not signify absolute nothingness, but represents instead some arbitrary level to which other quantities are compared. The following examples show that the reference level is always the zero point on the dB scale.

$$\text{\# dB IL} = 10 \log \frac{10^{-16} \text{ watt/cm}^2}{10^{-16} \text{ watt/cm}^2} \qquad \text{\# dB SPL} = 20 \log \frac{20 \ \mu\text{Pa}}{20 \ \mu\text{Pa}}$$
$$= 10 \log (1) \qquad\qquad\qquad\qquad = 20 \log (1)$$
$$= (10)(0) \qquad\qquad\qquad\qquad\quad = (20)(0)$$
$$= 0 \text{ dB IL} \qquad\qquad\qquad\qquad\quad = 0 \text{ dB SPL}$$

(Note: the log of 1 is zero since $10^0 = 1$)

Because zero decibels stands for some definite sound magnitude, negative decibel values can occur for stimuli that are *attenuated*, or made less intense than the reference level. An illustrative example is shown below:

$$\text{\# dB IL} = 10 \log \frac{10^{-18} \text{ w/cm}^2}{10^{-16} \text{ w/cm}^2}$$
$$= 10 \log (10^{-2})$$
$$= 10 (-2)$$
$$= -20 \text{ dB IL}$$

DECIBELS OF GAIN

The system known as *decibels gain* is often used to describe the action of an electronic amplifier, such as a hi-fi set or a hearing aid. Gain itself may be thought of in terms of the numerical ratio which is formed by comparing the output of a system to its input. It is a simple matter to transform this relationship into decibel notation:

$$\text{Gain} = \frac{\text{Output Amplitude}}{\text{Input Amplitude}}; \quad \text{dB Gain} = 20 \log \frac{\text{Output Amplitude (volts)}}{\text{Input Amplitude (volts)}}$$

The outputs and inputs to electronic devices are often measured in terms of signal *voltages*. Voltage and its unit, the *volt*, are the electrical counterparts (i.e., analogies) to pressure and micropascals, respectively. It is therefore appropriate to use the coefficient of 20 in this dB Gain equation.

Examples

The identical one volt sinusoidal signal has been introduced to each of the electronic systems shown in Figure I-12. A 10-fold increase in voltage occurs as the stimulus passes through the amplifier in I-12A. This corresponds to a gain of 20 decibels. The device shown in Figure I-12B had no effect upon the tone and thus passes the signal with *unity* or zero dB gain (i.e., the output voltage equals the input, reference, voltage level). In Figure I-12C, the voltage output from the attenuator is only half as great as the input. This reduction in voltage may be described either as a "negative gain" or an *attenuation* of six decibels.

All of the decibel systems discussed so far have had fixed reference values to which various observed stimuli magnitudes have been compared. A number of decibel systems used in the Hearing Sciences employ reference levels which change from one test frequency to the next (see Laboratory Experiment II-6 for details).

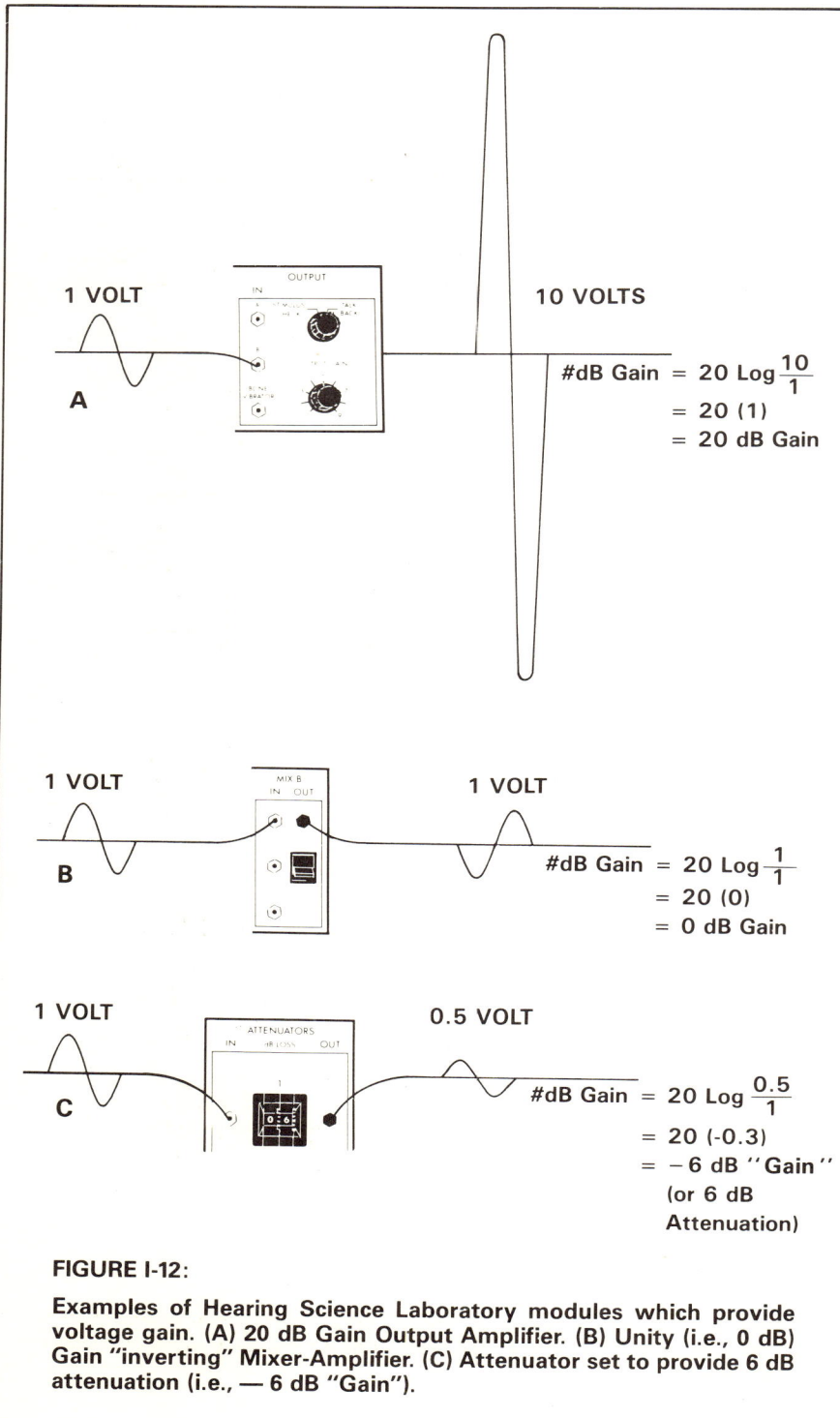

FIGURE I-12:
Examples of Hearing Science Laboratory modules which provide voltage gain. (A) 20 dB Gain Output Amplifier. (B) Unity (i.e., 0 dB) Gain "inverting" Mixer-Amplifier. (C) Attenuator set to provide 6 dB attenuation (i.e., — 6 dB "Gain").

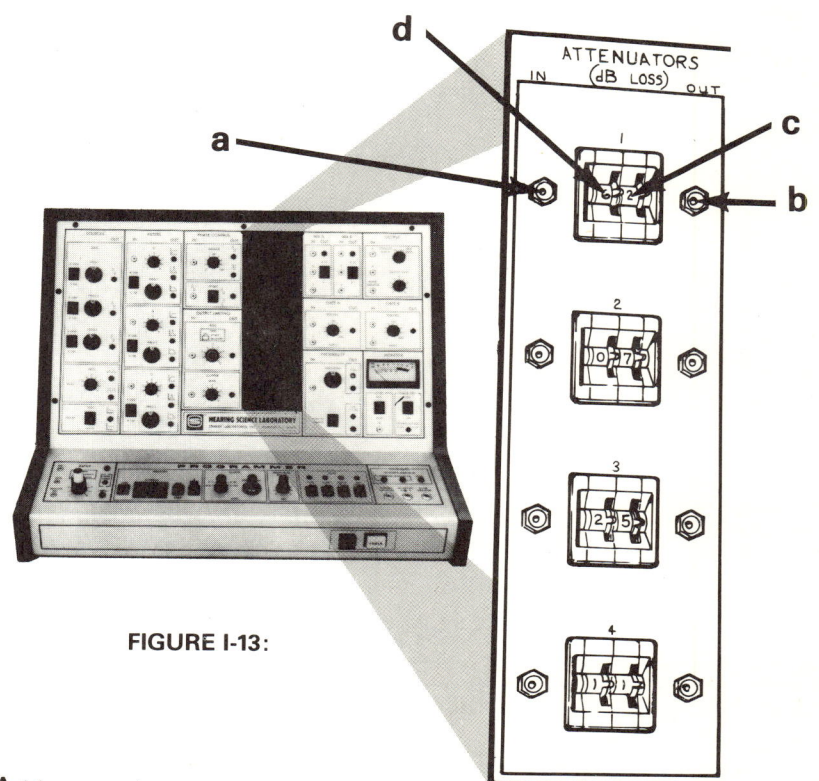

FIGURE I-13:

Attenuators

The Hearing Science Laboratory contains four calibrated step Attenuators (see Figure I-13). Each Attenuator may be used to control the voltage level (and ultimately the Sound Pressure Level) of a signal reaching the listener's ears. This may be accomplished over a 69 decibel range in steps of 1 and 10 decibels. Attenuation is accomplished by routing a single patchcord between the black Output Jack from any signal source or processor to the white Input Jack (I-13a) of an Attenuator. If both rotary thumb wheel controls of an Attenuator are set to zero, the test signal will emerge from the black Attenuator Output Jack (I-13b) unaltered in any way (i.e., with zero dB attenuation or unity gain). Non-zero Attenuator settings reflect the number of decibels by which the test signal voltage and thus the corresponding sound pressure level output from the headphones or loudspeakers have been reduced. It should be clear that a higher Attenuator setting creates a greater loss in signal strength. Note that the rotary thumb wheel control which governs individual decibel steps (I-13c) rotates freely from zero to nine and back again to zero, whereas the 10 decibel step control (I-13d) has been designed not to go below zero or above six. Do not try to force the control beyond the limits of these stops.

LABORATORY INSTRUMENTATION: PRINCIPLES AND FUNCTIONS

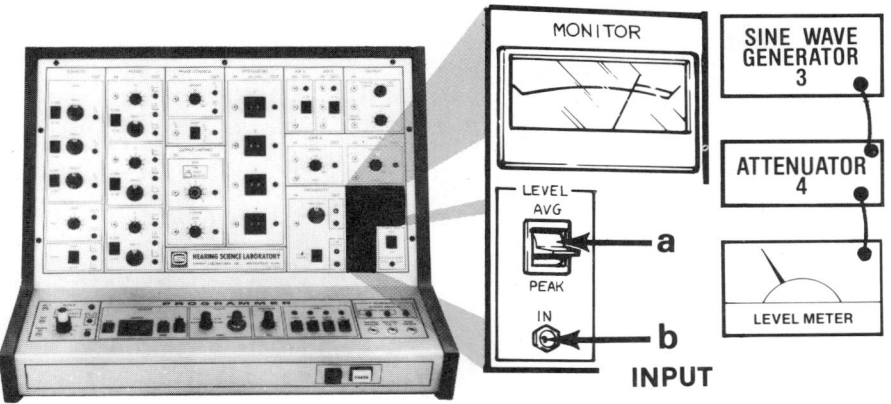

FIGURE I-14:

Monitor Level Meter

The relative magnitude of any stimulus produced by the Hearing Science Laboratory may be measured by means of the Monitor Level Meter, located at the right side of the front panel (see Figure I-14). A switch (I-14a) has been provided below the meter which permits one to examine either the relative *peak* or *average* voltage values of a signal (see Laboratory Experiment I-4 for details). The Monitor Level Meter should always be used in conjunction with a separate Attenuator as diagrammed in Figure I-14 so that no test signal level will exceed the full-scale deflection of the meter. The large scale provided on the meter face permits readings to be made directly in decibels of voltage. A ten-fold increase in signal voltage, for example, would correspond to a 20 decibel increase in the meter reading.

COMBINING SIGNALS TO FORM COMPLEX SOUNDS

Sound waves interfere with one another as they travel through a medium. The sound pressure created by two or more interacting waves will be equal to the algebraic sum of the individual wave amplitudes at any given instant in time or location in space (see Laboratory Experiment I-1). Consider the example of two sine waves that meet in space. If both waves are exactly zero degrees in-phase and possess identical frequencies and amplitudes, their sound pressures will *reinforce* each other and create a resultant pressure whose maximum is twice the maximum of the original amplitude of either wave alone (see Figure I-15A).

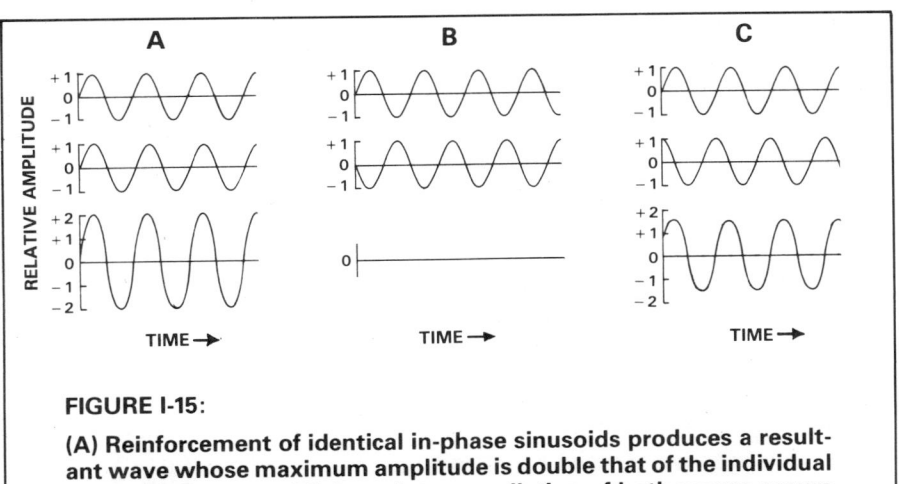

FIGURE I-15:

(A) Reinforcement of identical in-phase sinusoids produces a resultant wave whose maximum amplitude is double that of the individual component waves. (B) Complete cancellation of both waves occurs when they share a 180° phase relationship. (C) Partial reinforcement created by two waves 90° out-of-phase with each other.

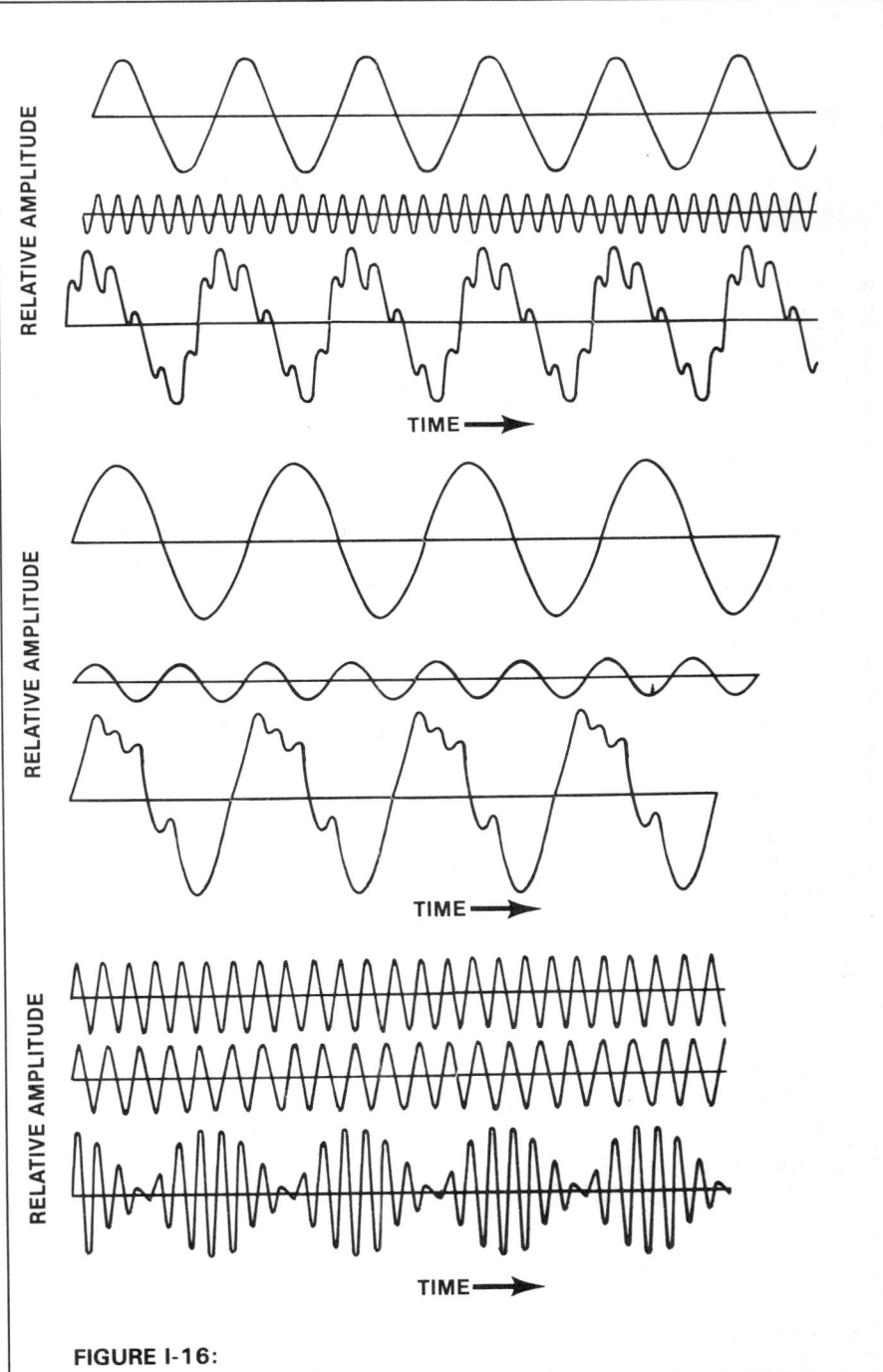

FIGURE I-16:

The frequencies, magnitudes, and instantaneous phase relationships of the component signals govern the particular complex waveform that is synthesized.

If, however, the two waves are 180 degrees out of phase with each other, the compressions on one wave will coincide with the rarefactions on the other as shown in Figure I-15B. The combined amplitudes of the two signals will produce an algrebraic sum of zero. Complete *cancellation* of both original sound signals will occur in this case, and the ambient, or background, air pressure will remain at its normal, undisturbed state. Virtually any intermediate resultant pressure value is possible, depending upon the particular amplitudes and phase relationships of the waves combining at each instant in time. Figure I-15C, for example, illustrates how two identical waves, 90° out of phase with each other, produce a resultant wave that is 1.41 times greater in amplitude than either original component. Figure I-16 shows several examples of the resultant waves created by the combination of sinusoids having dissimilar frequencies, magnitudes, and instantaneous phase relationships. The complex waveform patterns that are produced periodically repeat themselves like sinusoids but will be perceived by listeners to have different sound qualities from a simple pure tone. Experiments in the hearing and speech sciences often require the synthesis of several different sinusoids into a complex waveform or the combination of several complex signals with each other.

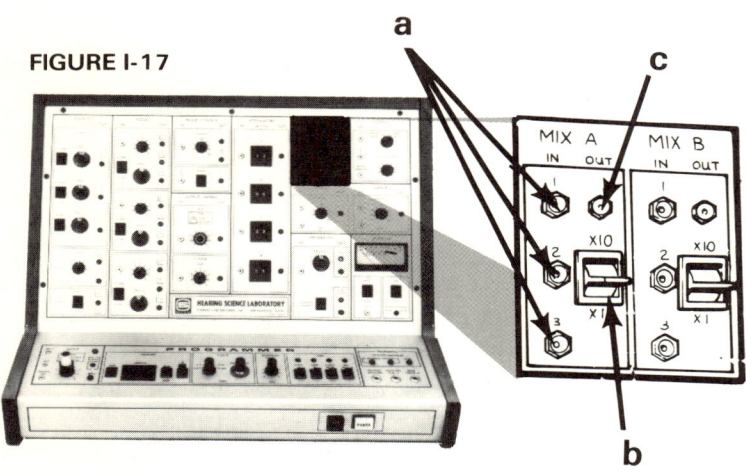

FIGURE I-17

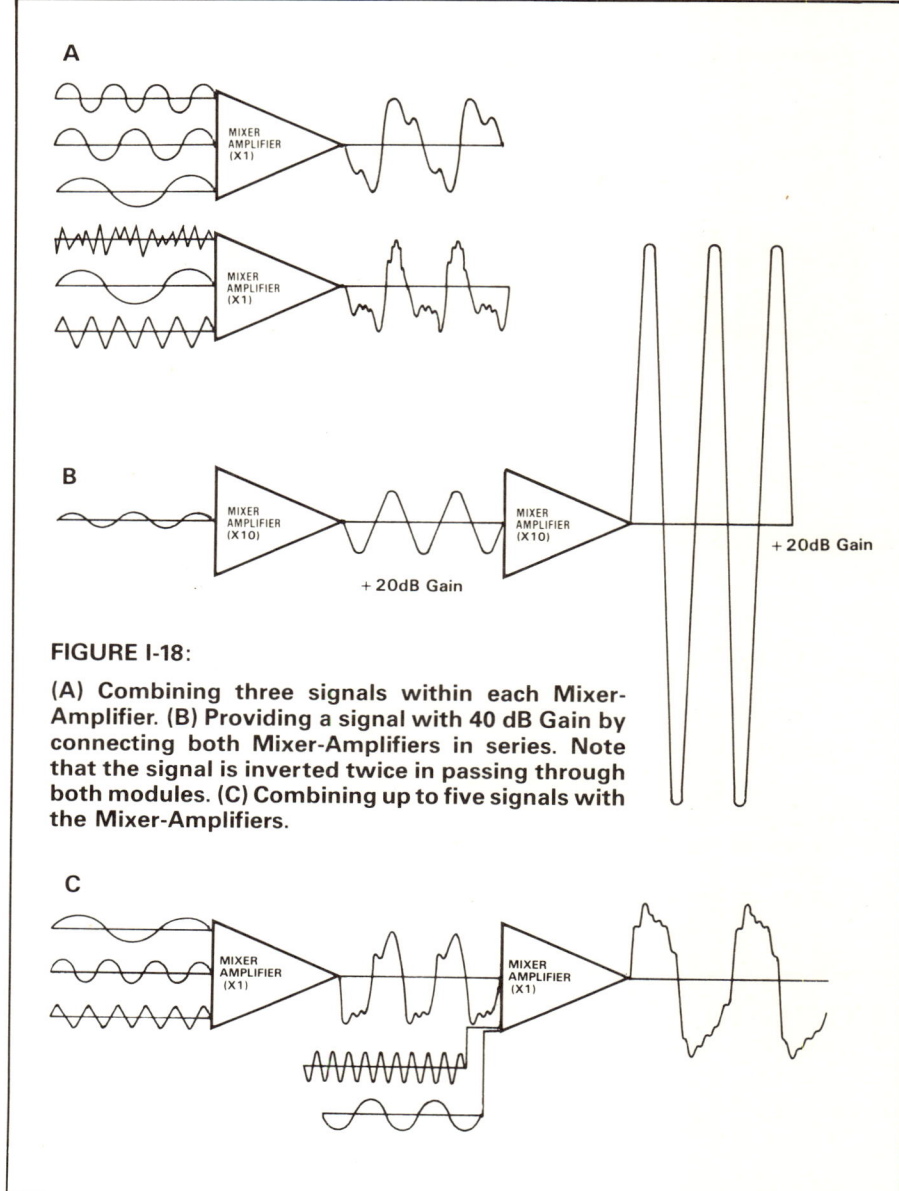

FIGURE I-18:

(A) Combining three signals within each Mixer-Amplifier. (B) Providing a signal with 40 dB Gain by connecting both Mixer-Amplifiers in series. Note that the signal is inverted twice in passing through both modules. (C) Combining up to five signals with the Mixer-Amplifiers.

Mixer-Amplifiers

The two Mixer-Amplifiers (Figure I-17) on the Hearing Science Laboratory permit a wide range of stimuli combinations to be made. Each of the three white Mixer Input Jacks (I-17a) is electronically isolated from the others so that no input stimulus can alter any other input signal component until the algebraic mixing process can take place. When the Mixer-Amplifier Gain Switch (I-17b) is set to the *X* 1 position, signals will emerge from the black Output Jack (I-17c) of the module unaltered in signal magnitude (i.e., with unity or zero dB Gain). Setting the switch to the *X* 10 position will give each signal that enters the Mixer a ten-fold increase in voltage which corresponds to 20 decibels of gain, as was shown in Figure I-12A. A total of 40 decibels of signal gain can be achieved by routing signals through two Mixer-Amplifiers connected *in series* (i.e., the output of one is connected to the input of the second). These configurations, as well as several other Mixer-Amplifier applications, are shown in Figure I-18. (Note: Each HSL Mixer is an "inverting amplifier" and may be used in the same manner as the Phase Control Modules shown in Figures I-7 and I-8 to alter the phase relationship of input signals by 180°. The experimenter should be alert to the fact that a 180° phase shift will occur any time these modules are used for signal mixing.)

PERIODIC COMPLEX SOUNDS

The French physicist John Baptiste Fourier (1768-1830) showed that all complex waveforms could be "analyzed" into a series of individual sine waves. That is, all complex waves can be thought of as complicated combinations of sinusoids. Conversely, Fourier's mathematical techniques can also be used to predict the exact complex waveform that can be "synthesized" from a group of individual sine waves added together. Fourier's analysis is sometimes referred to as "harmonic analysis" because the sine wave components in many complex musical sounds have frequencies

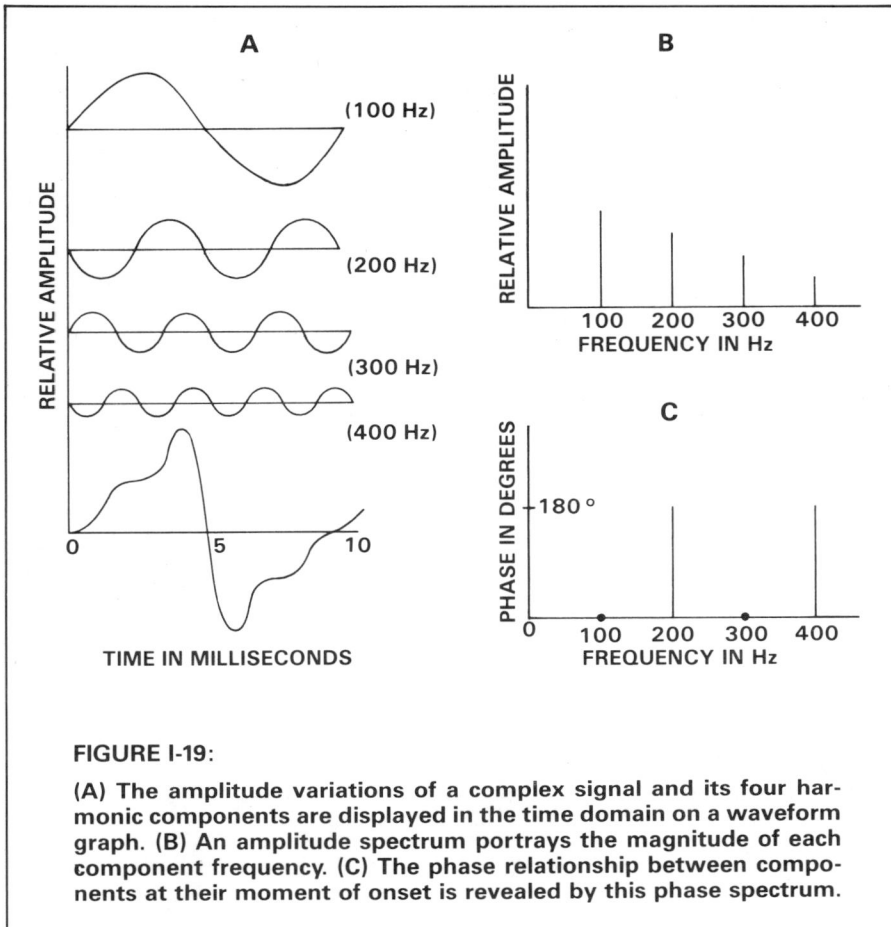

FIGURE I-19:

(A) The amplitude variations of a complex signal and its four harmonic components are displayed in the time domain on a waveform graph. (B) An amplitude spectrum portrays the magnitude of each component frequency. (C) The phase relationship between components at their moment of onset is revealed by this phase spectrum.

precise information about the frequencies, amplitudes, and phase relationships of the individual ingredients which combine to create the complex waveform but does not reveal the resultant summation of these components.

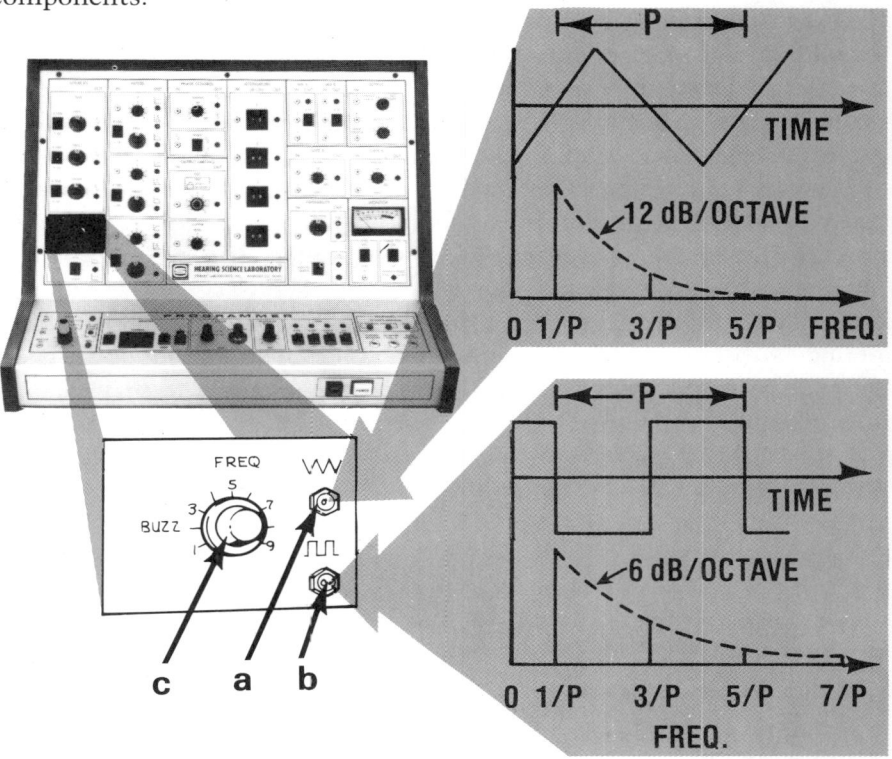

FIGURE I-20:

"Buzz" Generator

The waveforms and corresponding line spectra of the signals that are obtained from the two Output Jacks of the HSL "Buzz" generator are shown in Figure I-20a and b. Note that both the *triangle wave* and *square wave* stimuli contain the odd numbered harmonics of the fundamental tone in the series. The difference in wave shape between the two signals is due, as always, to amplitude and/or phase differences between their component frequencies. In this case, the harmonics for the triangle wave decrease in energy more rapidly at higher frequencies than do their square wave counterparts. Both of these harmonically rich signals are similar in some respects to the buzzing sound created by the human larynx during *phonation* (i.e., the production of vocal sounds) and may be used to create "synthetic" vowels as in Laboratory Experiment VIII-1. The fundamental frequencies of both signals may be varied simultaneously by Frequency Control Knob (I-20c) from 10 to 1000 Hz. The front panel scale markings range from 1 to 9 and serve as relative frequency landmarks.

APERIODIC COMPLEX SOUNDS (NOISE)

A vast number of environmental and speech sounds possess waveform patterns that do not repeat themselves from one moment to the next. Such *aperiodic* signals may be comprised of a random and ever-changing mixture of many thousands of frequency components which do not share any simple harmonic relationship to each other. The numerous components of an aperiodic complex sound cannot be represented with the individual vertical lines of a *line spectrum*. The concentration and distribution of energy

which are related to each other in a special and orderly fashion. Specifically, the frequency components can be whole number (i.e., integer) multiples or *harmonics* of the *fundamental*, or lowest frequency, tone in the musical sound. For example, the complex waveform shown in Figure I-19A consists of 100 Hz, 200 Hz, 300 Hz, and 400 Hz tones. The first harmonic is simply 1 X 100 Hz, or the fundamental frequency itself. The second, third, and fourth harmonics are 200, 300, and 400 Hz, respectively. The precise relationships of the frequency components in a complex wave are not readily apparent from a *waveform graph* which portrays changes in the magnitude of a sound in the *time domain* (i.e., on an instant-to-instant basis) as in Figure I-19A. An analysis of a complex wave in the *frequency domain* may conveniently be shown on a graph called a *spectrum*. The amplitude and frequency of each sine wave component is indicated, respectively, by the size and position along the horizontal axis for each vertical line on the *amplitude spectrum* shown in Figure I-19B. The phase relationships between the various frequency components in the complex sound, at the moment of onset for the wave or any other instant in time, may be displayed on a *phase spectrum* as illustrated in Figure I-19C. There are advantages and limitations to each type of graph. The waveform graph is valuable for studying changes in the resultant waveform amplitude and shape and sound pressure changes produced by components as time passes, but reveals few details about the individual signal frequencies within a complex wave. The spectrum graph, on the other hand, is very useful for portraying for the frequencies in an aperiodic sound are displayed on a *continuous spectrum.* Figures I-21A and B show, respectively, the waveform and continuous amplitude spectrum produced by a hiss-like "S" sound.

Aperiodic sounds are generally perceived to be more "noise-like" in their subjective quality than periodic complex waves, which often have a definite "tonality." The signal shown in Figure I-21 is commonly called *white noise,* after its visual counterpart "white light," but contains an essentially random mixture of tones rather than colors. When the multitude of ever-changing amplitude variations of the components in white noise are algebraically summed over a long time, the resultant continuous spectrum forms a straight line like that shown in Figure I-21B. This cumulative *long-term spectrum* of white noise reveals that an equal amount of energy is contained within any given equal band of frequencies. The sound energy within, for example, every 100 Hz increment is equivalent to that of any

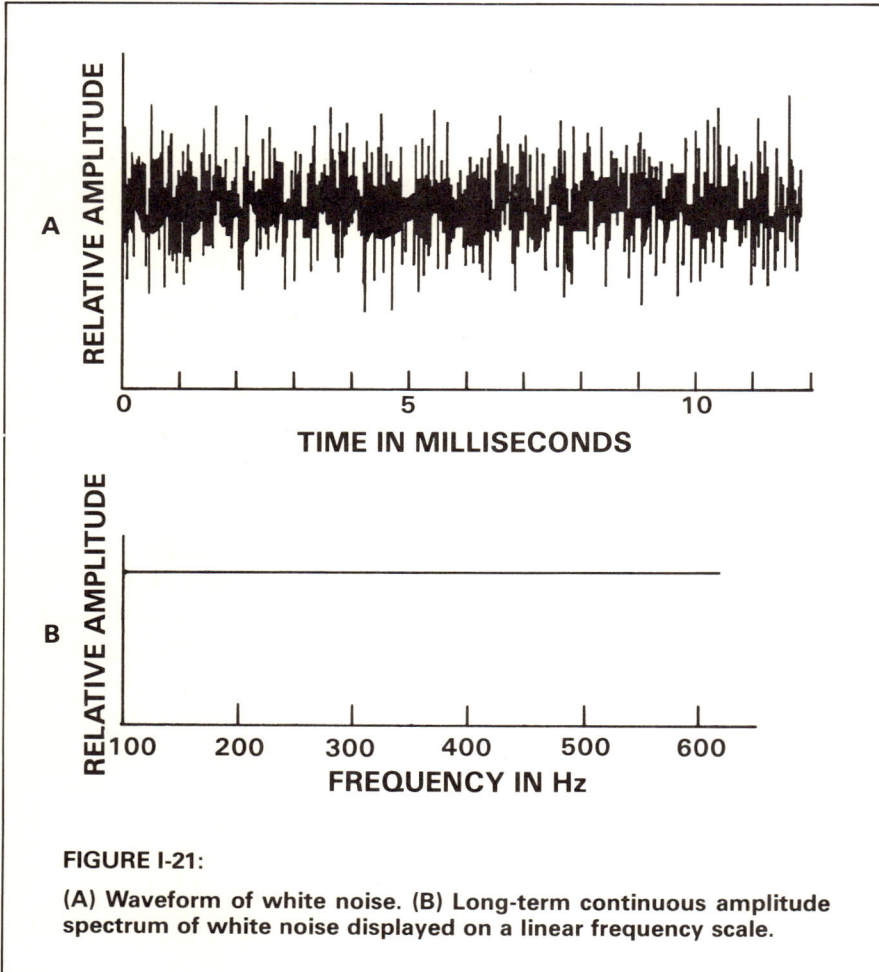

FIGURE I-21:

(A) Waveform of white noise. (B) Long-term continuous amplitude spectrum of white noise displayed on a linear frequency scale.

other 100 Hz increment. As with sound pressures or intensities, it is often more convenient to represent frequency units on a logarithmic rather than a linear scale. When, however, the energy contained in white noise is plotted on such a graph, its continuous spectrum looks quite different (compare Figures I-22 with I-21B). Note that each division of the logarithmic scale is twice the value of the one below or one-half the value of the one above itself

on the scale (i.e., the base number of the scale is 2). Such a doubling or halving in frequency is called an *octave* difference, and it should be clear that each octave increment will contain twice the number of hertz and hence twice the sound energy of the preceding octave. From the earlier discussion on decibels, we saw that a doubling in sound energy gave rise to

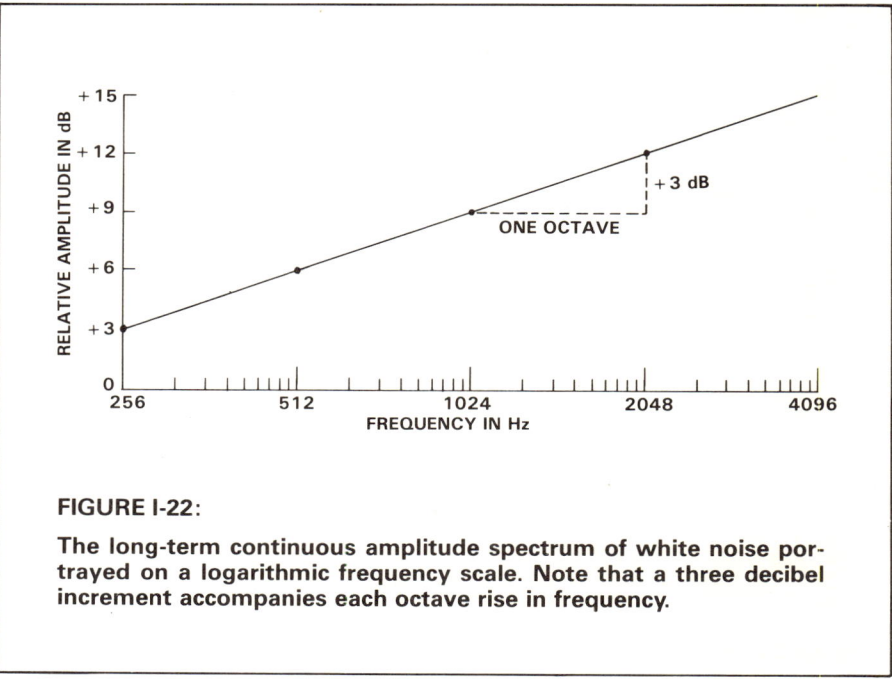

FIGURE I-22:

The long-term continuous amplitude spectrum of white noise portrayed on a logarithmic frequency scale. Note that a three decibel increment accompanies each octave rise in frequency.

a 3 dB increment. The continuous spectrum in Figure I-22 illustrates this fact and rises at the rate of 3 dB per octave. This example of how different displays can be plotted from the same stimuli should underscore the fact that a meaningful interpretation of a graph cannot be made without a clear understanding of the measures, units, and scales which have been employed.

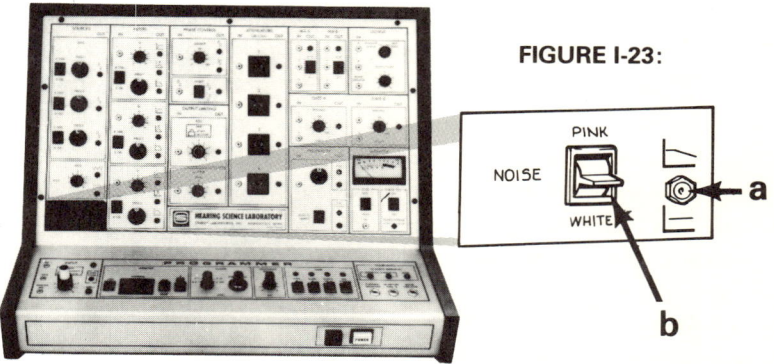

FIGURE I-23:

Noise Generator

Two types of noise can be produced at the black Output Jack of the Hearing Science Laboratory Noise Generator (Figure I-23a). White noise, of the type described above, can be obtained at the Output Jack by placing the Noise Selector Switch (I-23b) to the downward, "White" position. Placing this switch upward to the "Pink" position activates a special filtering circuit which modifies the normal 3 dB per octave rise in energy of white noise into a uniform, *equal-energy per octave* stimulus called *pink noise*. The spectral characteristics of pink noise are shown on both linear and

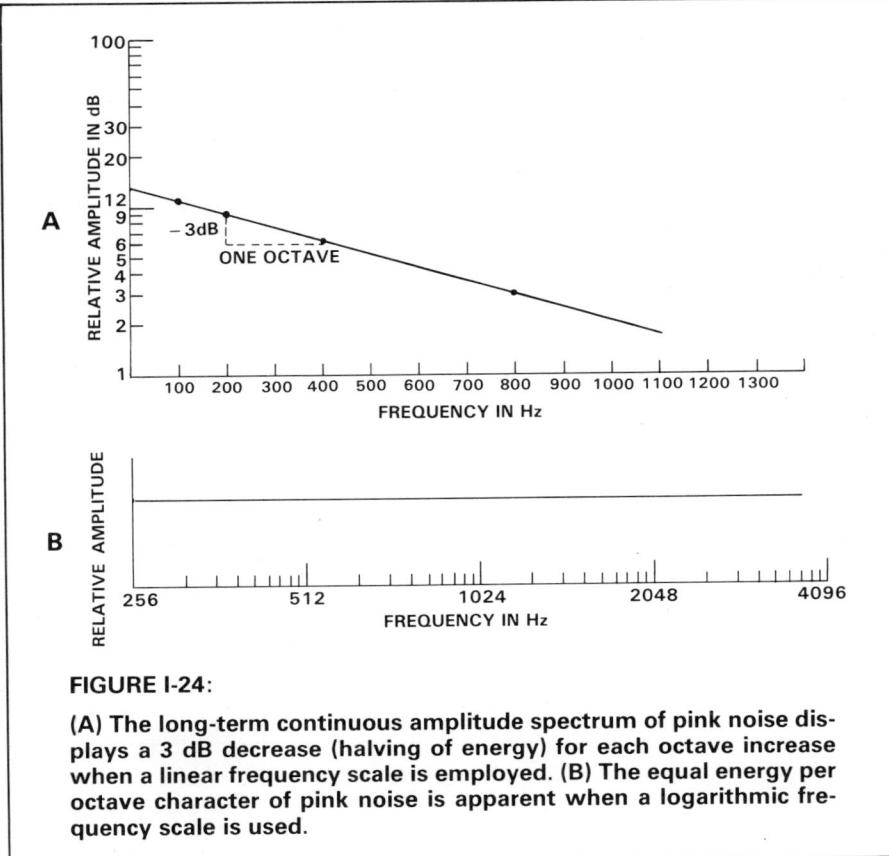

FIGURE I-24:

(A) The long-term continuous amplitude spectrum of pink noise displays a 3 dB decrease (halving of energy) for each octave increase when a linear frequency scale is employed. (B) The equal energy per octave character of pink noise is apparent when a logarithmic frequency scale is used.

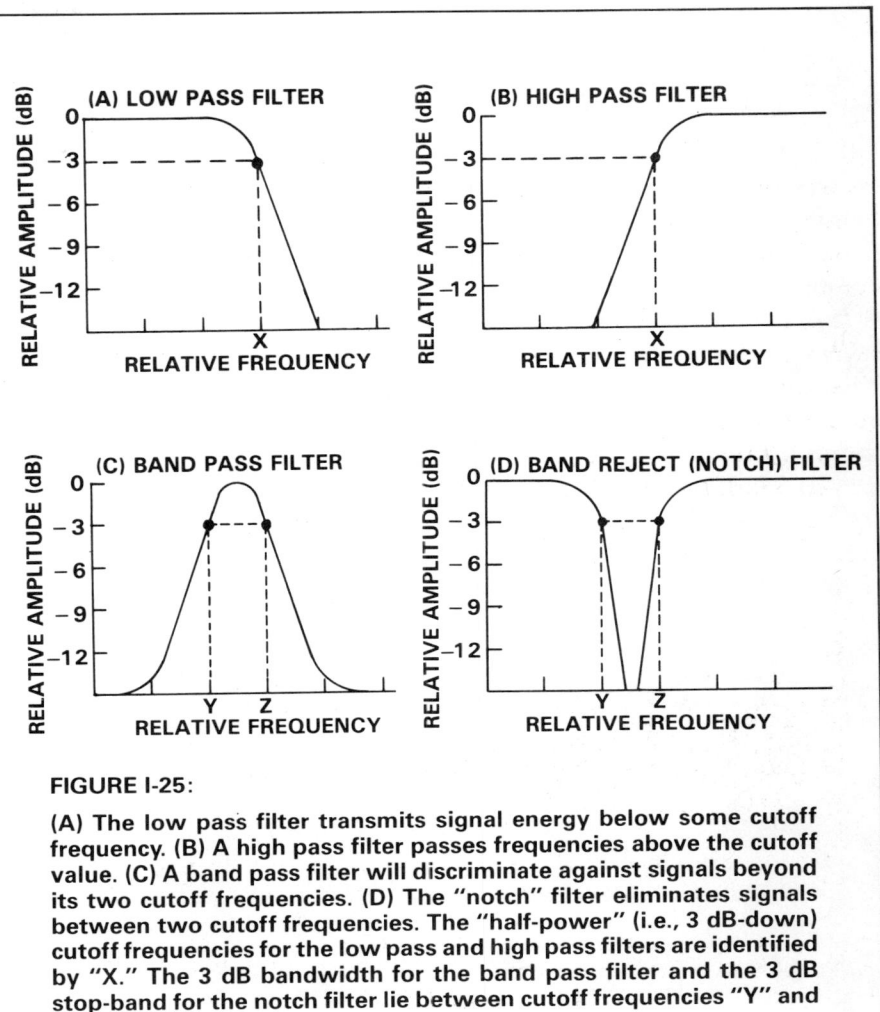

FIGURE I-25:

(A) The low pass filter transmits signal energy below some cutoff frequency. (B) A high pass filter passes frequencies above the cutoff value. (C) A band pass filter will discriminate against signals beyond its two cutoff frequencies. (D) The "notch" filter eliminates signals between two cutoff frequencies. The "half-power" (i.e., 3 dB-down) cutoff frequencies for the low pass and high pass filters are identified by "X." The 3 dB bandwidth for the band pass filter and the 3 dB stop-band for the notch filter lie between cutoff frequencies "Y" and "Z."

logarithmic scales in Figure I-24A and B, respectively, and reveal the presence of a higher concentration of energy for the low frequencies than is found in white noise. Such low frequency noise closely approximates a variety of naturally occurring environmental sounds and is often used in hi-fi and audio testing applications.

BASIC CONCEPTS OF FILTERING

The alteration of the spectral content of complex sounds is a routine need in hearing and speech science experiments. A *filter* is a device which selectively reduces the energy of certain signal frequencies while permitting others to pass through with little or no attenuation. The creation of pink noise, mentioned above, requires the use of a *low pass filter* which can discriminate against or "reject" signals above some *cutoff frequency*. A different operation is performed by a *high pass filter*, which rejects frequencies below the cutoff. By connecting a low and high pass filter together in *series* (i.e., the output of one device is routed to the input of the other), a *band pass filter* can be formed. Such a device will permit a band of frequencies between two cutoff values to be passed while rejecting frequencies which fall both below the lower cutoff and above the upper cutoff limits. It is also possible to eliminate a band of frequencies between two cutoff limits. Such a *band reject*, or "notch," filter can be created by connecting the inputs of both a high and low pass filter together and electrically combining their outputs to form what is known as a *parallel* configuration. The performance characteristics of these four fundamental types of filters are summarized in Figure I-25. No filters, other than the hypothetically ideal ones shown in Figure I-26, are capable of totally eliminating all signal ener-

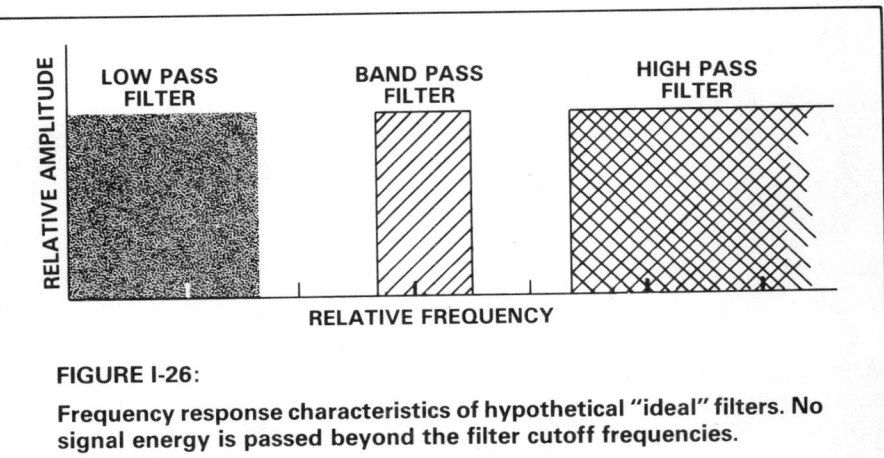

FIGURE I-26:

Frequency response characteristics of hypothetical "ideal" filters. No signal energy is passed beyond the filter cutoff frequencies.

gies beyond their cutoff frequencies. One practical and common engineering convention is to describe the cutoff frequency of a filter as the point at which a signal has lost half its power in passing through the device and therefore been attenuated by 3 dB. This so-called "3 dB down-point" is indicated for each of the filter types in Figure I-25. The difference, in hertz, between the upper and lower 3 dB cutoff frequencies defines the *bandwidth* or *passband* of a band pass filter and the *stop band* of a notch filter. The degree to which a filter attenuates frequencies above or below its cutoff frequency is called the *roll-off rate* and is expressed in terms of *decibels per octave (dB/oct)*. In figure I-27, the roll-offs and bandwidths for several different filters are shown. Note that the relatively *narrow bandwidth* filter (curve I in Figure I-27B) is far more restrictive in the frequencies it passes in comparison to the performance of the *wide band* filter shown in curve II of the same figure. This relative *selectivity* of a filter may be defined by its *quality* or "Q" factor, which is formed by the ratio of the filter's *center frequency* to its bandwidth. The center frequency itself is defined as the *geometric mean* of the upper and lower cutoff frequencies such that:

$$\frac{\text{Upper } F_{3dB}}{\text{geometric mean}} = \frac{\text{geometric mean}}{\text{Lower } F_{3dB}}$$

For this filter, the center frequency would be:

$$\text{Geometric Mean of Filter Cutoffs} = \sqrt{(\text{Upper } F_{3dB})(\text{Lower } F_{3dB})}$$

and the "Q" of the bandpass becomes:

$$Q = \frac{\text{Center frequency}}{\text{bandwidth}}$$

$$= \frac{\sqrt{(\text{Upper } F_{3dB})(\text{Lower } F_{3dB})}}{\text{Upper } F_{3dB} - \text{Lower } F_{3dB}}$$

It should be clear from the numerical examples shown in Figure I-27B that the more narrow the bandwidth of a filter, the smaller the denominator shown above and the higher the numerical value of "Q." The ability of a high Q (narrow band) filter to pass only a restricted range of frequencies makes it a very useful tool in the analysis of complex sounds. One filter with a variable center frequency or several narrow band filters, each having a different center frequency, could be used to perform an analysis of the sound's components (see Laboratory Experiment I-2). A trade-off exists, however, between the frequency selectivity of a filter and its ability to quickly respond to the abrupt and ever-changing amplitude variations in complex signals, such as speech. This trade-off relationship, shown in the equation below, should be recognized as another expression of the intimate link between time and frequency described earlier on page 4. The frequency-time trading relationship that exists in filters may be linked to a fundamental concept known as *resonance*. All objects tend to have a natural or *resonant frequency* at which they vibrate with a maximum amplitude. Any effort to force an object to vibrate at a frequency other than its resonant frequency will meet with additional opposition to vibration from the object itself. The exact nature of this internal opposition or *impedance*, as well as the resonant frequency of a vibrating system, depends upon such physical characteristics as the mass and relative elasticity of a mechanically vibrating object or the particular choice of circuit components in an electronic system that produces oscillations. These mechanical and electrical factors govern the responsiveness of a resonator, such as a bandpass filter, to the frequency and time characteristics of different signals.

It takes a certain amount of time for a resonator to fully respond to an oscillating signal (i.e., for an oscillation to build up to and decay from its maximum amplitude). This filter *response time* gets longer as the bandwidth of the system gets smaller. As we shall see in Laboratory Exper-

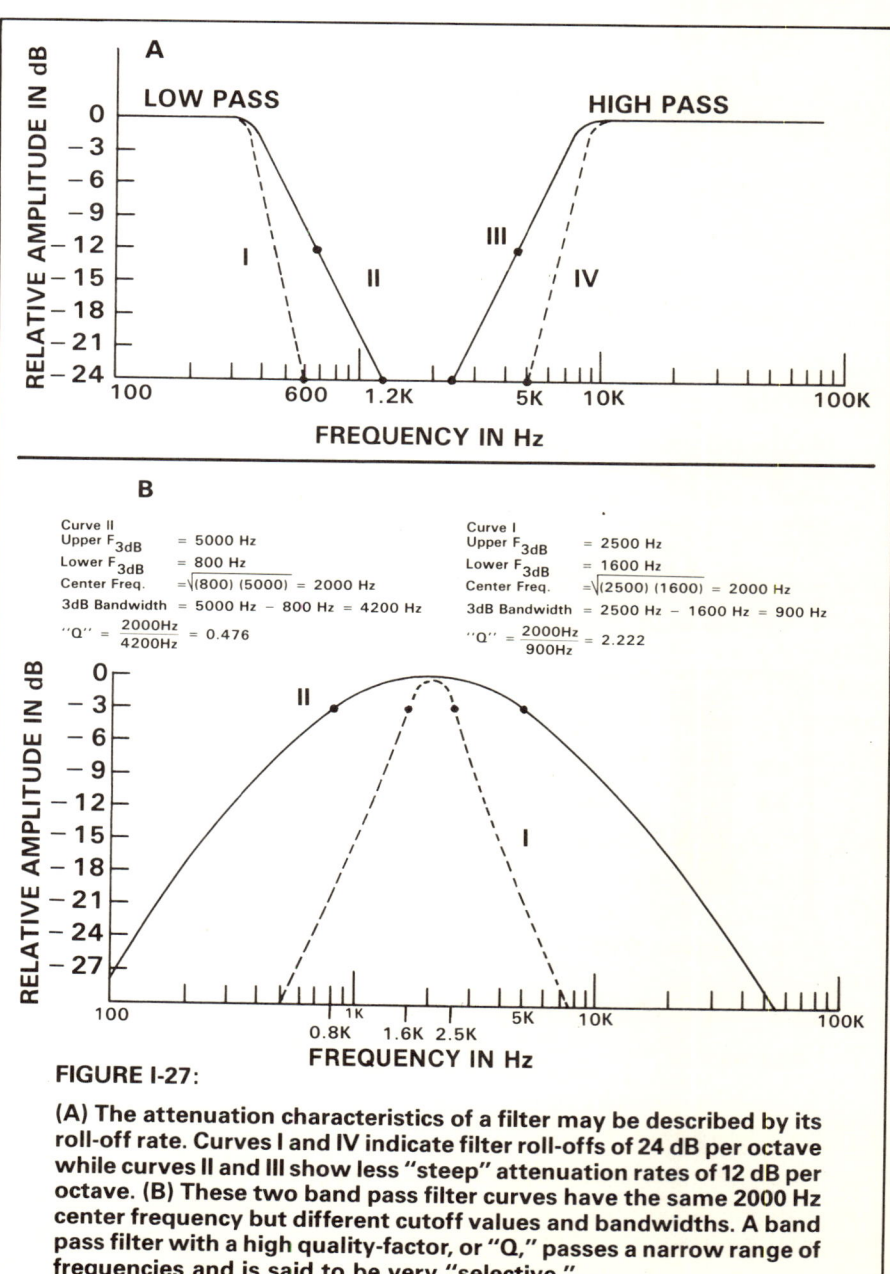

FIGURE I-27:

(A) The attenuation characteristics of a filter may be described by its roll-off rate. Curves I and IV indicate filter roll-offs of 24 dB per octave while curves II and III show less "steep" attenuation rates of 12 dB per octave. (B) These two band pass filter curves have the same 2000 Hz center frequency but different cutoff values and bandwidths. A band pass filter with a high quality-factor, or "Q," passes a narrow range of frequencies and is said to be very "selective."

LABORATORY INSTRUMENTATION: PRINCIPLES AND FUNCTIONS

iment V-2, a sinusoid which is abruptly switched on and off contains additional energy at frequencies above and below the tone frequency during the instant of signal *onset* and *offset*. A wide band filter will quickly respond to these different frequencies and pass their energies. But a very narrow band filter, with the same center frequency as the pure tone signal, will reject the frequencies in the initial portion of the stimulus and begin to pass energy only during the subsequent tonal portion of the signal. The numerical examples shown below illustrate this issue.

Filter Response Time (in seconds) $\simeq \dfrac{1}{\text{Bandwidth in Hz}}$

Relatively Wideband Filter: $T \simeq \dfrac{1}{5000 \text{ Hz}} \simeq 0.0002$ second

Relatively Narrowband Filter: $T \simeq \dfrac{1}{50 \text{ Hz}} \simeq 0.02$ second

filter may be selected by means of the Frequency Range Switch (I-28e) and the Variable Frequency Control Knob (I-28f). The selectivity of the bandpass filter function is governed by the Q Control Knob (I-28g). Rotating this control clockwise to higher Q dial settings will increase the selectivity of the bandpass filter. NOTE: Varying the Q control setting will also affect the characteristics of the high pass and low pass filter outputs in the

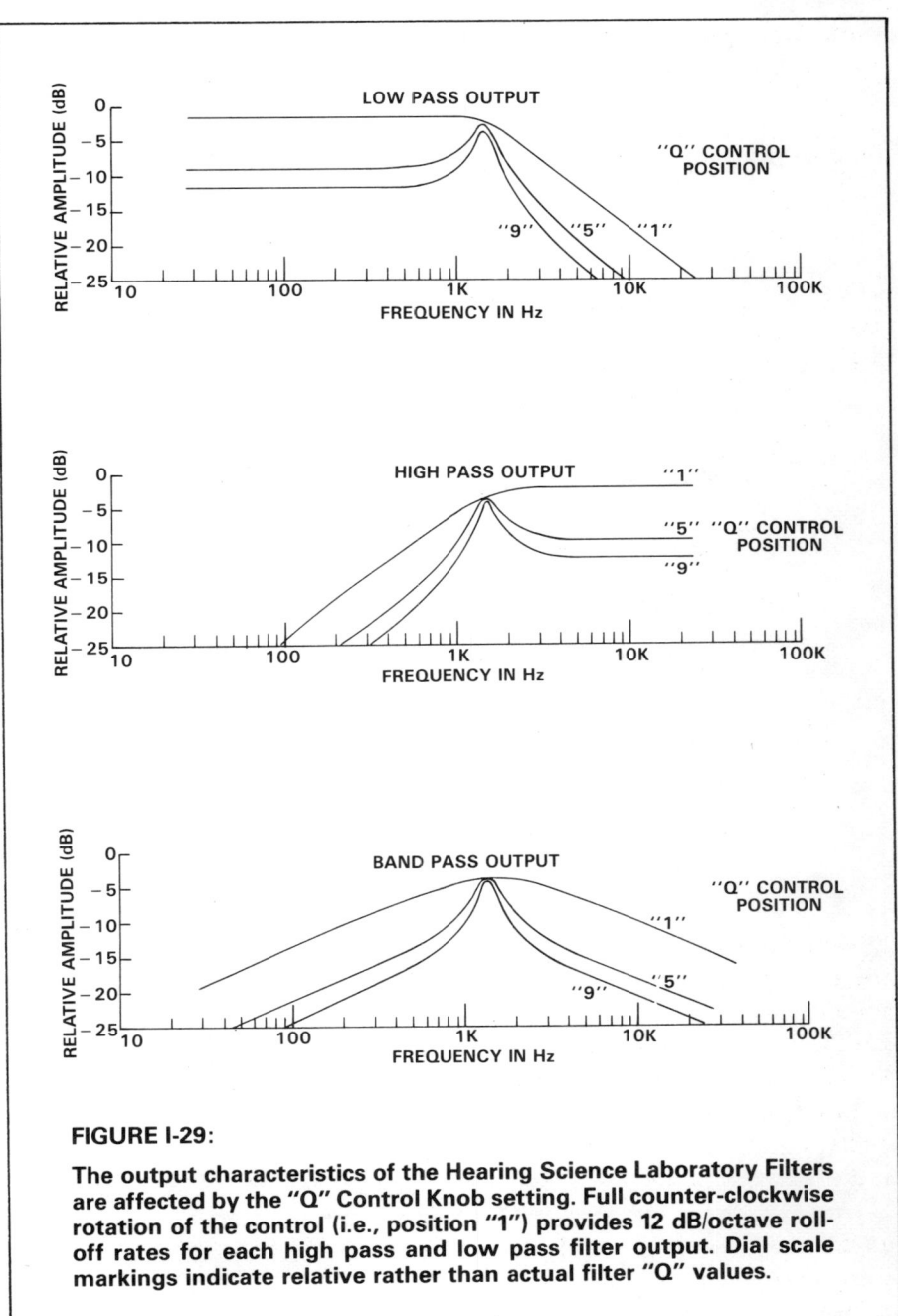

FIGURE I-29:

The output characteristics of the Hearing Science Laboratory Filters are affected by the "Q" Control Knob setting. Full counter-clockwise rotation of the control (i.e., position "1") provides 12 dB/octave roll-off rates for each high pass and low pass filter output. Dial scale markings indicate relative rather than actual filter "Q" values.

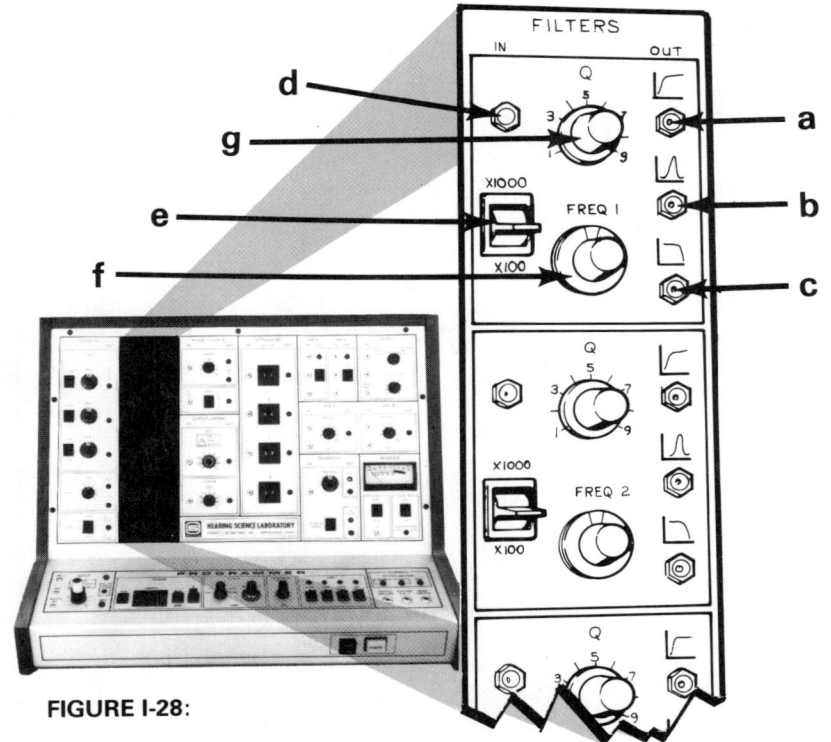

FIGURE I-28:

Filter Operation

There are three sets of filters on the Hearing Science Laboratory (see Figure I-28). Each Filter Set provides separate Output Jacks for high pass, band pass, and low pass filter functions (I-28a, b, and c, respectively) for signals that are routed to the white Input Jack (I-28d). The cutoff frequencies of the high and low pass filters as well as the center frequency of the bandpass

manner shown in Figure I-29. A recommended method for obtaining a variety of different low and high pass filter roll-off rates and cutoff frequencies is to *cascade* one filter with another (i.e., to connect the output of one filter to the input of another). Several applications of this technique are illustrated in Figure I-30.

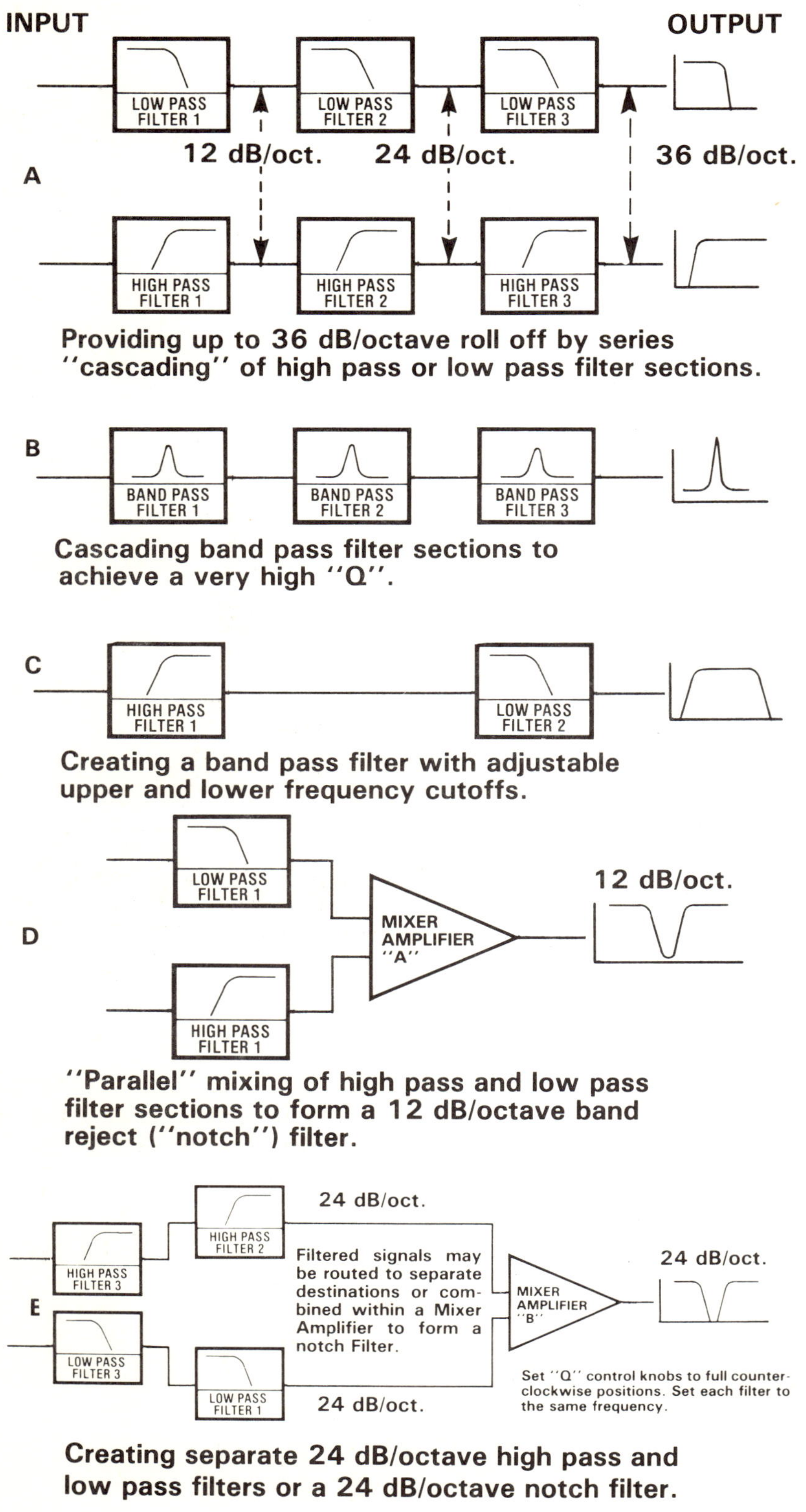

SWITCHING OF SIGNALS

The trade-off between the time and frequency characteristics of filters mentioned earlier is but one example of the numerous interactions that can occur between different acoustic and psychoacoustic variables. Several experiments to be described later in this text, for example, deal with the influence of stimulus duration upon perceived detectability, pitch, loudness, quality, speech intelligibility, and location of sounds in space. The very sequence and manner in which signals are permitted to switch on and off may also have great influence on experimental results and interpretations (see Laboratory Experiment V-2 on the rise and fall of waveforms for more details).

The important function of turning audio signals on and off in a controlled fashion is performed by devices known as *Electronic Switches,* or "Gates."

FIGURE I-30:
A variety of filter configurations can be obtained through series and parallel cascading of several filter sections.

- **A** Providing up to 36 dB/octave roll off by series "cascading" of high pass or low pass filter sections.
- **B** Cascading band pass filter sections to achieve a very high "Q".
- **C** Creating a band pass filter with adjustable upper and lower frequency cutoffs.
- **D** "Parallel" mixing of high pass and low pass filter sections to form a 12 dB/octave band reject ("notch") filter.
- **E** Creating separate 24 dB/octave high pass and low pass filters or a 24 dB/octave notch filter.

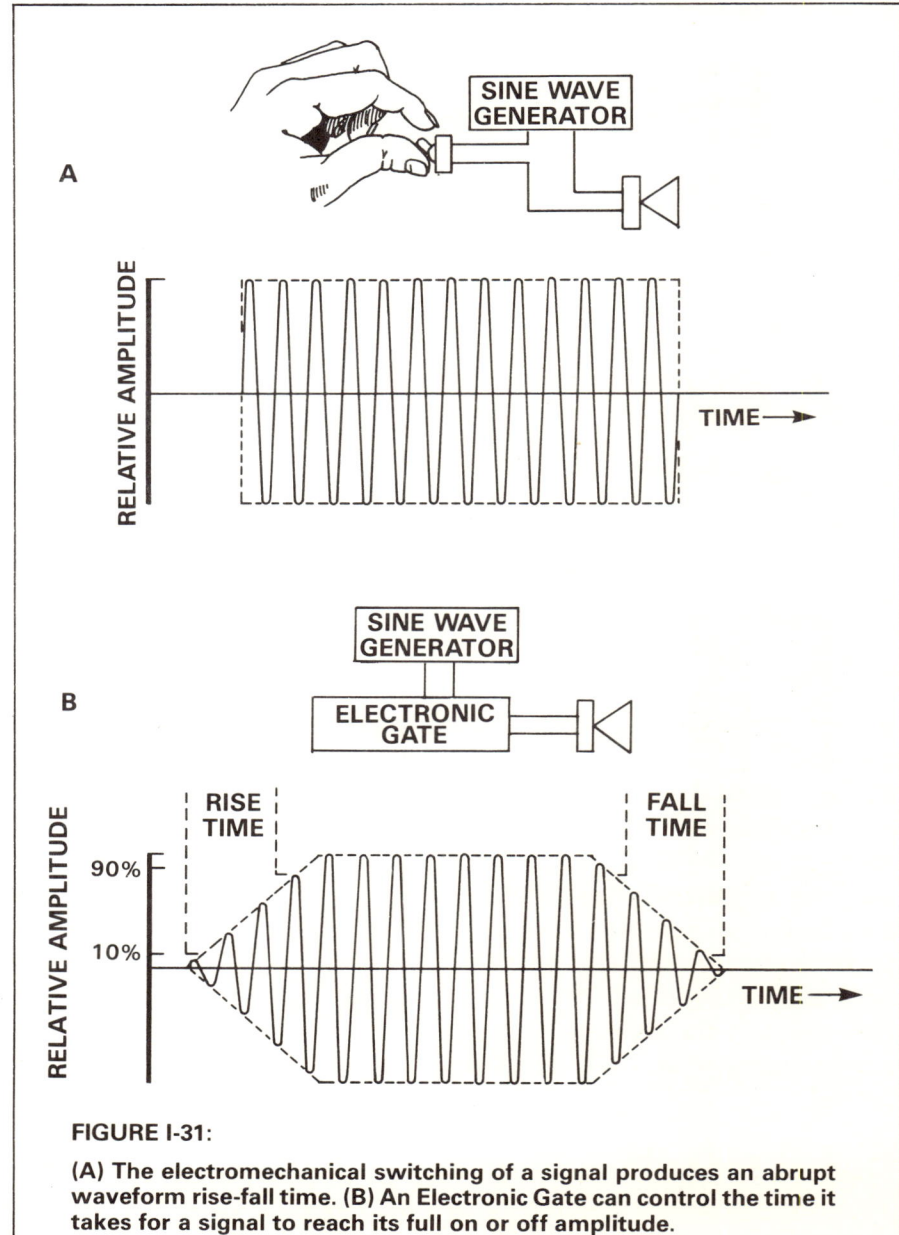

FIGURE I-31:
(A) The electromechanical switching of a signal produces an abrupt waveform rise-fall time. (B) An Electronic Gate can control the time it takes for a signal to reach its full on or off amplitude.

LABORATORY INSTRUMENTATION: PRINCIPLES AND FUNCTIONS

Figure I-31A shows the basic waveform of a sinusoid that is turned on and off by the mechanical closure and opening of the electrical contacts in an ordinary switch. Note that the onset and offset of the signal are very abrupt and the waveform rises to and falls from its greatest magnitude virtually instantaneously. The more gradual *rise-fall* times for the signal shown in Figure I-31B are achieved by routing the sinusoid through a variable *Electronic Gate*. The time required for the waveform to increase from 10% to 90% of its *full-on Amplitude* is commonly defined as the *rise-time* of the signal. The corresponding *fall-time*, or "decay," of the stimulus is that period between the reduction of the signal amplitude from 90% to 10% of its full-on value. The dashed outline which connects points of maximum positive and negative amplitudes on each of the signals in Figure I-31 is called the *envelope* of the waveform. It provides a convenient display of how the overall magnitude of a stimulus varies with the passage of time.

the onset, offset, and duration of the signals that are routed to the Gates. The Digital Event Programmer is divided into several sections which perform the following functions:

1. The Programmer Memory (Figure I-33a) contains 100 locations, or "Addresses," numbered 0 thru 99, in which one may store instructional commands that turn the Electronic Gates on and off.

2. The Data Entry Switches (I-33b) govern which Electronic Gates receive the "on" or "off" instructional commands at any given memory addresses.

3. The Programmer Clock (I-33c) repetitively cycles through all 100 memory addresses at a controlled rate.

4. The Response Delay module (I-33d) is capable of stopping the Programmer Clock up to 5 seconds per address at any desired memory location (see page 20).

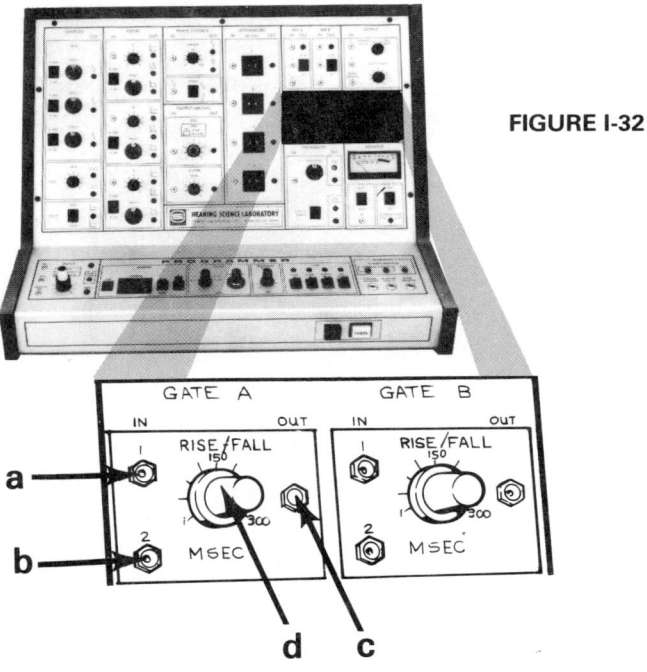

FIGURE I-32:

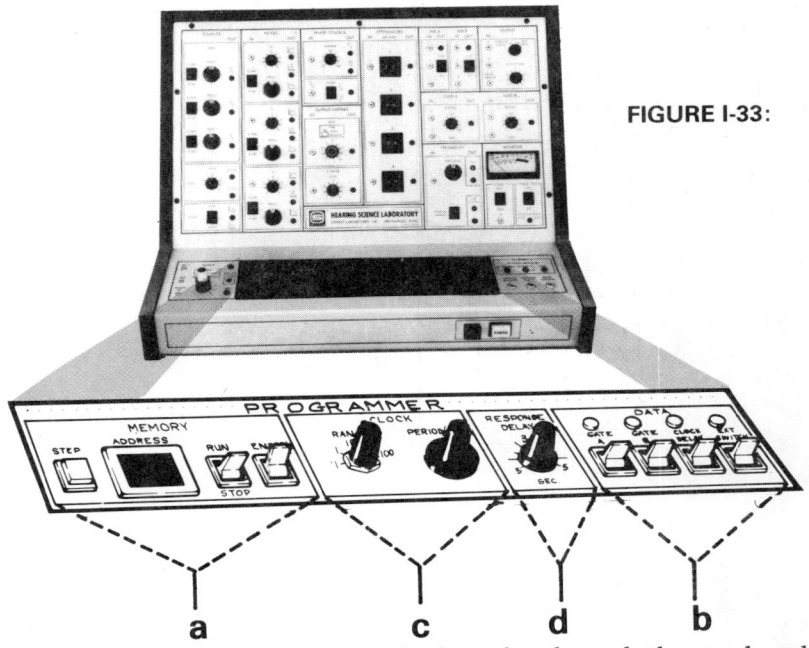

FIGURE I-33:

Programmable Electronic Gates

The Hearing Science Laboratory contains two Programmable Electronic Gates (Figure I-32) which may be used to switch stimuli on and off in a controlled manner. The white Input Jacks (I-32a, b) of each Electronic Gate are electronically isolated from one another so that two separate input signals may be "mixed" together at each gate. The rise-fall time of the gated signals that emerge from the Output Jack (I-32c) may be varied from approximately one millisecond to 300 milliseconds by means of the Control Knob shown in Figure I-32d. The programmable features of the Electronic Gates permit the creation of virtually any desired stimulus durations or sequencing without the need for external logic circuitry or computer control.

Digital Event Programmer

This high degree of flexibility in creating stimuli sequences is achieved through the use of a Digital Event Programmer (Figure I-33) that controls

The rate at which the Programmer Clock cycles through the one hundred memory addresses governs the amount of time that is "assigned" to each individual address. If, for example, it takes 100 milliseconds for the clock

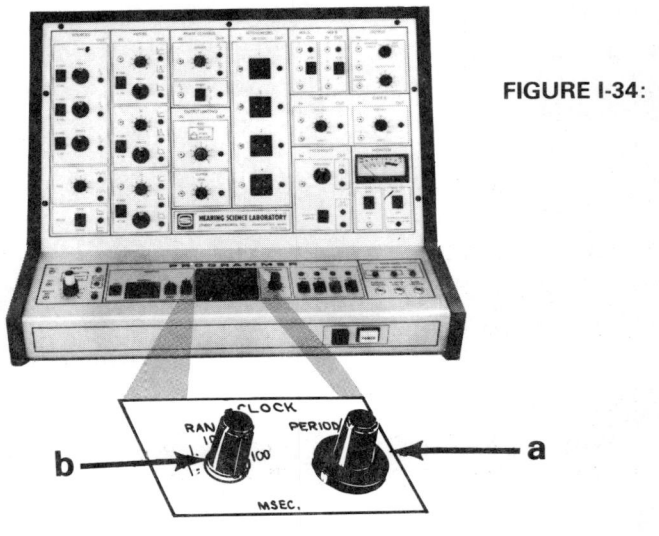

FIGURE I-34:

to cycle completely, each address will have a duration of 1 millisecond. Individual memory address durations ranging from 0.1 millisecond to one second may be selected by appropriate adjustment of the continuously variable Period/Step Control (Figure I-34a) and its accompanying four position Range Switch (I-34b). Sample clock settings are shown below:

Sample Clock Settings

Range Switch	Period/Step Control	Duration Per Memory Address	Total Duration of One Clock Cycle (individual address duration $\times$ 100 addresses)
X 0.1	10	1 millisecond	100 milliseconds
X 1	1	1 millisecond	100 milliseconds
X 10	3	30 milliseconds	3 seconds
X 100	5	0.5 seconds	50 seconds

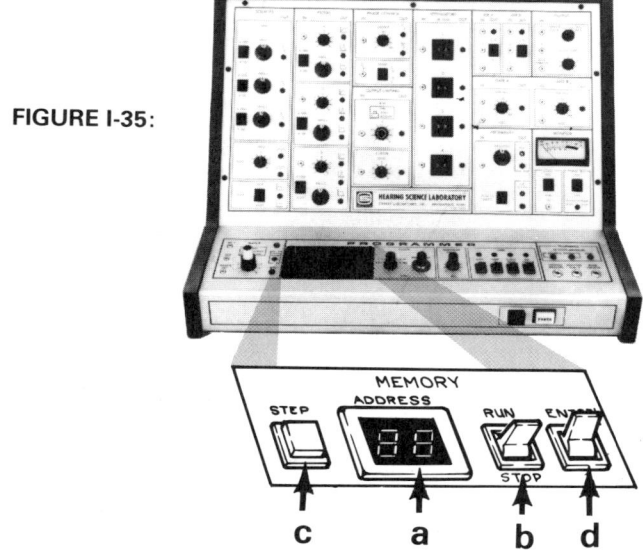

FIGURE I-35:

A Digital Display (I-35a) provides a numerical readout of the particular Programmer Memory Address in use. Any desired memory address may be quickly reached by placing the Clock Run/Stop Switch (I-35b) to the "Stop" position and repeatedly tapping the Step Button (I-35c) which advances the Programmer Memory, one Address at a time. Instructional commands for each Memory Address are recorded or erased when the spring-loaded Enter Switch (I-35d) is used in conjunction with the Data Entry Controls described below.

Entering Commands

The Digital Event Programmer issues two kinds of instructional commands to the Electronic Gates: "switch on" or "switch off." The total amount of time that a Gate, and the signal it switches, remains on or off depends upon the number of memory addresses which receive the switching command and the time value assigned to each memory address by the Programmer Clock setting. The "switch-on" command for Gate "A" is initiated by first placing the Gate "A" Data Entry Switch (I-36a) in the upward

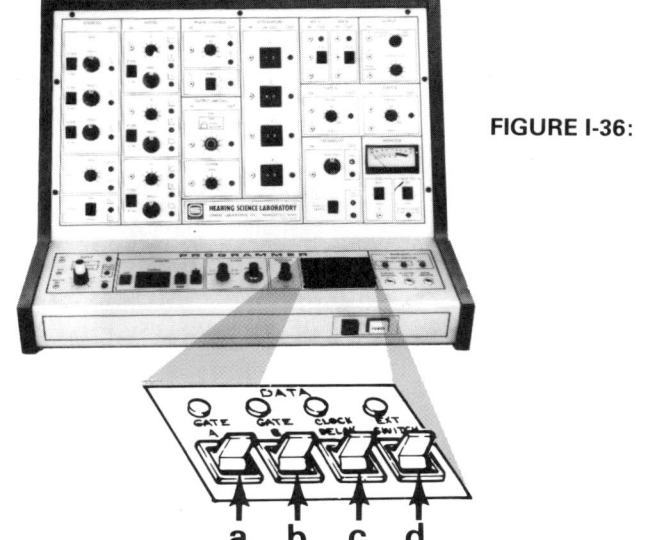

FIGURE I-36:

position and then depressing the spring return Enter Switch (I-35d). The light emitting diode (LED) located above the Gate "A" Data Switch will illuminate, indicating that Gate "A" has been turned on, thereby permitting input signals to pass through the module. Placing a Data Switch to its downward position and depressing the Enter Switch causes the LED to turn off and erases the command at that particular memory address. Gate "B" will go on when its corresponding Data Switch (I-36b) is in the upward position and the Enter switch is depressed. Both Gates will turn on or off simultaneously if both their Data Switches are in the up or down positions, respectively, and the Enter Switch is depressed. It is possible to enter or erase commands for all 100 Programmer addresses quickly by positioning a Data Switch up or down, respectively, and depressing the Enter Switch while the Clock is running (i.e., with the Run/Stop Switch, I-35b, in the "Run" position).

Special Programmer Functions

The Hearing Science Laboratory Event Programmer contains two special function data memories in addition to those which control Electronic Gates "A" and "B." These additional memories control the Clock Delay and External Switch channels. Placing the Clock Delay Switch (I-36c) to its upward position and depressing the Memory Enter Switch (I-35d) will cause the Clock to pause each time it recycles to the particular memory address which contains the delay command. The duration of this pause may be varied from roughly 0.5 to 5 seconds by means of the Response Delay Control Knob (Figure I-33d). Delays longer than 5 seconds may be obtained by programming two or more delay addresses in succession. One may use the clock delay memory function to provide sufficient time between test trials, conditions, and comparisons, as well as an adequate answering interval for subject responses.

Setting the External Switch Lever (I-36d) to its upward position and entering the instructional command on this fourth memory channel causes an electro-mechanical relay switch closure to occur and electrically connect together the two External Switch Jacks (I-37a, b). This additional switching function may serve as a third programmable Electronic Gate having an essentially instantaneous rise-fall time. Any signal routed to one of the two

LABORATORY INSTRUMENTATION: PRINCIPLES AND FUNCTIONS

FIGURE I-38: SAMPLE PROGRAMMING INSTRUCTIONS

In each of the examples shown below, a pure tone signal has been selected as the input for Gate "A" and a noise signal has been routed to Gate "B." The outputs from the two Gates may be combined within a Mixer-Amplifier and delivered to a single headphone or sent to two separate output transducers.

A) Alternating 5 millisecond stimuli.

B) Alternating 15 millisecond signals with 10 millisecond interstimuli silent intervals.

C) Simultaneous 20 millisecond signals with 30 millisecond interstimuli silent intervals.

D) 15 millisecond noise burst between 40 millisecond interrupted tone bursts; followed by 2.5 second silent pause.

E) 15 millisecond tone "pip" embedded within a 150 millisecond noise burst; followed by 1 second silent pause.

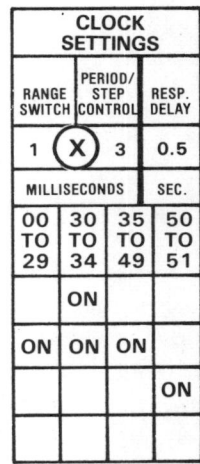

F) Program and corresponding waveforms for creating the entire sequence of stimuli events ("A" through "E") on a single memory cycle. Note the addition of clock pauses between each stimulus sequence. The 1 second warning light command follows completed programmer cycle.

External Switch Jacks will emerge at the other jack when an "on" command is entered into the External Switch memory channel. The External Switch Memory channel may also be used to achieve programmer control over devices such as external warning lights, buzzers, and operant conditioning equipment. For example, a bulb and battery (or power supply) connected in series with the External Switch jacks can serve as a pre-test warning light.

(CAUTION: This switching function is designed for low voltage applications only. DO NOT attempt to switch voltages greater than 12 volts at 500 milliamperes [6 watts].)

Any combination of on-off commands may be entered or erased from the four Programmer channels by appropriate settings of the four Data Entry Switches (Figure I-36). The sample programming instructions shown in Figure I-38 illustrate several of the limitless sequences that are possible. Each experiment in this text that utilizes the Digital Event Programmer includes such a table of recommended instructional commands and Clock settings for establishing a particular sequence of experimental events. The programming suggestions represent only one alternative to the many formats which may be appropriate for achieving the desired conditions.

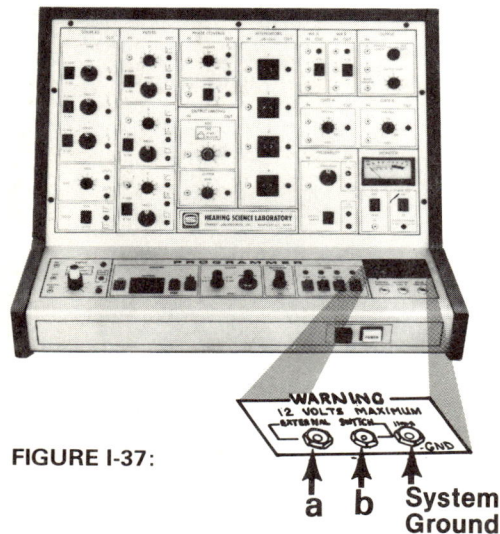

FIGURE I-37:

Probability Gating

A number of psychoacoustic experiments require that stimuli be delivered to a subject on a probabilistic basis. In Laboratory Experiment II-3, for example, the likelihood that a tone will be presented within some formally defined observation time period must be varied from 10% to 90% of the total number of test trials. In Laboratory Experiment II-5, a test tone must occur in one of two listening periods on a random basis (i.e., with a 50% probability of appearing in either observation interval). The Probability Gate shown in Figure I-39 may be used to achieve this type of control over the stimulus delivery schedule. Any signal routed to the white Input Jack (I-39a) will appear at the P(A) Output Jack when its neighboring green (upper) LED is lit (I-39b) or at the P(B) (1-P{A}) Output Jack when the yellow (lower) LED is lit (I-39c). The setting of the Probability Weighting Control Knob (I-39d) governs the percentage likelihood that the input signal will emerge at the P(A) Output Jack. When the control dial reading is 3, for example, and the momentary Sample Button (I-39e) is tapped before each experimental test trial, an input signal will appear at the P(A) Output Jack roughly 30% of the time and at the P(B) Output Jack 70% of the time (i.e., with a probability of 100% - P{A}).

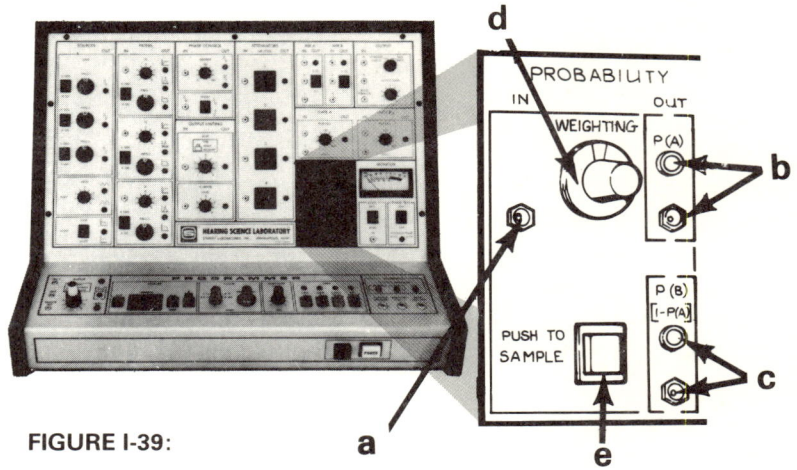

FIGURE I-39:

STIMULI AMPLIFICATION AND TRANSDUCTION

Input Preamplifiers

Speech sounds are important and widely used stimuli in the study of the processes of hearing and communication. For the majority of experiments in which speech stimuli are used, it is necessary to convert the acoustic energy of spoken sounds into an electrical signal so that it may be controlled or altered electronically. The process by which one type of energy is transformed into another is called *transduction*. A microphone is a *transducer* which changes the acoustic energy of sound into its electrical counterpart. The signal voltages produced by a microphone are typically quite small in magnitude and require some form of *amplification* before further processing takes place. The Input Preamplifier (Figure I-40) on the Hearing Science Laboratory is designed to provide up to sixty decibels of gain for

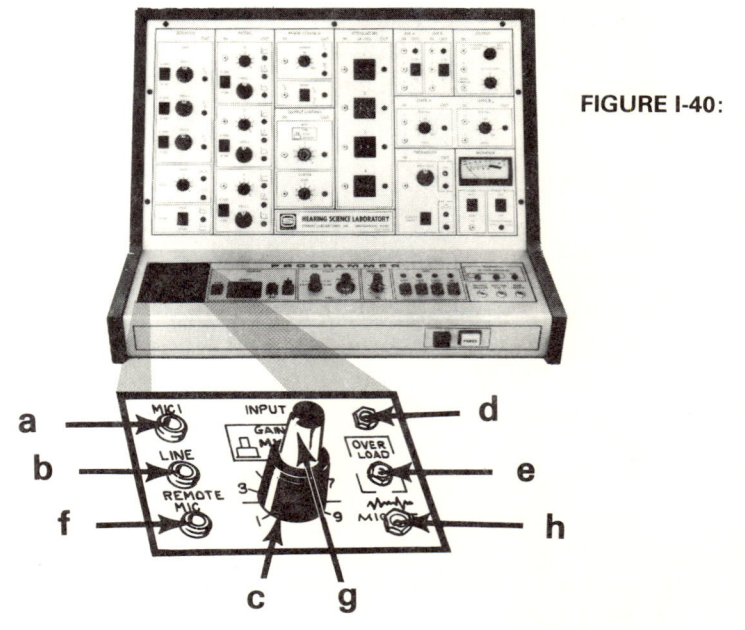

FIGURE I-40:

LABORATORY INSTRUMENTATION: PRINCIPLES AND FUNCTIONS

low impedance microphone signals or pre-recorded sound stimuli which are delivered to the miniature phone jacks located at the extreme left hand side of the front panel (I-40a, b). The amplification of these input signal levels may be varied by means of the large diameter black Mic 1/Line Gain Control Knob (I-40c). These signals may then be routed from the black Output Jack (I-40d) of the Preamplifier module to any of the various white input jacks on the HSL in accordance with the requirements of a particular experiment or demonstration. The red LED Overload Indicator (I-40e) will flash on if excessive amplification or too large a signal has been applied to the preamplifier module, causing the stimulus waveform to distort. When this occurs, one should either increase the distance between the sound source and the microphone, lower the Gain Control Knob setting, or attenuate the sound source. Signals from a second microphone may be sent to the Remote Microphone Input Jack (I-40f) for talkback purposes between the subject and the experimenter or when studies and demonstrations require two independent microphones. A second Preamplifier, electronically identical to the one for the Mic 1/Line input stimuli, has been included in the HSL for remote microphone applications. The gain of this duplicate preamplifier may be adjusted via the narrow diameter grey Talkback Gain Control Knob (I-40g). The signals from this second preamplifier channel emerge from a second Output Jack (I-40h) and are also internally wired to channel "A" of the Output Amplifiers for talkback purposes described below.

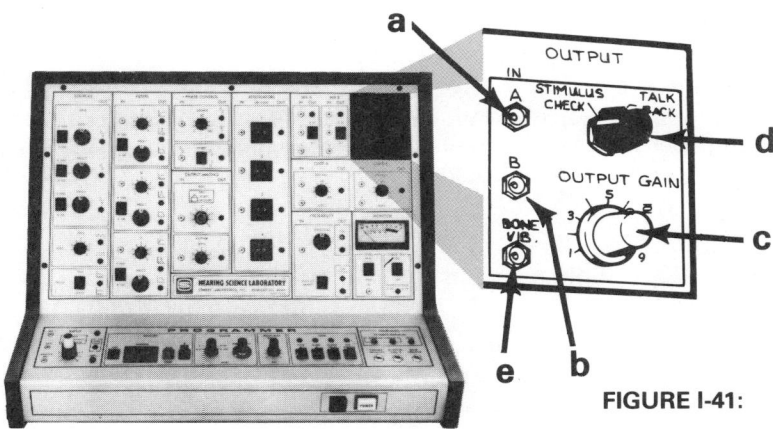

FIGURE I-41:

Output Amplifiers

After the various test stimuli have been produced and electronically processed on the Hearing Science Laboratory, they are ready to be presented to the listener. This is achieved by transducing the electrical signals into sounds through the use of *headphones, loudspeakers,* or a *bone conduction vibrator*. Each of these types of transducers requires a somewhat different amount of electrical energy in order to produce a sufficiently strong sound output for demonstrations and experiments. The Output Module (Figure I-41) located at the upper right hand corner of the front panel contains several independent amplifiers that are designed to power a variety of transducers. If, for example, there is a need to deliver test sounds from a single headphone or loudspeaker, simply route the chosen electrical stimulus, via a patch cord, to either of the white Input Jacks shown in Figure I-41a and b. Both of these jacks lead to identical *Power Amplifiers* whose outputs are internally connected to the Phones/Speaker Jack located at the lower right hand corner of the front panel (Figure I-42a). A pair of *low impedance* loudspeakers (≤16 ohms) or *high impedance* headphones (≥300 ohms), such as those phones provided with the HSL, may be connected to the Phones/Speaker Jack. CAUTION: Do not attempt to plug headphones having an impedance below 300 ohms into the Phone/Speaker Jack as this may cause excessively loud signal levels to be delivered to the listener. The Phone/Speaker Jack has a special narrow diameter (0.210 inch) to prevent the accidental use of improper headphones. A spare plug which accommodates the Phones/Speaker Jack has been included in the patch cord kit for those who wish to connect *sound field loudspeakers* to the HSL. A maximum of one watt RMS may be obtained from each Output Power Amplifier channel. The gain of both amplifier channels is simultaneously varied by identical amounts through the adjustment of the Output Gain Control Knob (Figure I-41c).

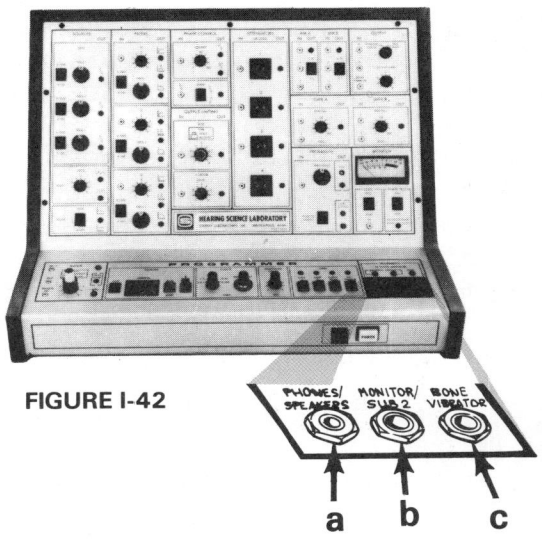

FIGURE I-42

The two-position switch shown in Figure I-41d controls the routing of signals to a second headphone jack labeled Monitor/Subj 2 (see Figure I-42b). This jack will accommodate a standard 0.250 inch diameter *stereo phone plug* and may be freely used with any low impedance headphones. When the "Stimulus Check" switch position is selected, those headphones connected to the Monitor/Subj 2 Jack will permit the experimenter to monitor the precise stimuli that are being delivered to the test subject's own headphones via the Phones/Speaker Jack. This feature eliminates the need for the experimenter to enter a remote test room and actually listen to the subject's headphones for a spot check of the stimuli. If desired, this switch setting may also be used to present the stimuli to an additional test subject. When the "Talkback" switch position is selected, signals sent to the Remote Microphone Preamplifier (Figure I-40f) will automatically be connected to one of the experimenter's monitor headphones. This allows the test subject to talk back to the experimenter (see Figure I-43A). For two-way intercom communication between experimenter and listener, the tester would deliver his or her own speech to the subject in the manner shown in Figure I-43B. Figure I-43C shows one possible configuration that permits the performance of experiments requiring that the signals from two independent microphones be routed separately to each ear.

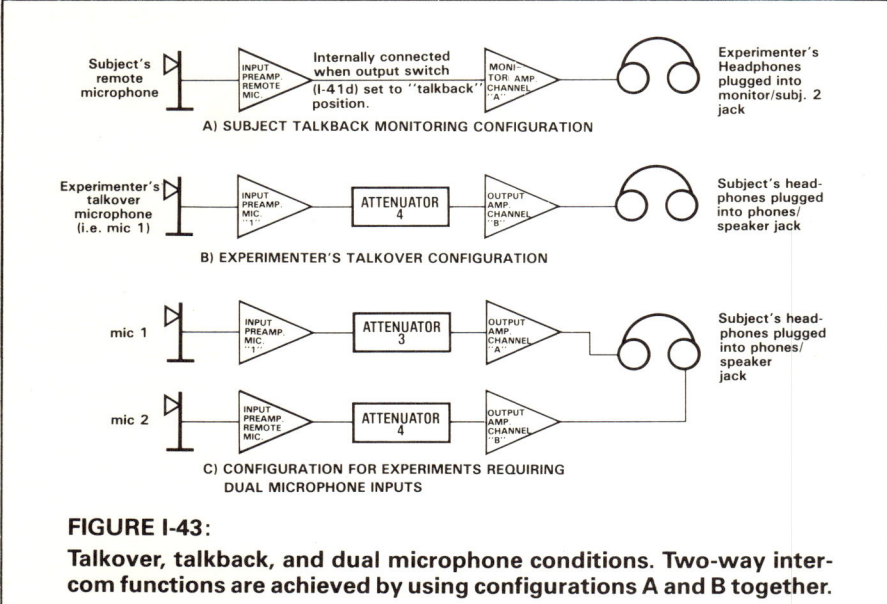

FIGURE I-43:
Talkover, talkback, and dual microphone conditions. Two-way intercom functions are achieved by using configurations A and B together.

Bone Vibrator Amplifier

Any of the signals produced by the Hearing Science Laboratory may be presented to a subject by means of a *bone conduction vibrator*. This device is commonly used in clinical audiometry to stimulate a listener's auditory system by coupling acoustic energy directly to the bones of the skull. These skull vibrations are transmitted through a variety of complex pathways and processes to the inner ear of a listener where the mechanical disturbances are transduced into the neural impulses that are ultimately perceived as sound by the brain. Differences between the detection of sounds delivered by *bone conduction* and by *air conduction* (i.e., listening via headphones or loudspeakers) are of importance to the clinical diagnosis of hearing disorders. An independent Bone Vibrator Output Amplifier is included in the Output Module of the Hearing Science Laboratory. Signals routed to the white Bone Vibrator Input Jack indicated in Figure I-41e will be amplified and delivered to the Bone Vibrator Output Jack shown in Figure I-42c. This jack will accommodate most clinical bone vibrators. Level control of the bone vibrator signals is readily provided by first passing the test signal through any of the four rotary thumbwheel attenuators on the HSL before connecting the stimulus to the Bone Vibrator Input Jack as shown in Figure I-44.

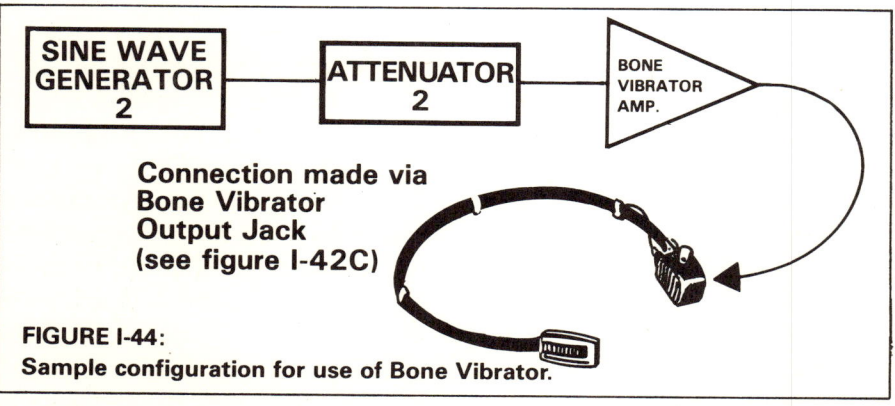

FIGURE I-44:
Sample configuration for use of Bone Vibrator.

OUTPUT LIMITATION

There are physical limits to the maximum output of any electronic amplifier. These limitations are governed by such factors as the amplifier's specific circuit design, complement of components, and power supply capabilities. The graph shown in Figure I-45 displays the output performance of a common type of amplifier for a variety of pure tone input signal levels. Note that as the input to the device is increased from an initially low level, a corresponding rise occurs in the amplifier's output magnitude. For the particular amplifier illustrated, we observe that the output voltage is consistently twice the level of the input (i.e., the system gain is fixed at two

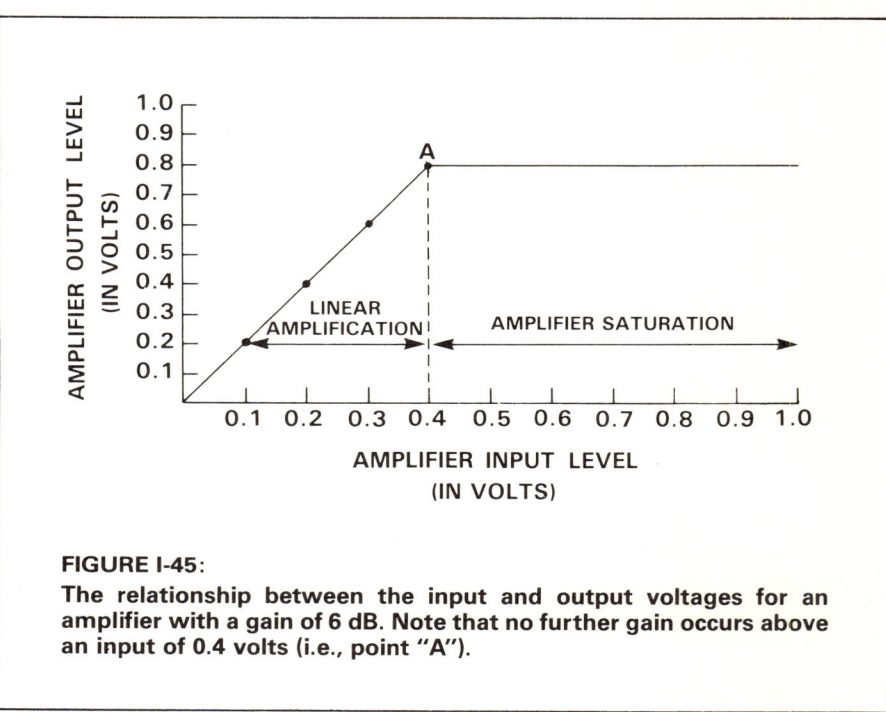

FIGURE I-45:
The relationship between the input and output voltages for an amplifier with a gain of 6 dB. Note that no further gain occurs above an input of 0.4 volts (i.e., point "A").

to one, or 6 dB). This relationship holds true up to the *maximum power output* or *saturation output level* of the amplifier. This is indicated as point "A" on the graph. Any increase in the input signal strength past this point produces no additional output amplification because the inherent maximum power limits of the amplifier have been reached. When input levels are kept below this saturation point, the amplifier produces an accurate enlarged replica of the original input signal waveform (see Figure I-46A). The operation of the amplifier beyond its saturation point, however, will cause a number of the largest waveform amplitude peaks and valleys to be *clipped* at the maximum output level. This "clipping" is shown in Figure I-46B. This type of waveform *distortion* typically adds an unpleasant sound quality to the test signal. Such *peak clipping* may occur if any of the individual or combination of Preamplifiers, Mixer-Amplifiers, or Output Amplifiers on the HSL are set to excessively high levels. This situation is easily remedied by lowering the signal level at the offending "overdriven" amplifier stage or by attenuating the signal through one of the four rotary thumbwheel Attenuators.

Although peak clipping does have a detrimental effect upon sound quality, numerous experiments have shown that it will not seriously interfere with

LABORATORY INSTRUMENTATION: PRINCIPLES AND FUNCTIONS

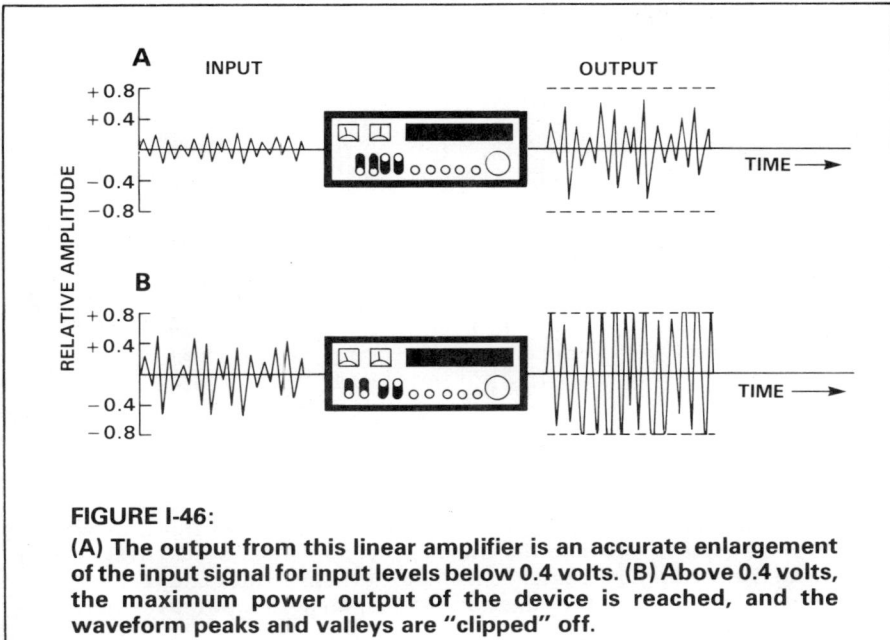

FIGURE I-46:
(A) The output from this linear amplifier is an accurate enlargement of the input signal for input levels below 0.4 volts. (B) Above 0.4 volts, the maximum power output of the device is reached, and the waveform peaks and valleys are "clipped" off.

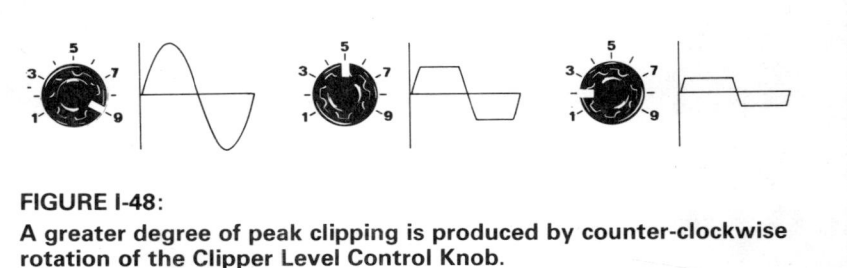

FIGURE I-48:
A greater degree of peak clipping is produced by counter-clockwise rotation of the Clipper Level Control Knob.

a listener's ability to discriminate speech sounds. This holds true for "symmetrical" peak clipping but not for "asymmetric" or "center" clipping (see Laboratory Experiments VIII-6 thru VIII-9). Peak clipping provides a simple yet effective means of limiting the maximum sound power output from a hearing aid amplifier without seriously affecting speech intelligibility. This is an especially important consideration, for many hearing impaired listeners cannot tolerate sound pressures above some specific level.

the minimum clipping effect on the signal. A counter-clockwise rotation of the knob will increasingly clip more of the signal waveform peaks and valleys in the manner shown in Figure I-48.

Automatic Gain Control

Automatic Gain Control (AGC) is another technique that is used to limit the maximum output of an amplifier. When the input signal to an amplifier exceeds some pre-established level, an AGC circuit will detect this condition and reduce the gain of the system. If the input signal drops below that preset level, the AGC circuit will permit the amplifier gain to return to its normal value. The location of the AGC module on the Hearing Science Laboratory is shown in Figure I-49. Figure I-50 displays the manner in which the AGC module processes a pure tone signal that is routed to the

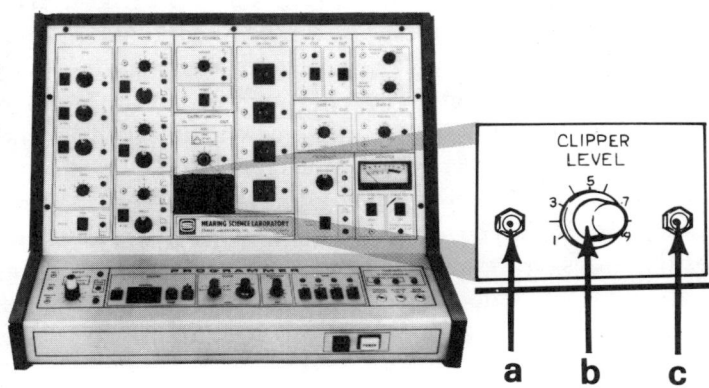

FIGURE I-47:

Adjustable Peak Clipper

A Peak Clipper featuring variable clipping level has been included in the Hearing Science Laboratory as shown in Figure I-47. Any stimulus connected to this module's white Input Jack (I-47a) will undergo a degree of peak clipping that is governed by the setting of the Clipper Level Control Knob (I-47b). The processed signal will emerge from the black Output Jack (I-47c). Adjusting the Clipper Level Control Knob fully clockwise exerts

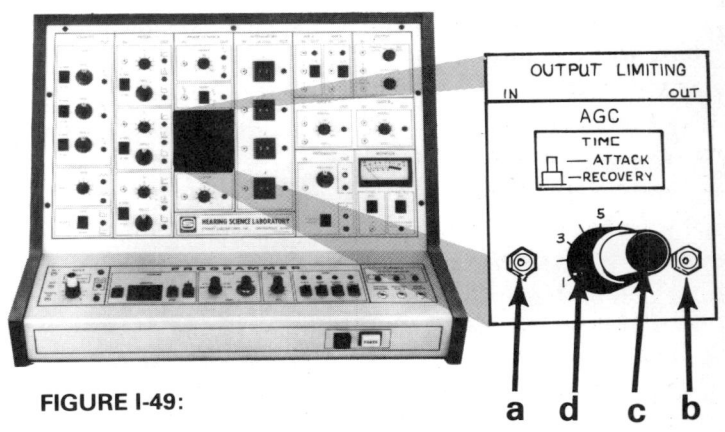

FIGURE I-49:

white Input Jack (Figure I-49a). Each point on the curve represents the signal voltage that emerges from the black Output Jack (Figure I-49b) for a particular input voltage level. After transduction by headphones or loudspeakers, these voltage changes will be mirrored by corresponding changes in output sound pressure level. Note that for input signals levels less than 60 millivolts, each change of input voltage produces ten times as much of a change in output voltage. This ten to one gain in voltage (20dB) forms a *linear*, or straight-line, relationship when plotted on the graph (compare with Figure I-45). Above the 60 millivolts landmark (graph point "A") variously known as the *AGC threshold* or *lower AGC limit*, continued increases in input levels produce corresponding, but ever smaller, increases in output level until input signals reach 100 millivolts. For increases in

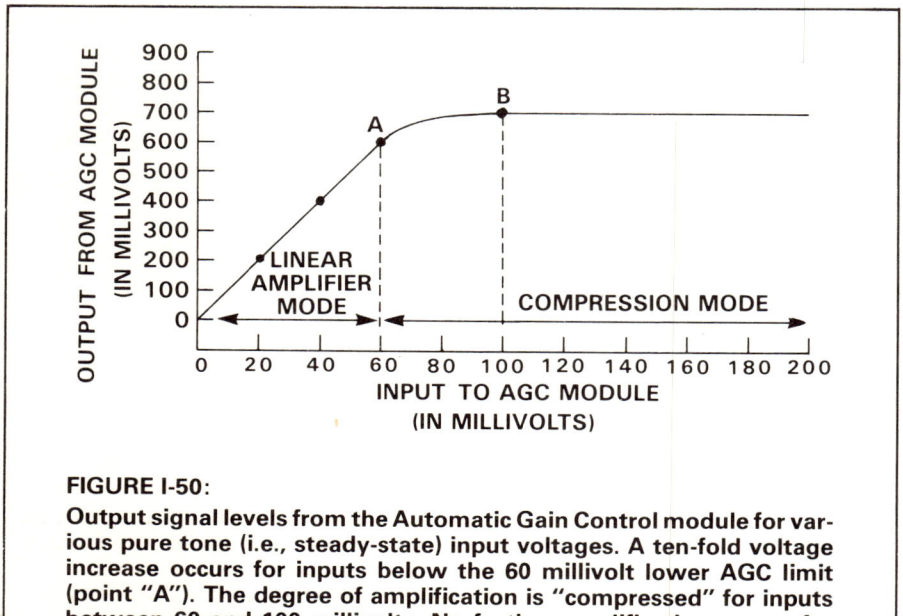

FIGURE I-50:
Output signal levels from the Automatic Gain Control module for various pure tone (i.e., steady-state) input voltages. A ten-fold voltage increase occurs for inputs below the 60 millivolt lower AGC limit (point "A"). The degree of amplification is "compressed" for inputs between 60 and 100 millivolts. No further amplification occurs for inputs above 100 millivolts.

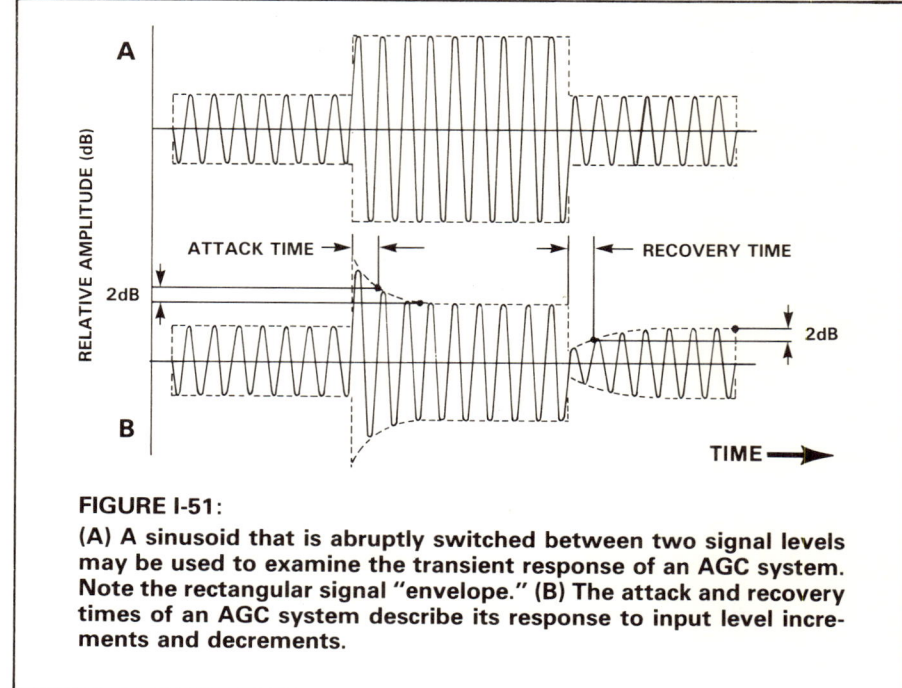

FIGURE I-51:
(A) A sinusoid that is abruptly switched between two signal levels may be used to examine the transient response of an AGC system. Note the rectangular signal "envelope." (B) The attack and recovery times of an AGC system describe its response to input level increments and decrements.

input levels above 100 millivolts ("B" on the curve), no further signal gain is provided by the AGC amplifier circuit, and the output level from the system remains fixed.

Unlike peak clipping methods, AGC systems preserve the original signal waveform shape essentially intact and do not chop off amplitude peaks and valleys. There are, however, other forms of signal distortions that are produced by AGC methods and variables. After three decades of practical applications and research with AGC, questions remain as to the precise nature and extent of the technique's ability to satisfy the listening needs of the hearing impaired. Figure I-51 illustrates the effects of AGC on a *transient* signal waveform that changes from one moment to the next. Unlike the non-varying, *steady-state*, pure tone signal used to obtain the preceding *input-output* graph, the sinusoid shown in Figure I-51A is being switched abruptly from one amplitude level to another. Figure I-51B shows the effects of an AGC system upon such an input signal. Every AGC circuit requires a certain amount of time to "sense" that a signal has exceeded the lower AGC threshold as well as to react to the change by reducing the system gain. During that brief time, the intense signal will be further increased by the normal gain of the amplifier. This appears on the waveform graph as a brief amplitude "spike" called *overshoot*. The time interval required by an AGC circuit to react to an abrupt signal amplitude change and reduce the amplifier gain to a specified stable level is called the *attack time*. The small diameter gray control knob shown in Figure I-49c may be used to vary the attack time of the AGC module from roughly ten to five hundred milliseconds.

The counterpart to attack time is known as *recovery time* or *release time*. This is the interval required by the AGC circuit to sense the abrupt reduction of an input signal level and restore the system gain, and its corresponding output level, to a specified stable level. Note from Figure I-51B that there is also a momentary *undershoot* during which the AGC circuit overreacts to the smaller signal by excessively lowering its level. Current standards have placed the specified levels which define the attack and recovery times of hearing aid AGC circuits to be within two decibels of the steady state levels for the larger (80 dB) and smaller (55 dB) standard input test signals, respectively. The large diameter black knob shown in Figure I-49d will vary the AGC recovery time from approximately ten to three hundred milliseconds. Both the attack and recovery times increase as their control knobs are rotated clockwise. Additional details about automatic gain control are contained within Laboratory Experiments VIII-12 and VIII-13.

Demonstrations and Experiments Part II

Fundamental Concepts

I

EXPERIMENT I-1: LAW OF SUPERPOSITION (INTERFERENCE)

Purpose:
To demonstrate the reinforcement and cancellation of pairs of waveforms which share differing phase relationships.

Background Principle:
The multitude of sound waves within our environment continually encounter one another as they travel from their generating sources. Interactions between these waves produce sounds whose amplitude, at each point in time and space, is equal to the algebraic summation of the constituent waveform magnitudes. This phenomenon, known as *interference* or the *law of superposition*, was illustrated earlier in Figure I-15. Each pair of sinusoidal waveforms in Figure I-15A was identical in frequency and maximum amplitude. When, in addition, the compressions and rarefactions of one component waveform coincided in space and time with corresponding points on the other wave, the two signals were in phase with each other (see page 5 regarding the concept of phase). Both stimuli combined to form a resultant wave that had the identical frequency as the original stimuli, but twice their maximum amplitudes. Such an increased, or reinforced, resultant wave does not occur when the two components shown in Figure I-15B combine. Since both waves are out of phase by one half period (i.e., by 180°) at each instant in time, cancellation occurs, the algebraic sum of the two magnitudes is zero, and no sound is produced. Varying degrees of partial reinforcement or cancellation will result when the two waves shown in Figure I-15C, for example, are out of phase by 90° (i.e., ¼ period) and yield a resultant whose maximum amplitude is 1.41 times the magnitude of either original component (i.e., 3 dB greater).

Procedure:
Two identical frequency sinusoids can be produced by splitting the output signal from one Sine Wave Generator into two separate components. In order to alter the phase relationship between the two waveforms, the pure tone stimulus must be routed through the Adjustable Phase Shifter. Both the reference and phase-shifted outputs from this module are then sent to separate Attenuators so that the magnitude of each component may be adjusted independently. The components are combined within a Mixer-Amplifier and the resultant signal is delivered to an Output Amplifier channel and headphone. The amplitude of either stimulus component, or the resultant waveform, may be monitored with the Level Meter by connecting, in turn, the "dashed" circuit wires labeled "A", "B", and "C" on the front panel wiring guide and block diagram. Attenuator #3 should be initially set to provide fairly high attenuation (e.g., 50 or 60 dB) in order to prevent too large a signal level from entering the Meter circuit. After the Meter patch cord is attached to the desired signal jack, reduce the Attenuator setting until a satisfactory meter reading is obtained. If an oscilloscope is available, one may attach its input probe to the meter test points so that the stimuli waveforms may be observed.

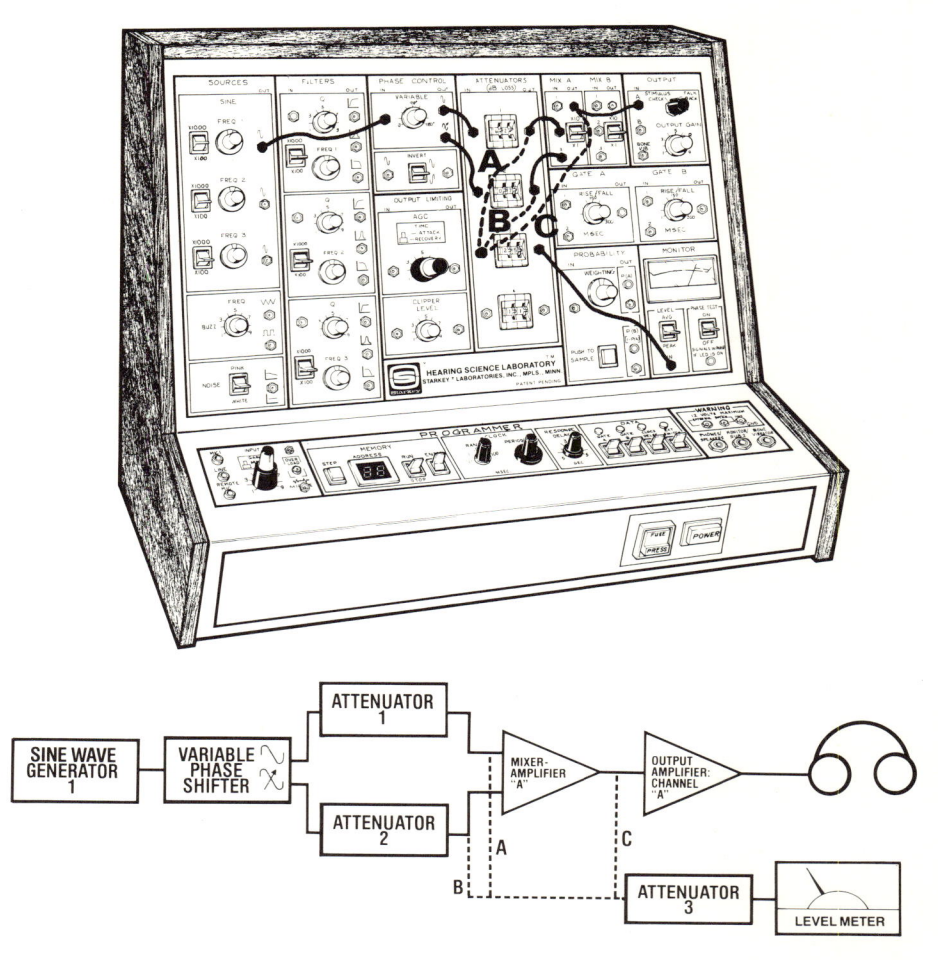

Exercises:
(1) Adjust the Frequency Control Knob and Range Switch to provide a signal frequency near 1000 Hz. Set Attenuators #1 and #2 to identical levels (e.g., 15 dB attenuation each). Alternately connect the Level Meter patch cord to those two Input Jacks where the signals enter the Mixer-Amplifier (i.e., connections marked "A" and "B" on the wiring guide). Confirm that each signal produces an equal reading upon the Meter. Next, connect the Meter patch cord to the Output Jack of the Mixer-Amplifier and note the magnitude in dB of the combined signals (wire "C"). Vary the Adjustable Phase Shifter Control Knob and record the Meter readings for several phase settings. Do the signals completely reinforce and cancel each other at the 0° and 180° phase settings, respectively? Can you account for the fact that the resultant tone may still be faintly perceptible even though the Meter shows no reading?

(2) Repeat exercise #1 with dissimilar Attenuator settings (e.g., 5 and 15 dB). Note that even when both signals are 180° out-of-phase, a resultant wave is clearly formed. Can you explain the reasons for this "partial cancellation"?

NOTES:

Selected References:

Durrant, J.D. and Lovrinic, J.H. (1977). *Bases of hearing science.* pp. 32-33. Williams and Wilkins, Baltimore, Maryland.

von Helmholtz, H. (1863). *On the sensation of tone as a physiological basis for the theory of music.* (First American ed. of the second English ed. of the fourth German ed.) Dover, New York, 1954.

Green, D.M. (1976). *An introduction to hearing.* Chapter 1. Lawrence Erlbaum Assoc., Hillsdale, New Jersey.

Mee, F.G. (1967). *Sound,* (2nd ed.). pp. 22-24. Heinemann Educational Books, Ltd., London.

Roederer, J.G. (1975). *Introduction to the physics and psychophysics of music,* (2nd ed.). Ch. II, III, V. Springer-Verlag, New York.

Wood, A. (1966). *Acoustics.* Ch. VIII. Dover, New York.

EXPERIMENT I-2: FOURIER'S THEOREM

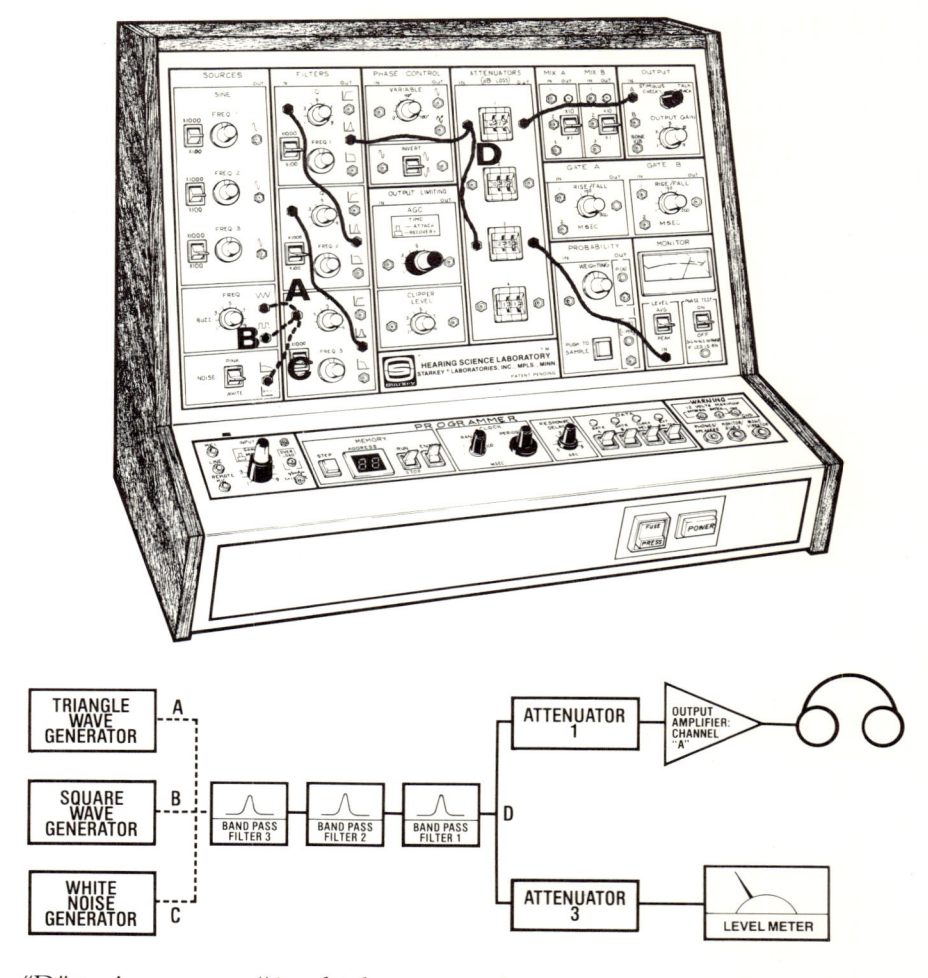

Purpose:
To isolate individual pure tone components within a complex sound.

Background Principle:
Sounds with sinusoidal waveforms are rarely produced within our everyday environment. Almost all naturally occurring sounds possess complex waveforms which may be examined with devices that display the magnitude of a stimulus as time passes (i.e., on an *oscilloscope*). The periodically repeating pattern shown in Figure "A" represents the waveform of the English vowel sound "ah" (/a/) when uttered by a male speaker. As discussed in the first section of this text, the French physicist Fourier showed that any complex periodic waveform is actually composed of a series of individual sine waves whose frequencies and phases were related to each other in a simple mathematical manner. Fourier's techniques may also be used to analyze a non-periodic waveshape such as that produced by the English "sh" ([ʃ]) shown in Figure "B." One can verify the presence of discrete pure tone frequencies within complex sounds by electronically filtering out all but selected tone components from the stimulus.

Procedure:
An extremely selective narrow bandpass filter can be created by connecting several bandpass filters together in a series, or cascaded, configuration. This means that the output of one filter is routed to the input of another (review Figure I-30 for other cascading applications). A choice of several complex sounds may be analyzed by routing the input wire of Filter #3 along paths "A", "B", or "C" shown in the wiring guide and block diagram. For maximum selectivity, rotate each Filter "Q" Control to the fully clockwise position. Note that the final Filter output is sent to two separate Attenuators. This arrangement permits the adjustment of the signal strength reaching both the Level Meter as well as the Output Amplifier channel and headphone.

Exercises:
(1) Connect circuit wire "B" between the Square Wave Output Jack and the input to Filter #3. Adjust the Frequency Control Knob to position 5 which corresponds to approximately 100 Hz. Set each of the three filters to an initial frequency control setting that is roughly the same as the "Buzz" Source. Route the Meter-Attenuator input wire "D" to the bandpass Output Jack of each Filter, one at a time. Adjust the Frequency Control Knob of each Filter until a maximum Meter reading is obtained. Since the maximum output of a bandpass filter occurs at its center frequency, this simple technique may be used to guarantee that each of the filters is tuned to the same center frequency. After this initial calibration exercise, connect wire "D" to Attenuator #1, which receives the output from the three cascaded filters as shown in the wiring guide and block diagram. Adjust Attenuator #3 until the Meter reads zero dB and then record both Attenuator and Meter levels on Table I below. Locate additional Filter frequency settings that produce noticeable Meter readings. Remember to recalibrate all three Filters for each new frequency setting. Record the relative signal levels (in dB) present at each new frequency and plot your data points in the form of a line spectrum on the set of axes provided below. Do your findings match the spectrum shown earlier in Figure I-20? If not, can you identify those variables which may have influenced your results?

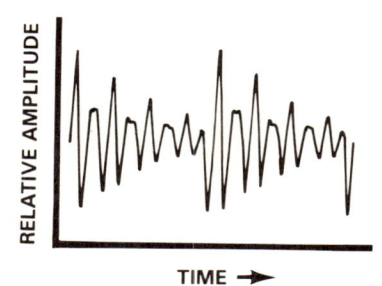

FIGURE A: The periodic waveform of the vowel /a/ as in "ah." (After Denes and Pinson, 1973).

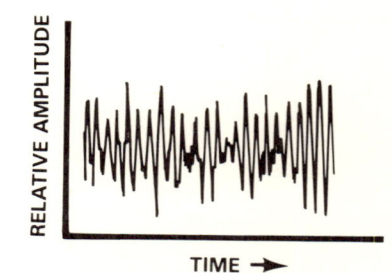

FIGURE B: The waveform of /ʃ/, as in "she," is aperiodic in nature. (After Denes and Pinson, 1973).

(2) Disconnect the circuit wire from the Square Wave Output Jack and insert it into the Triangle Wave Output Jack. Repeat exercise #1 and describe the differences between the spectra of the square and triangle waveforms.

(3) Connect the circuit wire "C" to the Noise Output Jack. Since it is not practical to measure every one of the near infinite pure tone components in white or pink noise, examine the energy that is present at a variety of frequencies, each an octave apart. Plot a continuous spectrum of the noise by connecting each tone magnitude value on your graph rather than drawing a separate vertical line for each. Plot your data points on the axes provided below. Compare and contrast the spectrum you obtained with those shown in Figures I-21, 22, and 24.

(4) If an oscilloscope is available, examine the waveform of narrow band noise as the Filter "Q" controls are adjusted. You will notice that the more narrow the bandwidth of the noise, the more its waveform will approximate that of a sinusoid which is slowly varying in frequency and amplitude. Compare the subjective quality of the noise before it enters Filter #3 and after it emerges from Filter #1.

NOTES:

TABLE 1

BANDPASS FILTER CENTER FREQUENCIES (in HZ)	RELATIVE AMPLITUDE OF FREQUENCY COMPONENT (i.e. ATTENUATOR #3 SETTING THAT PRODUCES ZERO dB METER READING)	METER READING (RECORD DEVIATION, IN dB, IF METER IS NOT AT ZERO)
(SQUARE WAVE SIGNAL)		
F 1:		
F 2:		
F 3:		
F 4:		
F 5:		
(TRIANGLE WAVE SIGNAL)		
F 1:		
F 2:		
F 3:		
F 4:		
F 5:		
(NOISE SIGNAL)		
F 1:		
F 2:		
F 3:		
F 4:		
F 5:		

Selected References:

Denes, P.B. and Pinson, E.N. (1973). *The speech chain; the physics and biology of spoken language.* Ch. III. Anchor Books, Garden City, New York.

von Helmholtz, H. (1863). *On the sensation of tone as a physiological basis for the theory of music.* (First American ed. of the second English ed. of the fourth German ed.) Dover, New York, 1954.

Kinsler, L.E. and Frey, A.R. (1962). *Fundamentals of acoustics,* (2nd ed.) Ch. I & II. Wiley, New York.

Moore, B.C.J. (1977). *Introduction to the psychology of hearing.* Chapter 1. University Park Press, Boston.

Papoulis, A. (1962). *The Fourier integral and its applications.* McGraw-Hill, New York.

Roederer, J.G. (1975). *Introduction to the physics and psychophysics of music,* (2nd ed.). pp. 106-109, Springer-Verlag, New York.

Wood, A. (1966). *Acoustics.* Dover, New York.

Wood, A.B. (1930). *A textbook of sound.* pp. 25-30. MacMillan Co., New York.

EXPERIMENT I-3: QUALITY OF SYNTHESIZED COMPLEX WAVES

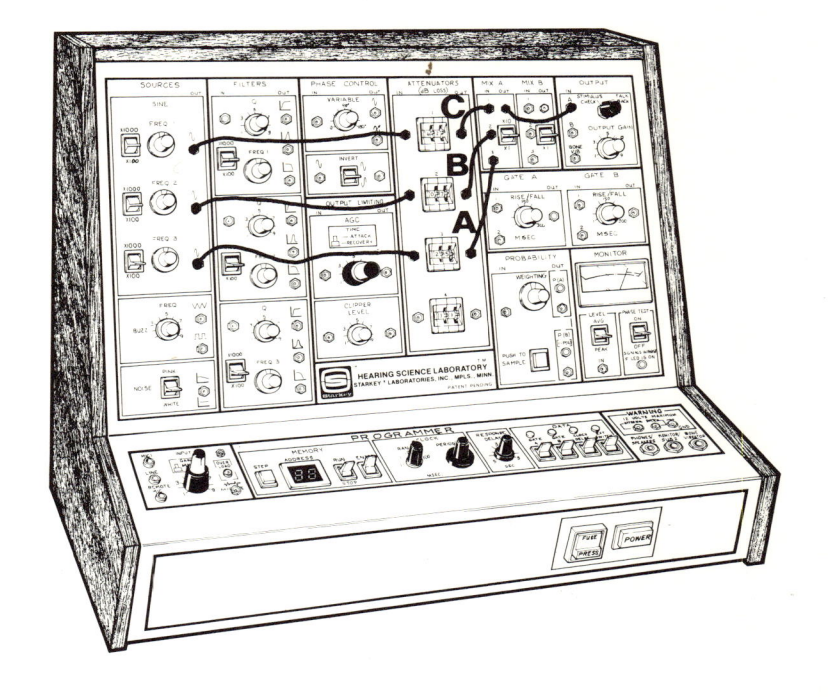

Purpose:
To explore the influence of spectrum upon the subjective quality of a sound.

Background Principle:
Words such as harsh, noisy, tonal, and shrill are commonly used to describe the quality of sounds. It is the specific characteristics of the sound's waveform that appear to influence our subjective perception of the stimulus quality. The resultant waveform of a complex sound is determined by the number and frequencies of the pure tone components within the signal as well as their respective magnitudes and phase relationships. In Figures I-15 and 16, shown earlier, we observed that a change in any of these component parameters will alter the resulting wave pattern. The question remains, however, as to the relative importance of one parameter over another in affecting resultant sound quality.

Procedure:
Note from the wiring guide and block diagram that each of the three pure tone signals is passed through separate Attenuators so that their amplitudes may be independently controlled. All three stimuli are mixed together within one Mixer-Amplifier whose output is routed to an Output Amplifier channel and headphone.

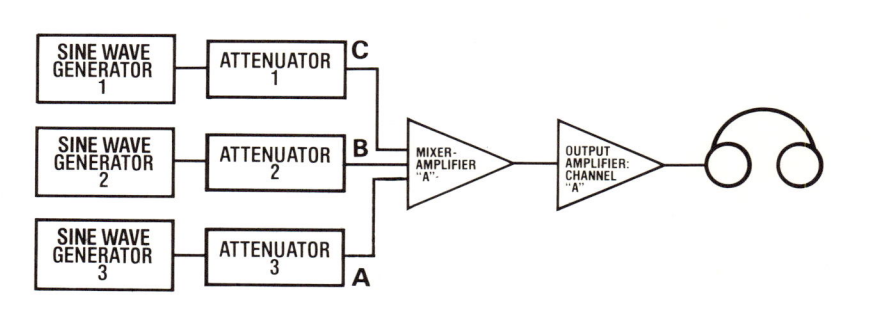

Exercises:
(1) Set all three Attenuators to identical levels (e.g., 15 dB). Adjust the three sine wave signals to be near the following frequencies:

F_1 : 200 Hz
F_2 : 1000 Hz
F_3 : 5000 Hz

Alternately connect and remove wires "A", "B", or "C" from the Mixer-Amplifier inputs and note the relative effect that each signal has upon the quality of the resultant wave. If available, attach an oscilloscope probe to the output of the Mixer-Amplifier so that the complex waveforms that are created may be observed. Does any one of the three frequencies seem to play a more prominent role in affecting the overall wave shape and quality?

(2) With all three signals mixed together, slowly vary the frequency and amplitude of an individual component and note the effects on overall sound quality and waveshape. Is one parameter more significant than the others in affecting the complex signal?

(3) Repeat exercises #1 and #2 for three frequencies that are more closely spaced (e.g., 200, 300, and 400 Hz; and 2000, 2500 and 3000 Hz) and note any differences.

NOTES:

Selected References:

von Bismarck, G. (1974a). Timbre of steady sounds: a factorial investigation of its verbal attributes. *Acustica*, **30**, 146-159.

von Bismarck, G. (1974b). Sharpness as an attribute of the timbre of steady sounds. *Acustica*, **30**, 159-172.

Jeans, J.H. (1937). *Science and music.* pp. 84-89. Cambridge University Press (republished by Dover, New York, 1968).

Olson, H.F. (1967). *Music, physics and engineering,* (2nd ed.). pp. 206-214. Dover, New York.

Plomp, R. and Steeneken, H.J.M. (1973). Place dependence of timbre in reverberant sound fields. *Acustica*, **28**, 50-59.

Roederer, J.G. (1975). *Introduction to the physics and psychophysics of music,* (2nd ed.). Ch. IV. Springer-Verlag, New York.

Wood, A. (1950). *The physics of music* (5th ed.). Methuen & Co., London.

EXPERIMENT I-4: PEAK, AVERAGE, AND RMS AMPLITUDE OF SIGNALS

Purpose:
To compare and contrast the common measures of signal amplitude.

Background Principle:
The magnitude of an acoustical signal or its electrical counterpart can be expressed by a variety of measures and units. *Amplitude*, mentioned on page 4, is a general term for sound magnitude and is also used to describe the physical displacement of a vibrating sound generator from its resting position. The *instantaneous amplitude* represents the magnitude of a changing signal at a particular point in time (e.g., points shown by dots in Figure "A"). The *peak* and *peak-to-peak* amplitudes shown in the figure are levels which are of importance for sound amplification and reproduction purposes. In Laboratory Experiments VIII-6 thru VIII-8, for example, we shall find that excessive peak signal amplitudes may create a *distortion* of the original waveform and an unpleasant sound quality. For most electrical and acoustical purposes, however, it is necessary to describe the overall *power* in a signal. Power is a measure of a sound's ability to do some amount of *work* in a given time period (i.e., to vibrate the molecules in the surrounding medium thereby generating heat). For any periodic symmetrical waveform like the sinusoid, however, it would not be meaningful to merely average instantaneous amplitudes over the entire waveform cycle in order to determine the overall signal power. It should be clear that the positive and negative waveform values would, in this case, cancel each other mathematically to yield an average power of zero.

The *root-mean-square (RMS) amplitude* of a signal is, however, an important measure that does reflect the power content of the stimulus. The term, RMS, relates to the statistical process from which the measure is derived. Specifically, the RMS amplitude is determined by first squaring the instantaneous waveform levels to remove their algebraic sign; then obtaining the *mean*, or average, of the squared values; and finally taking the square root of the mean. In the numerical examples shown below, several instantaneous amplitude values on the sinusoid in Figure "A" have been used to compute the average level and **approximate** RMS level.

	Sampled values from first cycle of sine wave in Figure "A"
AVERAGE AMPLITUDE (ARITHMETIC MEAN)	$= \dfrac{0 + 1 + 2 + 1 + 0 + (-1) + (-2) + (-1)}{8}$ $= 0$
ROOT-MEAN-SQUARE AMPLITUDE	$= \sqrt{\dfrac{(0)^2+(1)^2+(2)^2+(1)^2+(0)^2+(-1)^2+(-2)^2+(-1)^2}{8}}$ $= \sqrt{\dfrac{12}{8}} \quad = 1.22$

FIGURE A: The relationship between Peak (V_p), Peak-to-Peak ($V_{p\text{-}p}$), and Root-Mean-Square (V_{RMS}) amplitudes for a sine wave.

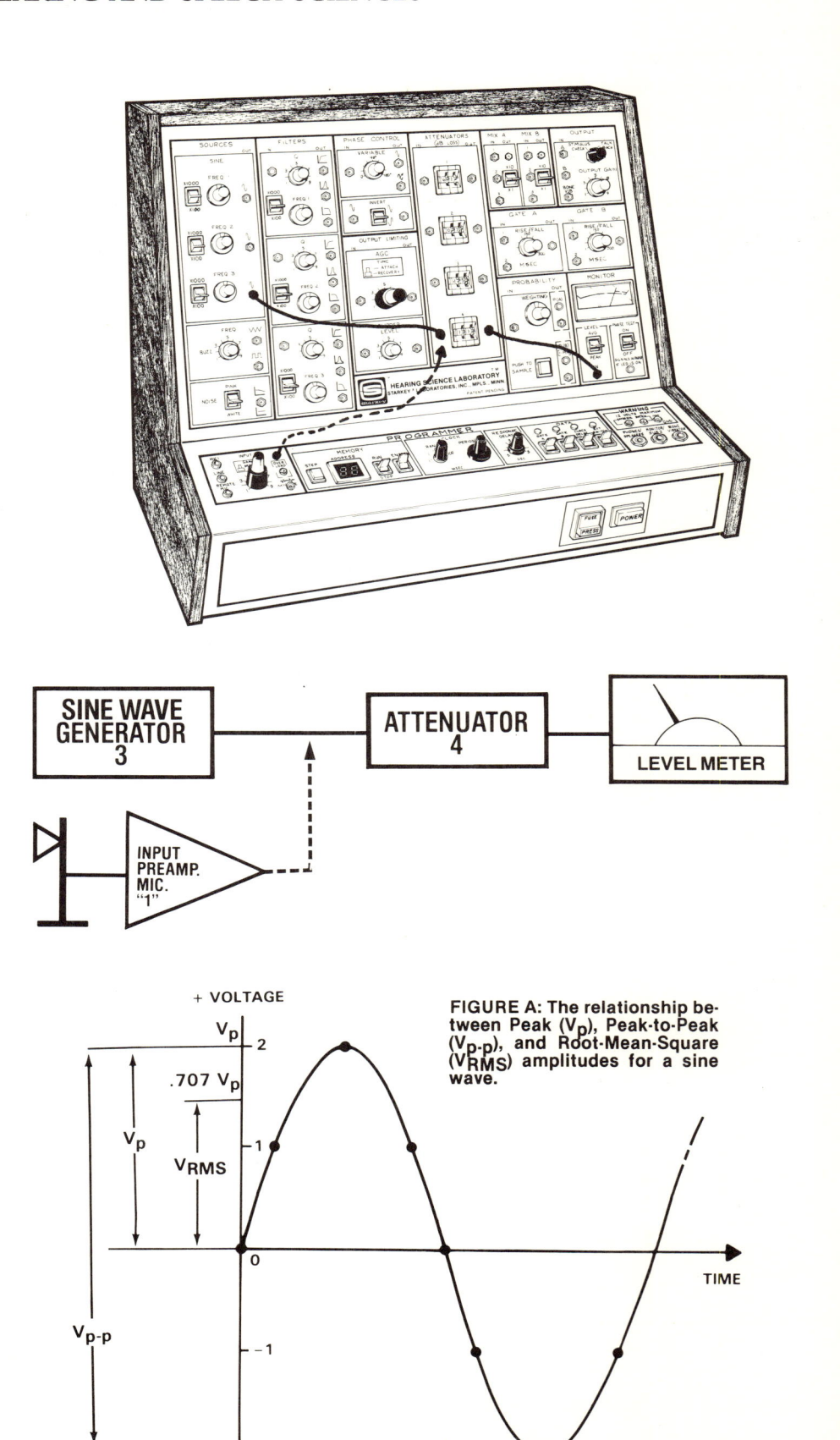

To determine the "true RMS" amplitude, an infinite number of waveform samples would have to be taken. RMS levels are relatively simple to compute and measure for sine waves but become extremely tedious and difficult to derive for more complex signals. With the appropriate calibration of the meter scale, a conventional type of monitoring *A.C. voltmeter* (i.e., one designed to respond to "alternating current" fluctuations) will show the RMS value of a **sinusoid** (see exercise #2). It is, however, important to note that only a *true RMS meter*, in which electronic circuits perform the mathematical steps described above, will accurately measure the root-mean-square level of a complex signal.

The elementary arithmetic relationships which link the various amplitude measures of a sinusoid are highlighted below and in Figure "A".

```
              FOR SINUSOIDAL SIGNALS
PEAK AMPLITUDE   =   0.5   X PEAK-TO-PEAK AMPLITUDE
PEAK AMPLITUDE   =   1.414 X RMS AMPLITUDE
RMS AMPLITUDE    =   0.707 X PEAK AMPLITUDE
RMS AMPLITUDE    =   0.353 X PEAK-TO-PEAK AMPLITUDE
```

Procedure:

A 1000 Hz signal from Sine Wave Generator #3 is sent through Attenuator #4 before being delivered to the Monitor Level Meter. The Attenuator should be set to a value that produces a meter scale reading near zero decibels.

Exercises:

(1) Alternate the Peak/Average Meter Switch from one position to another and note the difference in decibel levels. Use the arithmetical relationship between peak and RMS amplitude, listed above, to account for the dB change in the Meter reading.

(2) The signal amplitude emerging from the Sine Wave Generator is 2 volts RMS. Calculate the RMS and peak voltage equivalents for -10, -20, and -30 dB Meter scale readings.

(3) Re-route the input wire of Attenuator #4 to the Mic 1 Preamplifier Output Jack instead of Sine Wave Generator #3. Contrast the "ballistics" of the Meter movements for live speech signals when the Peak/Average Meter Switch position is changed. How do you account for the observed differences?

NOTES:

Selected References:

Durrant, J.D. and Lovrinic, J.H. (1977). *Bases of hearing science.* pp. 42-43. Williams and Wilkins, Baltimore.

Everitt, W.L. (1958). *Fundamentals of radio and electronics*, (2nd ed.). pp. 99-101. Prentice-Hall, Englewood Cliffs, New Jersey.

Grob, B. (1971). *Basic electronics.* Chapter 15. McGraw-Hill, New York.

Johnson, J.R. (1970). *Electric circuits: Part II, Alternating Current.* pp. 536-539. Holt, Rinehart and Winston, New York.

Punch, J.L. and Lawrence, W.F. (1977). Decibel notation with correlated and uncorrelated signals. *J. Amer. Audiol. Soc.*, **3**, 71-79.

EXPERIMENT I-5: REDUCTION OF ACOUSTIC FEEDBACK

Purpose:
To utilize a notch filter for the reduction of acoustic feedback in the presence of high gain amplification.

Background Principle:
Consider the situation shown in Figure "A" wherein a portion of the acoustic output of an amplifier is permitted to return to the input of the system and be re-amplified many times. Such *positive feedback* is not, as the name might imply, a desirable phenomenon. This feedback can cause the amplifier to produce a high level sinusoidal oscillation at a particular frequency. The characteristic "squeal," or "howl," associated with feedback in public address systems and hearing aids poses serious limitations to the amount of gain that the amplifier can provide. Common remedies for this problem include lowering the gain of the system or increasing the physical separation between the output and input transducers. In both instances, a less intense acoustic signal reaches the system input and is less likely to instigate feedback. The frequency content of the positive feedback will depend upon such factors as the length of the feedback path, the frequencies of any resonant peaks in the amplifier and, most important, whether or not the phase angle of the output signal arriving at the microphone promotes a reinforcement (i.e., amplification) of the signal. It is possible to reduce positive feedback by including a notch filter in the amplification system as shown in Figure "B." Such a device will prevent a narrow range of frequencies from passing through the amplifier and, thereby, if properly tuned, reject the feedback frequency itself while leaving the remainder of the signal intact.

Procedure:
The signals from a microphone are passed through the Mic. 1 Preamplifier and then delivered to the Input Jack of Filter #2. Set the Filter "Q" Control Knob to the fully counterclockwise position and combine both the high and low pass filter outputs within Mixer-Amplifier "A" to create an adjustable notch filter in the manner shown earlier in Figure I-30D. The Mixer signal is then routed through one Output Amplifier channel and headphone or loudspeaker.

Exercises:
(1) Produce acoustic feedback by placing the microphone close to the loudspeaker (or headphone) and increasing the gain of the amplification system. Gain may be varied with the Mic. 1 Preamplifier Gain Control Knob, Mixer-Amplifier Gain Switch, and the Output Amplifier Gain Control Knob. Vary the Filter Frequency Control Knob and Range Switch until the feedback is "nulled" or notched out completely.

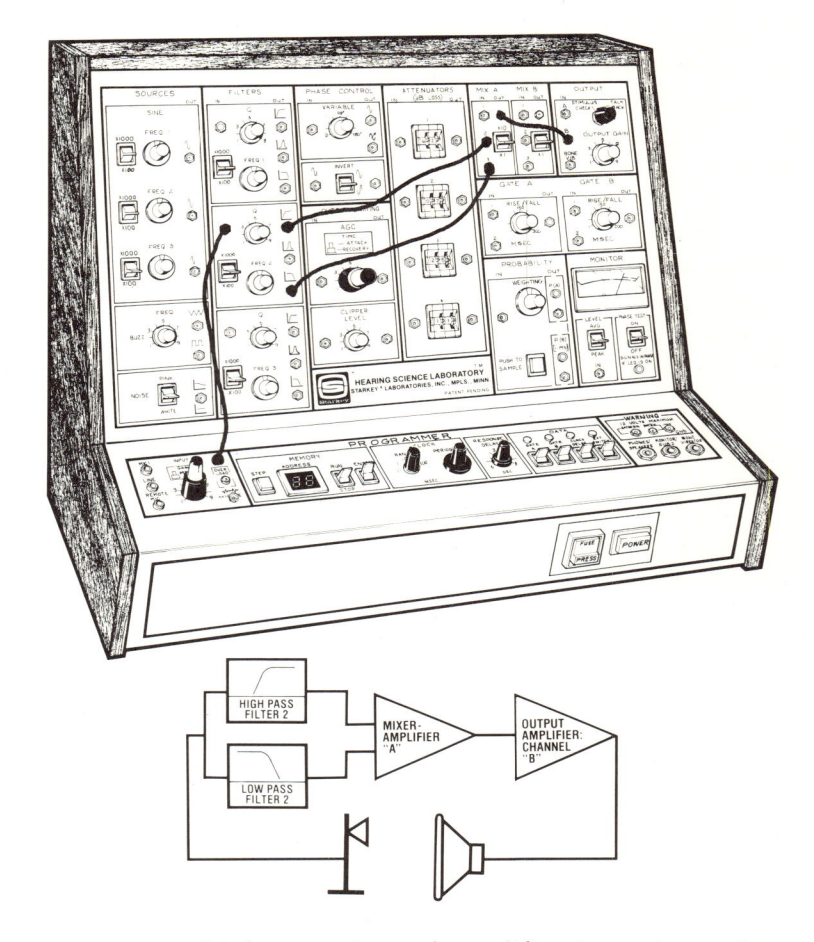

(2) Repeat exercise #1 for a variety of amplification gain settings and transducer separations. How do you account for the fact that the notch filter is unable to eliminate feedback at extremely high gain settings?

(3) Connect high pass and low pass filters in cascade, as shown earlier in Figure I-30E, to produce a notch filter with 24 dB/octave rolloff. Repeat exercises #1 and #2 and note if this "sharper" filter is more effective in reducing feedback than the one used in exercise #1.

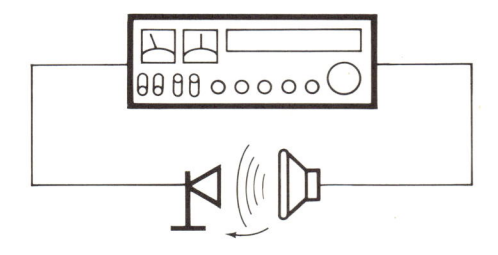

FIGURE A: Positive feedback occurs when the output from an amplifier is returned to the system input and is re-amplified many times.

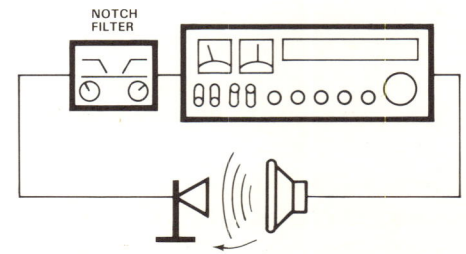

FIGURE B: One technique for reducing feedback utilizes a notch filter to reject the frequency of the offending "squeal."

NOTES:

Selected References:

Boner, C.P. and Boner, C.R. (1965a). A procedure for controling room-ring modes and feedback modes in sound systems with narrow-band filters. *J. Audio Eng. Soc.*, **13**, 297.

Boner, C.P. and Boner, C.R. (1965b). Minimizing feedback in sound systems and room-ring modes with passive networks. *J. Acoust. Soc. Am.*, **37**, 131-135.

Boner, C.P. and Boner, C.R. (1966). Behavior of sound system response immediately below feedback. *J. Audio Eng. Soc.*, **14**, 200.

Burkhard, M.D. (1963). A simplified frequency shifter for improving acoustic feedback stability. *J. Audio Eng. Soc.*, **11**, 234-237.

Connor, W.K. (1973). Experimental investigation of sound-system — room feedback. *J. Audio Eng. Soc.*, **21**, 27-32.

Prestigiacomo, A.J. and MacLean, D.J. (1962). A frequency shifter for improving acoustic feedback stability. *J. Audio Eng. Soc.*, **10**, 111.

Schroeder, M.R. (1962). Improvement of feedback stability of public address systems by frequency shifting. *J. Audio Eng. Soc.*, **10**, 109-110.

Schroeder, M.R. (1964). Improvement of acoustic-feedback stability by frequency shifting. *J. Acoust. Soc. Am.*, **36**, 1718-1724.

Schulein, R.B. (1976). Microphone considerations in feedback-prone environments. *J. Audio Eng. Soc.*, **24**, 434-444.

Waterhouse, R.V. (1965). Theory of howl-back in reverberant rooms. *J. Acoust. Soc. Am.*, **37**, 921-923.

Threshold of Audibility II

EXPERIMENT II-1: PSYCHOMETRIC FUNCTION FOR HUMAN HEARING

Purpose:
To examine the responses of a listener to pure tone stimuli of different magnitudes.

Background Principle:
In a primitive sense, the human hearing mechanism may be compared to a microphone as both devices are able to transduce the mechanical energy of sound vibrations into electricity. A simple experiment will reveal, however, that any notion of a rigidly fixed, absolute minimum threshold for detection does not accurately reflect the manner in which a listener responds to sound. Although it is possible to surgically enter the skull (indeed, it is actually done to certain animals and consenting humans) to attach electrodes to portions of the inner ear transducer and monitor the tiny "microphonic" voltages it produces, this objective measurement technique has understandably not "caught on" as a method of choice for routine hearing testing. After all, **hearing** is a sensation and must be experienced; it's more than a voltage reading.

What have evolved, instead, are procedures based upon models or theories of human hearing that rely upon the subjective reports of the listener as to when or what he or she has heard. One fundamental measure of hearing acuity is the determination of the minimum amount of sound pressure a listener requires for the detection of a pure tone stimulus.

Consider a listening situation in which the observer is asked to raise his hand each time he or she detects the presence of a tone. The test commences with a signal whose magnitude is so small that the subject fails to observe its occurrence. If the magnitude of the signal were to be increased in large steps of 10 decibels each, the listener is likely to respond in the manner shown by Figure "A". At first glance, these data would seem to indicate that the observer's hearing operates in an "all or nothing" fashion. Sound magnitudes smaller than the value of point "C" on the graph are not heard, while those tones above this sound pressure level are detected. But what of those signals whose magnitudes lie between levels "B" and "C"? If we present each test stimulus many times, we would find that the observer correctly detects a different percentage of the tones at each of the intermediate sound levels. The typical response pattern of human listeners in such an experiment may be represented by an S-shaped curve known as a *psychometric function* (see Figure "B"). This kind of performance suggests that human hearing is probabilistic in nature, with each sound pressure giving rise to a specific likelihood that a tone will be detected. (This is seen most clearly in the S-shaped regions of uncertainty in Figure "B.")

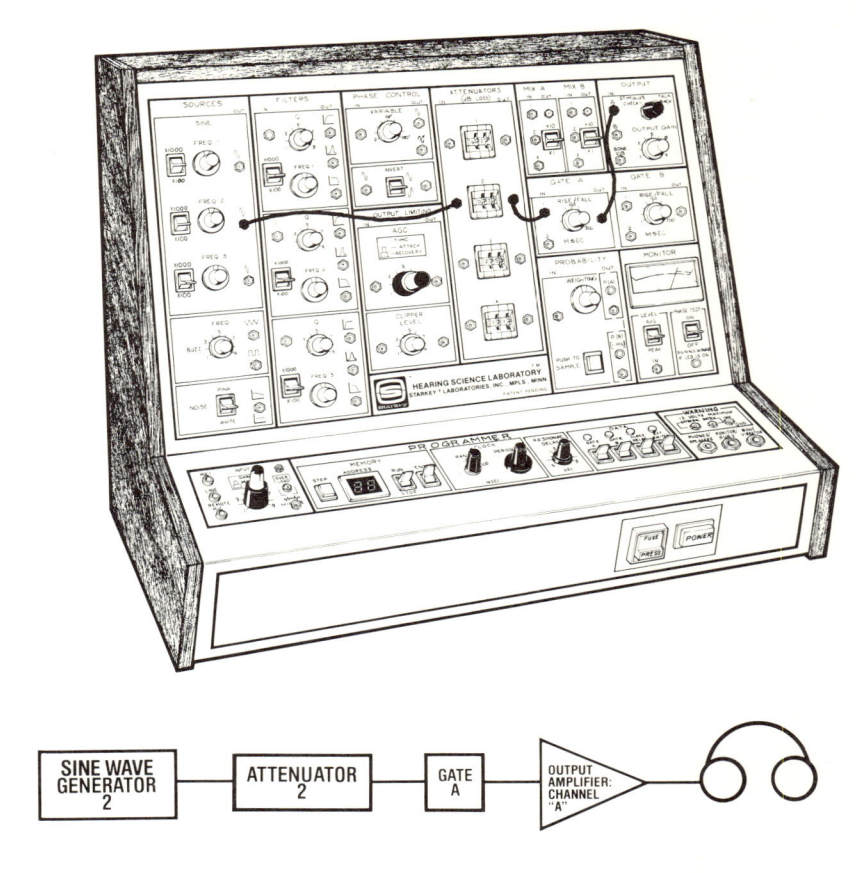

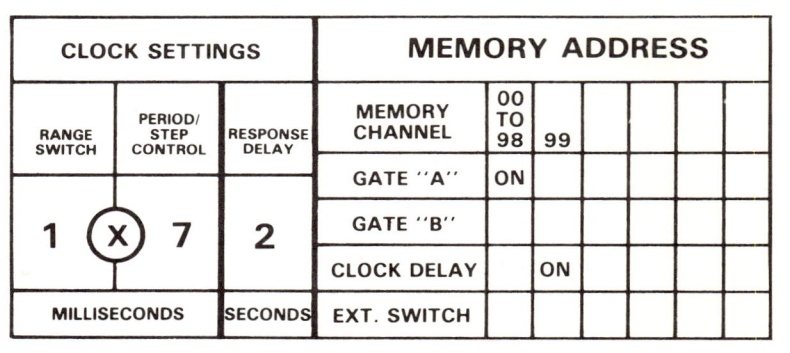

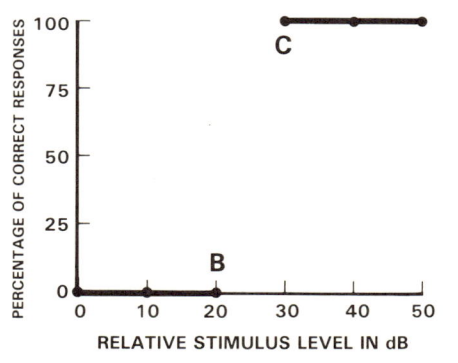

FIGURE A: A graphic representation of the notion that a subject responds in an "all or nothing" fashion.

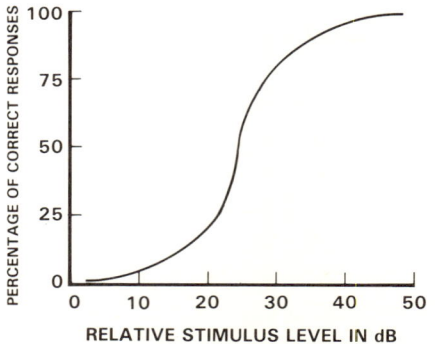

FIGURE B: The *ogive* (i.e., S-shaped) psychometric function reveals that a listener correctly responds to signals on a probabilistic basis. Note that higher level signals are more likely to be detected.

Procedure:

A pure tone signal is routed through an Attenuator, Electronic Gate, Output Amplifier channel, and headphone. The suggested Programmer instructions will permit the signal to be switched on for approximately 0.7 second. A two second pause is provided, after each test trial, by the Programmer Delay Channel. This silent interval should be ample for the subject to respond, either verbally or with a gesture, to the presence of the stimulus.

Exercises:

(1) Select an initial test tone frequency near 1000 hertz. Present the signal to the listener at the Attenuator settings indicated on Table I, below. Adjust the Output Amplifier Control Knob to position 3 for listeners with essentially normal hearing. For each test trial, deliver the stimulus ten times to the subject and record the percentage of correct responses obtained at the different sound magnitudes. Plot your data values on the axes provided in Figure "C" and compare with Figure "A."

(2) Repeat exercise #1 using Attenuator settings which lie between the levels of inaudibility and audibility for your particular listener. Use two decibel steps. Record and plot the data on Table II and Figure "D", respectively. Can you account for any differences between the shape of the psychometric function you obtained and the one shown in Figure "B"?

(3) Repeat exercise #2 for different tone frequencies. Does the basic shape of each psychometric function remain the same?

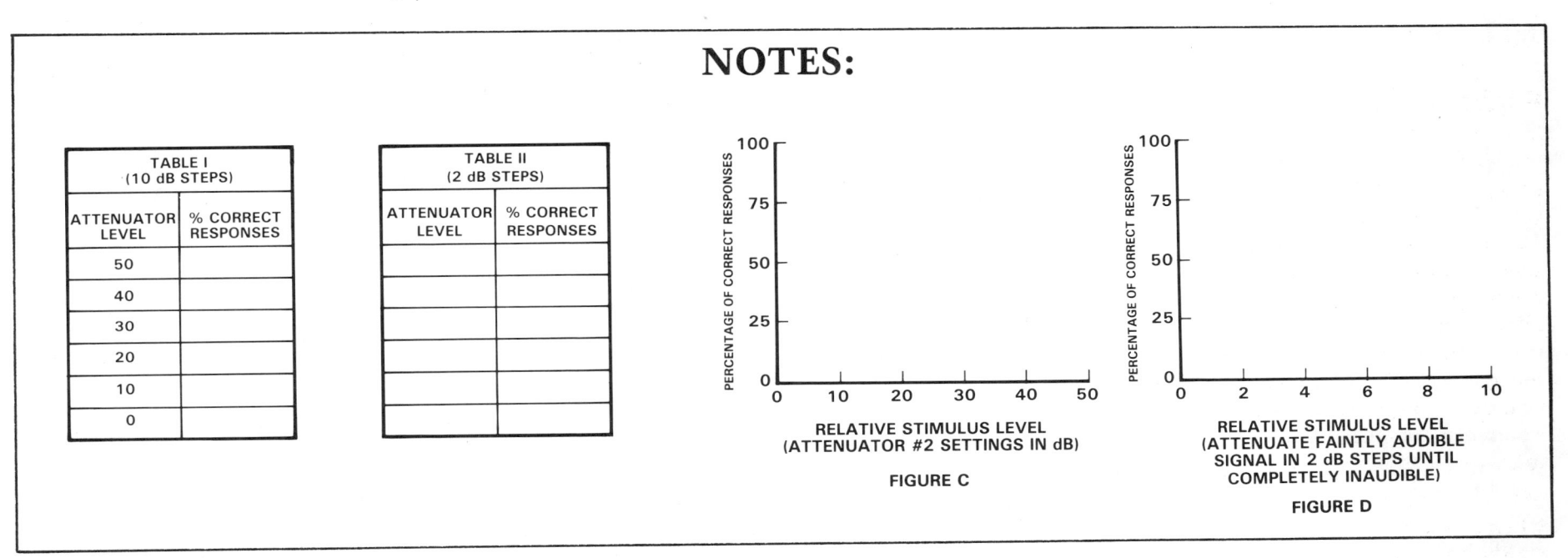

NOTES:

TABLE I (10 dB STEPS)

ATTENUATOR LEVEL	% CORRECT RESPONSES
50	
40	
30	
20	
10	
0	

TABLE II (2 dB STEPS)

ATTENUATOR LEVEL	% CORRECT RESPONSES

FIGURE C — RELATIVE STIMULUS LEVEL (ATTENUATOR #2 SETTINGS IN dB)

FIGURE D — RELATIVE STIMULUS LEVEL (ATTENUATE FAINTLY AUDIBLE SIGNAL IN 2 dB STEPS UNTIL COMPLETELY INAUDIBLE)

Selected References:

Corso, J. R. (1963). A theoretico-historical review of the threshold concept. *Psychol. Bull.*, **60**, 356-370.

Egan, J. P., Lindner, W. A., and McFadden, D. (1969). Masking-level differences and the form of the psychometric function. *Percept. Psychophys.*, **6**, 209-215.

Gescheider, G.A. (1976). *Psychophysics: Method and Theory*. Chapters 1-3. Lawrence Erlbaum Assoc., Hillsdale, New Jersey.

Green, D. M. (1960). Psychoacoustics and detection theory. *J. Acoust. Soc. Am.*, **32**, 1189-1203.

Green, D. M. (1966). Interaural phase effects in the masking of signals of different durations. *J. Acoust. Soc. Am.*, **39**, 720-724.

Green, D. M. and Swets, J. A. (1966). *Signal detection theory and psychophysics.* Chapters 7 and 8. Wiley, New York.

Krantz, D. H. (1969). Threshold theories of signal detection. *Psychol. Rev.*, **76**, 308-324.

Luce, R. D. (1960). Detection thresholds: a problem reconsidered. *Science*, **132**, 1495.

Luce, R. D. (1963). A threshold theory for simple detection experiments. *Psychol. Rev.*, **70**, 61-79.

Marks, L. E. and Stevens, J. C. (1968). The form of the psychophysical function near threshold. *Percept. Psychophys.*, **4**, 315-318.

Miller, G. A. and Garner, W. R. (1944). Effects of random presentation on the psychometric function: implications for quantal theory of discrimination. *Am. J. Psychol.*, **57**, 451-467.

Norman, D. A. (1963). Sensory thresholds and response bias. *J. Acoust. Soc. Am.*, **35**, 1432-1441.

Osman, E. (1975). Signal-noise duration, psychophysical procedure, interaural configuration, and the psychometric function. *J. Acoust. Soc. Am.*, **58**, 243-248.

Robinson, D.E. and Watson, C.S. (1972). Psychophysical methods in modern psychoacoustics. In J.V. Tobias (Ed.) *Foundations of modern auditory theory.* Vol. 2. Academic Press, New York.

Stevens, S.S. (1961). Is there a quantal threshold? In W.A. Rosenblith (Ed.) *Sensory communication.* MIT Press, Boston.

Swets, J.A. (1961). Is there a sensory threshold? *Science*, **134**, 168-177.

Zwislocki, J., Maire, F., Feldman, A.S., and Rubin, H. (1958). On the effect of practice and motivation on the threshold of audibility. *J. Acoust. Soc. Am.*, **30**, 254-262.

EXPERIMENT II-2: YES-NO PROCEDURE

Purpose:
To examine the detection performance of a listener who is informed precisely when to listen for the presence of a tone.

Background Principle:
If stimuli are delivered on a random basis to a subject, any variation in attentiveness may influence his detection performance upon his listening task. With the so-called *Yes-No procedure*, however, the test tone may be presented only during some formally defined period of time. The duration of this *observation interval* is often indicated by a flash of light which informs the observer precisely when to listen for the sound.

Unlike some conventional procedures (e.g., Experiment II-1) wherein the experimenter "sneaks up" upon the subject and delivers the test stimulus without warning, it is customary in a Yes-No task to alert the listener to the imminent approach of the observation interval with a brief tone, noise, or warning light. If the test tone is, in fact, introduced during the observation interval, and the subject correctly detects its presence, he is said to have scored a "hit," as opposed to a "miss," should he fail to discern its occurrence. The listener who reports hearing the tone when none was administered has reported a "false alarm," whereas a "correct rejection" would have been recorded had he properly reported the tone's absence. After the listener responds, he may be apprised as to whether or not the stimulus actually had been delivered. This simple feedback, coupled with the defined warning and observation intervals, effectively removes the subject's need for deciding when to listen during the experimental task and improves the reliability of the individual's responses from one test trial to the next. Figures "A" and "B" summarize the sequence of events and stimulus-response possibilities of the Yes-No procedure.

Procedure:
The first event in the Yes-No demonstration is the presentation of a warning noise burst that alerts the listener to the imminent approach of the observation interval. Note that the white noise signal output is first passed through an Attenuator so that it may be adjusted to a comfortable and non-fatiguing level. Electronic Gate "A" is programmed to switch the noise

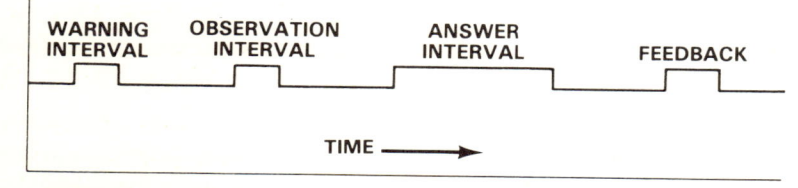

FIGURE A: A single trial of a typical Yes-No procedure has several formally defined time intervals. (Green and Swets, 1966).

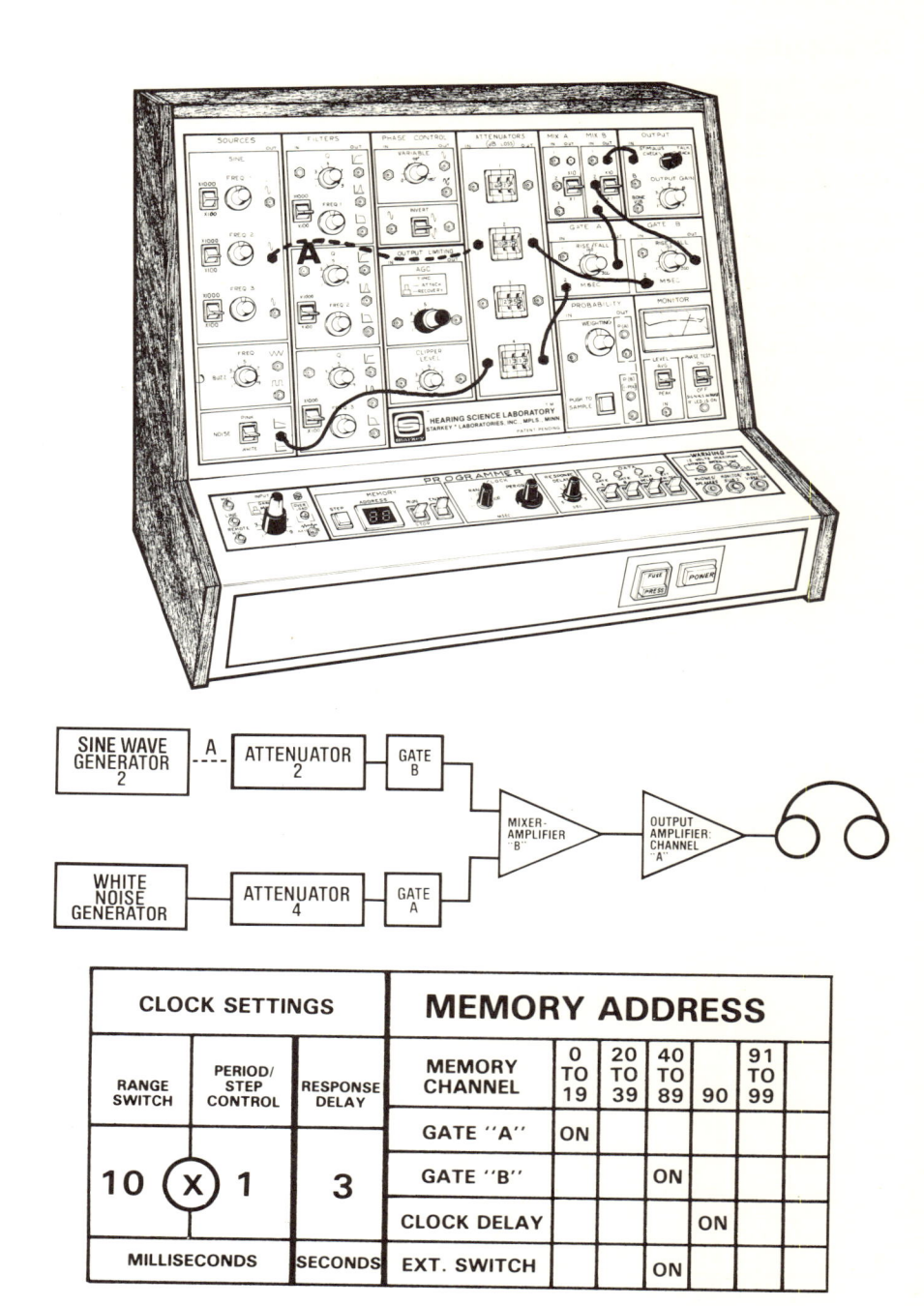

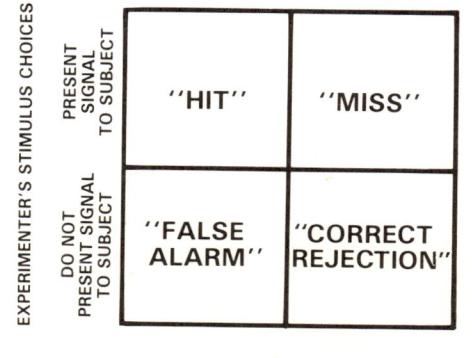

FIGURE B: The stimulus-response possibilities in the Yes-No procedure (After Green and Swets, 1966).

on and off just before the onset of the observation interval. The test tone is passed through Attenuator #2 and Electronic Gate "B". Both warning noise and test tone stimuli are combined within Mixer-Amplifier "B" and then routed to an Output Amplifier and headphone. It should be noted, within the suggested programming instructions, that the External Switch Channel is activated at the same time as Electronic Gate "B". By connecting a battery and bulb in series to the External Switch Jacks on the front panel, the onset and duration of the observation interval will be demarked by a light flash. The Programmer Delay Channel provides a momentary pause after each experimental sequence so that the subject has time to report whether the tone was presented. The duration of this pause may be adjusted by the Response Delay Control Knob and should be made long enough to permit the experimenter to inform the listener if the response was correct (e.g., 3 to 4 seconds). If the dashed wire "A", shown in the wiring guide, is disconnected, the tone will not be delivered during the observation interval.

Exercises:

(1) Adjust the test tone Attenuator and the Output Amplifier Control Knob to settings that render the tone just barely audible to the listener. Instruct the subject to confirm or deny the presence of the tone after each observation interval light flash. By alternately disconnecting and replacing the dashed circuit wire "A", each of the four response possibilities shown in Figure "B" can be obtained. If the subject always scores hits, decrease the magnitude of the tone so as to make detection more difficult.

(2) Examine the listener's detection performance when the warning noise is deleted from the experimental sequence. This can be achieved by unplugging the output wire from the Noise Generator. Is the warning stimulus helpful for detection?

(3) On a number of test trials, refrain from telling the listener whether his decisions were correct. Does the removal of this feedback appear to influence listener performance?

NOTES:

Selected References:

Carterette, E.C., Friedman, M.P., and Wymen, M.J. (1966). Feedback and psychophysical variables in signal detection. *J. Acoust. Soc. Am.*, **39**, 1051-1055.

Egan, J.P., Greenberg, G.Z., and Schulman, A.I. (1961). Operating characteristics, signal detectability, and the method of free response. *J. Acoust. Soc. Am.*, **33**, 993-1007.

Egan, J.P., Schulman, A.I., and Greenberg, G.Z. (1959). Operating characteristics determined by binary decisions and by ratings. *J. Acoust. Soc. Am.*, **31**, 768-773.

Green, D.M. and Swets, J.A. (1966). *Signal detection theory and psychophysics.* Chapter 2. Wiley, New York.

Robinson, D.E. and Watson, C.S. (1972). Psychophysical methods in modern psychoacoustics. In J.V. Tobias (Ed.) *Foundations of modern auditory theory.* Vol. 2. Academic Press, New York.

Swets, J.A., Tanner, W.P., Jr., and Birdsall, T.G. (1961). Decision processes in perception. *Psychol. Rev.*, **68**, 301-340.

Tanner, W.P., Jr. and Sorkin, R.D. (1972). The theory of signal detectability. In J.V. Tobias (Ed.) *Foundations of modern auditory theory.* Vol. 2. Academic Press, New York.

Watson, C.S. and Clopton, B.M. (1969). Motivated changes in auditory sensitivity in a simple detection task. *Percept. Psychophys.*, **5**, 281-287.

Watson, C.S. and Nichols, T.L. (1976). Detectability of auditory signals presented without defined observation intervals. *J. Acoust. Soc. Am.*, **59**, 655-668.

EXPERIMENT II-3: RECEIVER OPERATING CHARACTERISTIC

Purpose:
To manipulate a subject's decision-making criterion and note the corresponding change in detection performance.

Background Principle:
The Yes-No procedure described in Laboratory Experiment II-2 requires only the recording of a subject's hit and false alarm rates in order to completely specify his detection performance. To illustrate this point, consider a listener who is presented with 100 test trials in a Yes-No task, each of which contains a stimulus of some **fixed** magnitude. Should the subject correctly detect the presence of 60 of these tones (i.e., 60 hits), it is clear that he must have missed the remaining 40 stimuli. If we also presented 100 observation intervals which did not contain the signal, and the subject reports hearing a tone 35 times (i.e., 35 false alarms), then the correct rejections must number 65. It is customary to portray the percentage, or *probability*, of hits versus false alarms, respectively, upon a graph. It should be recognized from the illustrative example just described, in which a total of 200 trials were submitted to a listener, that only **one** data point upon Figure "A" has been generated (see graph point "A"). Further bits of performance data may be obtained (at the expense of many additional test trials) by manipulating the subject's criterion for deciding whether or not the tone had actually been presented during the observation intervals. One way of accomplishing this is to reward each hit by giving money to the subject and punish each false alarm by taking some away. If we specified, for instance, that there is only a 25% likelihood that a tone will be delivered during the observation intervals, we find that the listener becomes quite cautious about reporting the presence of the sound. Note that this conservatism is reflected in both lower false alarm and hit rates as well. In other words, a listener will be reluctant to report any positive response (see point "B" on Figure "A"). If, however, we inform the observer that there is a high probability of the tone's occurrence (e.g., 80% of the time), he will be emboldened to make frequent claims that the stimuli were presented, as shown by the higher hit and false alarm rates of graph point "C" on Figure "A." Continued alteration of the test instructions or response pay-offs and penalties will yield still other data values which may be connected by a smooth curve, known as a *Receiver Operating Characteristic (ROC)*. A listener who had been randomly guessing throughout the tests would have a fifty percent probability of being correct. This chance performance would be indicated by an ROC curve which formed a 45° diagonal line, as shown by the dashed line in Figure "A." Improvements in the listener's detection would be mirrored by ROC curves that arched closer to the upper left hand corner of the graph, where the percentage of hits is at a maximum and the number of false alarms is at a minimum. It is also possible to describe

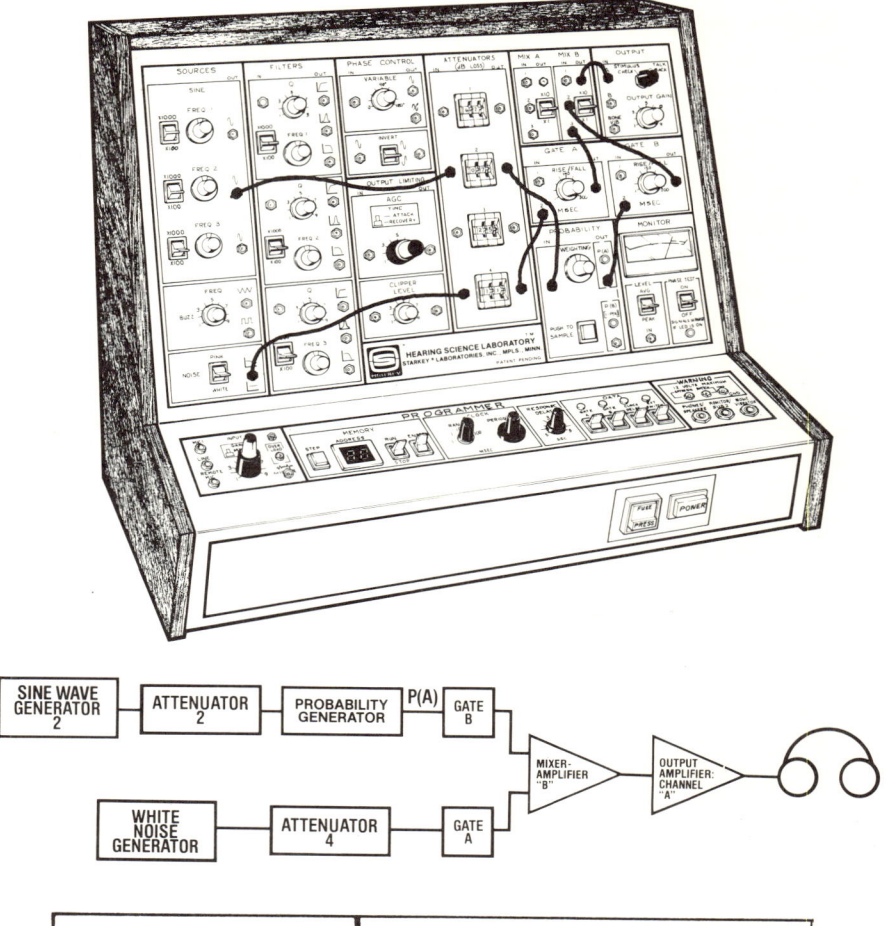

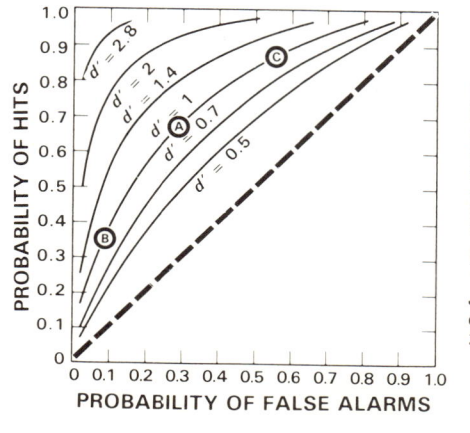

FIGURE A: The relationship between a subject's "hit" and "false alarm" rates is described by a receiver operating characteristic (ROC) curve. Changes in subject detection performance (as shown by different d' values and ROC curves) occur when the listener is informed of changes in the "likelihood" that a signal will be presented. Note that Percent Correct = Probability × 100. (After Swets, J.A., Tanner, W.P., Jr., and Birdsall, T.G. (1961). Decision processes in perception. *Psychol. Rev.*, 68, 301-340).

listener performance with a single mathematical quantity derived from the relative curvature and position of the ROC curve. This so called *detection index(d')* has been determined for various percentages of hits to false alarm ratios. The reader is directed to the references for the mathematical derivations of these concepts.

Procedure:

Note, from the wiring guide and block diagram, that an important addition has been made to the instrumentation used for the basic Yes-No listening task described in the preceding experiment. The test tone, emerging from its Attenuator, is now routed to the Probability Gate. The signal will appear at the P(A) Output Jack only when the green indicator light is on. By tapping the Sample Button once before each new experimental sequence of events, the tone will be delivered to Electronic Gate "B" on a probabilistic (i.e., percentage) basis which is determined by the Weighting Control Knob setting. If, for example, the Weighting Control is set to 8, the tone will appear at the P(A) Output Jack roughly 80 times out of 100 test trials. The suggested programming instructions are identical to those employed in Experiment II-2.

Exercises:

(1) Adjust the test tone Attenuator so that the signal is just barely audible to the listener. Instruct the subject that he or she will receive, or lose, a penny for each hit or false alarm, respectively. Inform the subject, prior to each group of test trials, exactly what percentage of the time the tone will be delivered (i.e., whatever the Weighting Control setting is). Tap the Sample Button before each test sequence and note the status of the green indicator light above the P(A) Output Jack. If it is lit, the tone will be delivered during the observation interval. Record stimuli presentation conditions as well as the subject's responses on a data sheet like the sample shown in Figure "B." Try several different Weighting Control settings for a particular test tone level and plot the percentages of listener hits and false alarms on a graph like that shown in Figure "A." Be sure to apprise the listener of each new Weighting Control setting which corresponds to the probability that the tone will occur during the observation interval. Connect the data points on the graph to form an ROC curve.

(2) Repeat exercise #1 for a variety of tone levels. Draw a complete set of ROC curves for the subject.

FIGURE B: Sample Data Sheet

TRIAL NUMBER	STIMULUS ALTERNATIVE	SUBJECT'S RESPONSE
1		
2		
3		
4		
5		
6		
7		
8		
9		
10		
etc.		

Check this column if signal is presented. Check this column if the subject reports hearing the tone.

NOTES:

Selected References:

Carterette, E.C. and Cole, M. (1962). Comparison of the receiver-operating characteristics received by ear and by eye. *J. Acoust. Soc. Am.*, **34,** 172-178.

Clarke, F.R. and Bilger, R.C. (1973). The theory of signal detectability and the measurement of hearing. In J. Jerger (Ed.) *Modern developments in audiology.* Academic Press, New York.

Green, D.M. and Swets, J.A. (1966). *Signal detection theory and psychophysics.* Wiley, New York.

Jeffress, L.A. (1964). Stimulus-oriented approach to detection. *J. Acoust. Soc. Am.*, **36,** 766-774.

Luce, R.D. (1963). A threshold theory for simple detection experiments. *Psychol. Rev.*, **70,** 61-79.

Markowitz, J. and Swets, J.A. (1967). Factors affecting the slope of empirical ROC curves: comparison of binary and rating responses. *Percept. Psychophys.*, **2,** 91-97.

Robinson, D.E. and Watson, C.S. (1972). Psychophysical methods in modern psychoacoustics. In J.V. Tobias (Ed.) *Foundations of modern auditory theory.* Vol. 2. Academic Press, New York.

Swets, J.A. (1959). Indices of signal detectability obtained with various psychophysical procedures. *J. Acoust. Soc. Am.*, **31,** 511-513.

Swets, J.A. (Ed.). (1964). *Signal detection and recognition by human observers: contemporary readings.* Wiley, New York.

Tanner, W.P., Jr. and Birdsall, T.G. (1958). Definitions of d' and η as psychophysical measures. *J. Acoust. Soc. Am.*, **30,** 922-928.

Tanner, W.P., Jr. and Sorkin, R.D. (1972). The theory of signal detectability. In J.V. Tobias (Ed.) *Foundations of modern auditory theory.* Vol. 2. Academic Press, New York.

EXPERIMENT II-4: ADAPTIVE TEST PROCEDURES

Purpose:
To estimate the location of the 50% probability of detection value upon an individual's psychometric function.

Background Principle:
Each of the detection procedures described so far has required the administration of a great many test stimuli to the subject. They are, therefore, somewhat uneconomical in the clinical setting. A practical alternative that has found wide applicability in the clinic and laboratory has been to define an individual's hearing threshold in terms of a single probability-of-correct-response point upon his psychometric function. Audiologists, for example, commonly utilize the 50% probability point as their measure of hearing sensitivity (i.e., the so-called *Audiometric Threshold*). The particular design of the psychophysical test employed enables one to estimate a specific point upon the psychometric function without advance knowledge of the exact configuration of the curve. In a broad class of test methods, known as *adaptive procedures,* the magnitude of a stimulus is varied throughout the course of the experiment. The preceding stimulus levels and subject responses are used to determine the magnitude of the next presentation. One of the most widely used techniques for estimating the 50% point, the Audiometric Threshold, is an adaptive procedure known as the *Method of Limits.* The experimenter may begin this test by presenting the first stimulus at a high level which is likely to be detected by the subject. If a correct response is obtained at this *initial value,* the magnitude of the following tone is diminished by a fixed amount, or *step.* Subsequent correct responses instigate further decreases in the signal strength until the listener makes his first error. This *reversal* in performance marks the end of the task. In the "ascending" form of this technique, an initial stimulus value is chosen that lies below the observer's threshold. The magnitude of the tone is increased in a stepwise manner, after each miss,

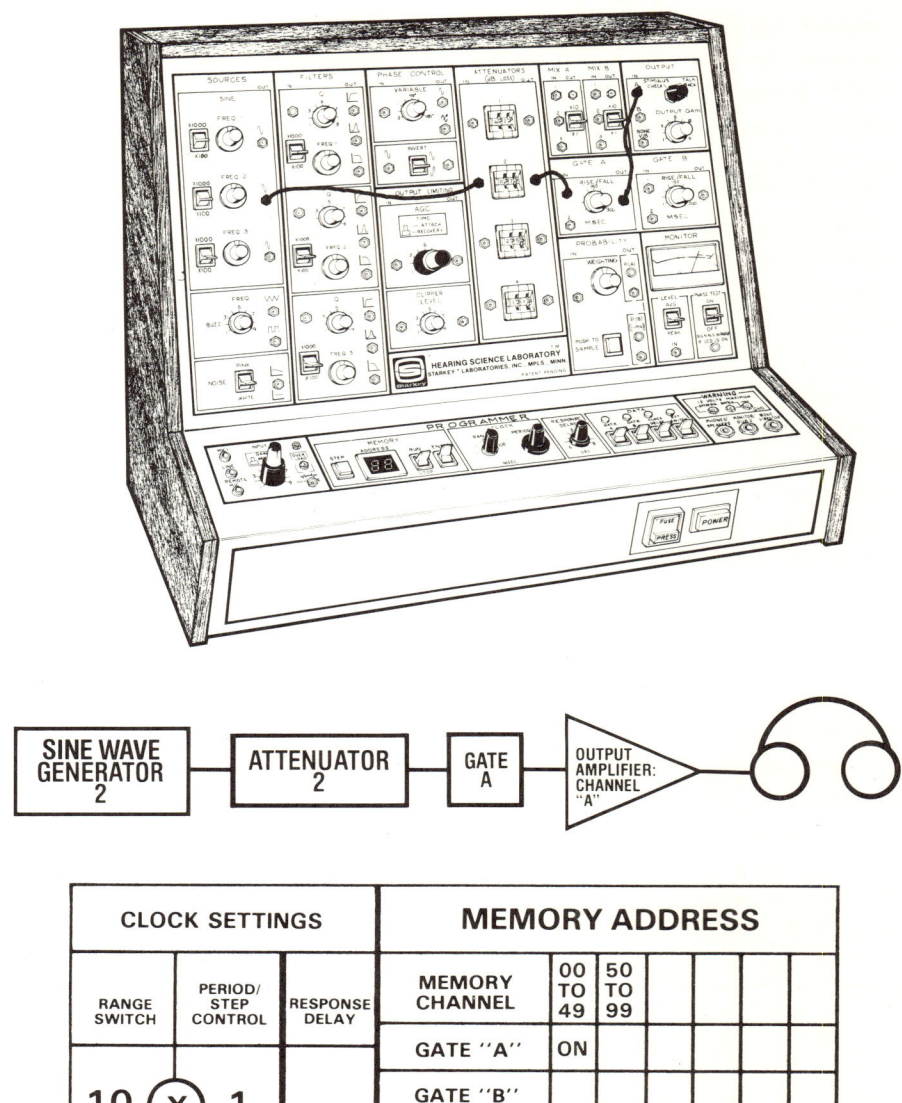

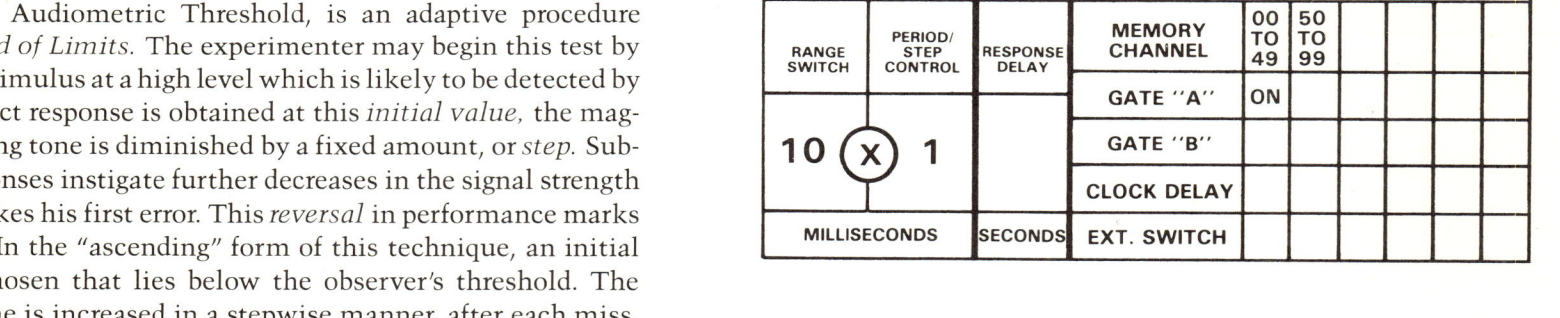

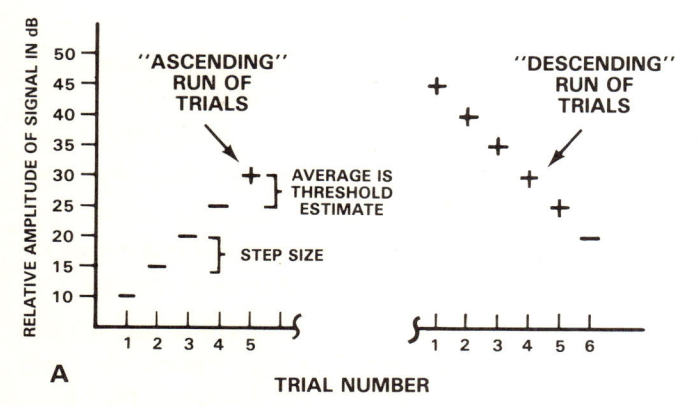

FIGURE A: Sample results illustrating the "ascending" and "descending" versions of the Method of Limits procedure.

FIGURE B: The hypothetical results from this up-down adaptive procedure indicate that the "Audiometric Threshold" for the subject is 33.1 dB.

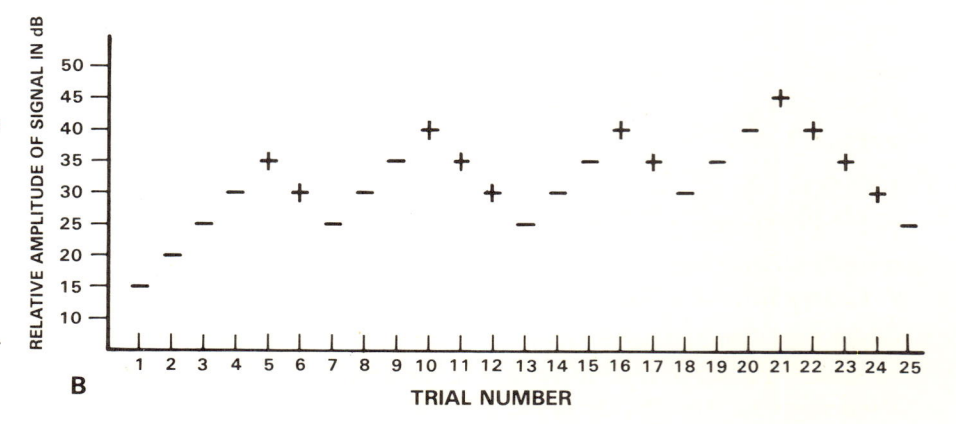

until a correct detection is achieved. The statistical estimate of the 50% threshold point may be obtained by averaging the values of the last two responses in each sequence. Figure "A" shows sample results from both of these "descending" and "ascending" versions of the Method of Limits procedure. Note from the graph that the hypothetical listener seems to perform better (i.e., he requires less sound magnitude to detect the stimulus) when descending, rather than ascending, steps are used. It is possible that the observer may derive some advantage from being alerted to the initial, relatively loud tone which may actually be "followed down" as it is made softer. Another popular method for estimating Audiometric Threshold extends the basic format of the method of limits task beyond the subject's first reversal point. This is the *up-down* technique and is illustrated in Figure "B". We see that, rather than terminate the test, each miss is followed by a stimulus increment while decrements in level are introduced after every hit. A series of steps in a particular direction is known as a *run*. In Figure "B", the trials numbered 1, 2, 3, 4, and 5, for example, comprise an upward run whereas trials 5, 6, and 7 make up a downward run. Note from Figure "B" that this type of up-down, or "staircase," technique effectively "stalks" a subject's threshold as it shifts about during the experiment. The choice of both the initial value and the step size are important factors in the up-down and method of limits tasks. Selecting an initial value that is distant from the observer's threshold, or choosing too small a step size, would waste test trials and time in the search for the subject's reversal points. Simple, yet accurate, estimates of the 50% probability of response threshold may be obtained by averaging the numerical values of the reversal peaks and valleys of the several different runs in the experiment. For the example shown in Figure "B", the peaks and valleys occur at trial numbers 5, 7, 10, 13, 16, 18, 21 and 25. Their stimuli levels are 35, 25, 40, 25, 40, 30, 45, and 25, respectively. (Note: it is customary to omit the first "practice run" from the threshold computation.) The average of the peaks and valleys (i.e., the Audiometric Threshold) in this example is equal to 33.1 dB.

Procedure:

An "interrupted" pure tone will serve as the test stimulus. Choose an initial frequency near 1000 Hz. The tone is passed through an Attenuator and Electronic Gate before entering one Output Amplifier and headphone. The suggested Programmer instructions permit the tone to be switched on for 0.5 second and off for 0.5 second, repeatedly. The Electronic Gate should be set to a rise-fall time of roughly 50 milliseconds.

Exercises:

(1) Select initial Output Amplifier and Attenuator settings that produce a clearly audible tone for the listener and then reduce the signal level in two decibel steps until the subject reports that the tone is no longer audible. Try the reverse, ascending version of the method of limits by starting the listening task at an initial level that is well below the subject's threshold. Are the subject's threshold levels the same for both methods?

(2) Repeat the ascending and descending method of limits tasks with the signal remaining continuously on. The signal will stay on if the Programmer Clock is stopped at any memory address between 00 and 49, which turns Electronic Gate "A" on. Are the threshold estimates different for the continuous and interrupted tone conditions?

(3) Repeat either the ascending or descending approach but do not end the task after the first reversal point. Continue to "bracket" the subject's threshold, using the up-down procedure described above. Is the threshold estimate obtained in this fashion the same as that obtained for any of the other techniques? How do you account for any differences?

NOTES:

Selected References:

Brownlee, K.A., Hodges, J.L., and Rosenblatt, M. (1953). The up and down method with small samples. *J. Am. Statist. Assoc.*, **48,** 262-277.

Cornsweet, T.N. (1962). The staircase method in psychophysics. *Am. J. Psychol.*, **75,** 485-491.

Guilford, J.P. (1954). *Psychometric methods.* McGraw-Hill, New York.

Kappauf, W.E. (1967). Use of an on-line computer for psychophysical testing with the up-and-down method. *Am. Psychol.*, **32,** 207-211.

Levitt, H. (1968). Testing for sequential dependencies. *J. Acoust. Soc. Am.*, **43,** 65-69.

Levitt, H. (1971). Transformed up-down methods in psychoacoustics. *J. Acoust. Soc. Am.*, **49,** 467-477.

Levitt, H. (1978). Adaptive testing in audiology. *Scand. Audiol. Suppl.*, **6,** 241-291.

Levitt, H. and Bock, D. (1967). A sequential programmer for psychophysical testing. *J. Acoust. Soc. Am.*, **42,** 911-913.

Levitt, H. and Rabiner, I.R. (1967). Use of a sequential strategy in intelligibility testing. *J. Acoust. Soc. Am.*, **42,** 609-612.

Manning, S.A. and Rosenstock, E.H. (1968). *Classical psychophysics and scaling.* McGraw-Hill, New York.

McNichol, D. (1972). *A primer of signal detection theory.* George Allen and Unwin, London.

Wetherill, G.B., and Levitt, H. (1965). Sequential estimation of points on a psychometric function. *Brit. J. Math. Statist. Psychol.*, **18,** 1-8.

EXPERIMENT II-5: TWO INTERVAL FORCED CHOICE PROCEDURE

Purpose:
To determine the 70.7% threshold point on an individual's psychometric function by using a two interval forced choice procedure.

Background Principle:
While the Yes-No procedure frees the listener from having to decide when to listen, he still must employ some criterion for deciding whether or not the tone was, in fact, presented at all during the observation interval. It is possible to minimize the variability associated with this decision making criterion by using what is known as a "forced choice" listening task. Compare the sequence of experimental events for a *Two Interval Forced Choice (2IFC) technique* (shown in Figure "A") with those of the Yes-No task described in Laboratory Experiment II-2. This new listening situation presents the subject with two observation intervals rather than one. The subject is informed that the test tone will always be presented within one of the two intervals and that it is his responsibility to identify that interval. The experimenter usually alternates the tone from one interval to the other on a random basis. A forced choice experiment may be constructed with any number of observation intervals but will ultimately be limited by the subject's ability to remember in which of the many listening periods the tone has occurred. Because a subject may achieve a 50% correct detection score by simply guessing in which of the two listening intervals the tone was presented, the experimenter must seek some threshold estimate greater than the 50% response value on the psychometric function. It is possible to estimate a number of different threshold response points with slight modifications of the basic Up-Down procedure. One such *transformed Up-Down* strategy which establishes the 70.7% response point requires that the experimenter wait for two correct detections in a row before decreasing the magnitude of the stimulus; as in the simple up-down method, any subject error must be followed by an increase in signal

FIGURE A: A single trial of a typical two interval forced choice (2IFC) procedure. (Green and Swets, 1966).

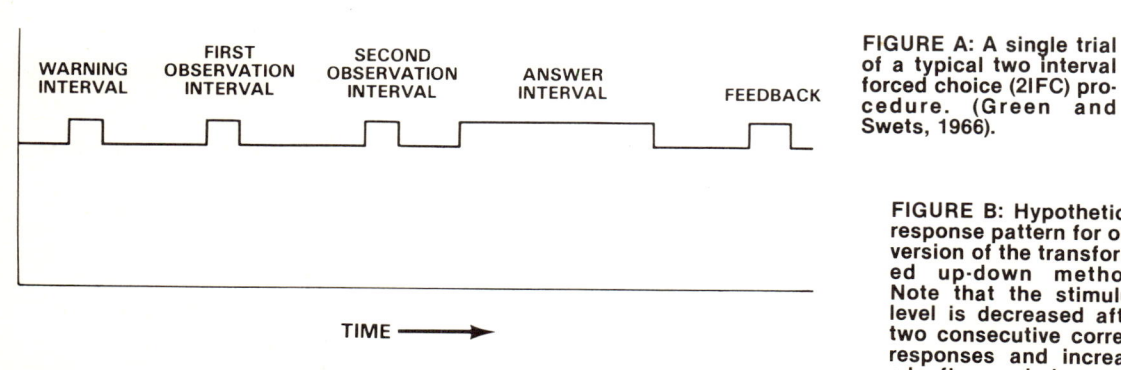

FIGURE B: Hypothetical response pattern for one version of the transformed up-down method. Note that the stimulus level is decreased after two consecutive correct responses and increased after each incorrect response. (Levitt, 1971).

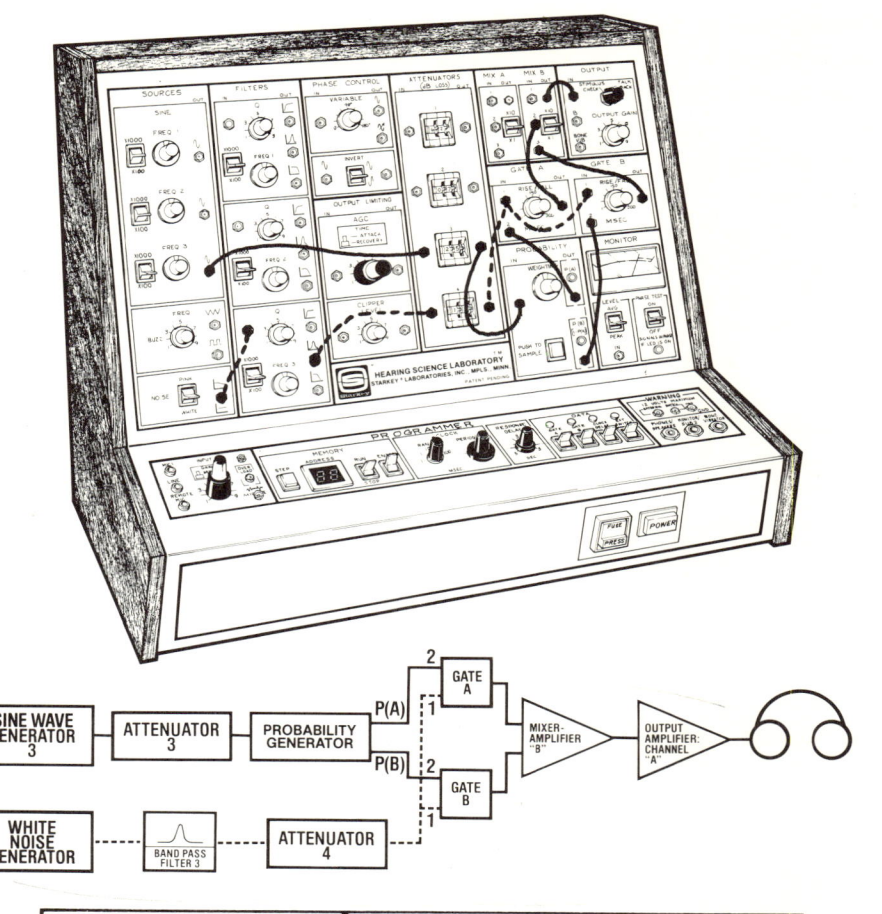

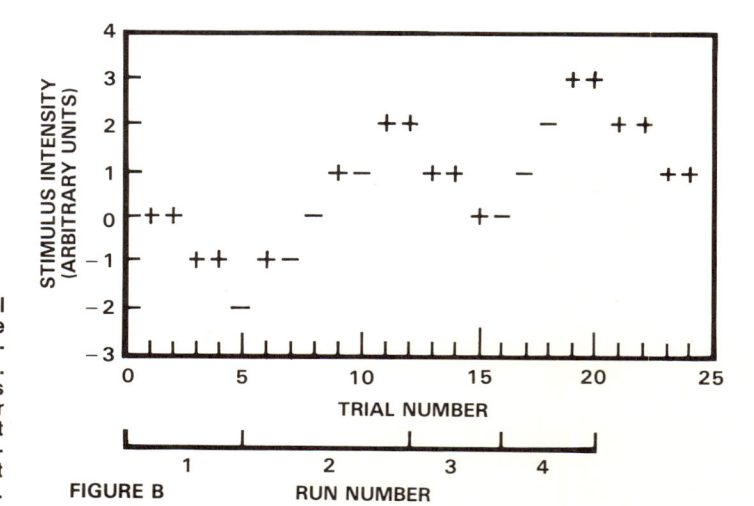

FIGURE A

FIGURE B

strength. A hypothetical series of test trials and subject responses are shown in Figure "B". As in the basic up-down method, it is possible to estimate the subject's threshold by averaging the peaks and valleys (i.e., the reversal points) of each run of trials. It is also possible to derive the measure of an individual's detection sensitivity, d', from the percentages of hits to misses that a subject scores (see Green and Swets, 1966).

Procedure:

The Electronic Gates are programmed to create two observation intervals followed by a momentary delay for the subject's response. The test tone is passed through an Attenuator and the Probability Gate. By adjusting the Weighting Control to a setting of "5" (i.e., 50%) and tapping the Sample Button before each new trial sequence, the tone will appear at the two Probability Gate Output Jacks on a random basis. When the signal emerges from the P(A) Jack, it will enter Electronic Gate "A" and, therefore, be delivered to the listener during the first observation interval. Probability Jack P(B) and Electronic Gate "B" govern the second observation interval. The Programmer External Switch channel will turn a light on during each observation interval if a bulb and battery are connected in series with the External Switch Output Jacks. An optional narrow band noise, centered around the test tone frequency, may also be used to denote the occurrence of the observation intervals and can be introduced by connecting the dashed circuit wires shown in the wiring guide and block diagram. Adding the noise, however, will change the basic listening task to that of a masked threshold experiment like those in section VI of this text. All signals are combined within a Mixer-Amplifier and sent to one Output Amplifier channel and headphone.

Exercises:

(1) Use an initial test tone frequency near 1000 Hz. Find the subject's threshold by using the 2IFC procedure described above. Plot the listener responses upon a graph like that shown in Figure "B."

(2) Repeat exercise #1 with the noise circuitry connected. How does the presence of the gated noise background affect the subject's responses?

(3) Repeat exercise #1 and after each response inform the subject whether he has chosen the correct interval. Does this kind of feedback affect the listener's performance in any way?

NOTES:

Selected References:

Campbell, R.A. (1963). Detection of a noise signal of varying duration. *J. Acoust. Soc. Am.*, **35**, 1732-1737.

Elliott, P.B. (1964). Tables of d'. In J.A. Swets (Ed.) *Signal detection and recognition by human observers.* pp. 651-684. Wiley, New York.

Green, D.M. and Swets, J.A. (1966). *Signal detection theory and psychophysics.* Wiley, New York.

Levitt, H. (1971). Transformed up-down methods in psychoacoustics. *J. Acoust. Soc. Am.*, **49**, 467-477.

Robinson, D.E. and Watson, C.S. (1972). Psychophysical methods in modern psychoacoustics. In J.V. Tobias (Ed.) *Foundations of modern auditory theory.* Vol. 2. Academic Press, New York.

Schacknow, P.N., and Barth, C.T. (1977). On the efficiency of 2IFC measurement. *J. Acoust. Soc. Am.*, **62 (S1)**, S96(A).

Tanner, W.P., Jr. and Sorkin, R.D. (1972). The theory of signal detectability. In J.V. Tobias (Ed.) *Foundations of modern auditory theory.* Vol. 2. Academic Press, New York.

Taylor, M.M. and Creelman, C.D. (1967). PEST: efficient estimates on probability functions. *J. Acoust. Soc. Am.*, **41**, 782-787.

Theodor, L.H. (1972). A neglected parameter: some comments on "A table for calculation of d' and β." *Psychol. Bull.*, **78**, 260-261.

EXPERIMENT II-6: HEARING THRESHOLD LEVELS AND THE AUDIOMETER

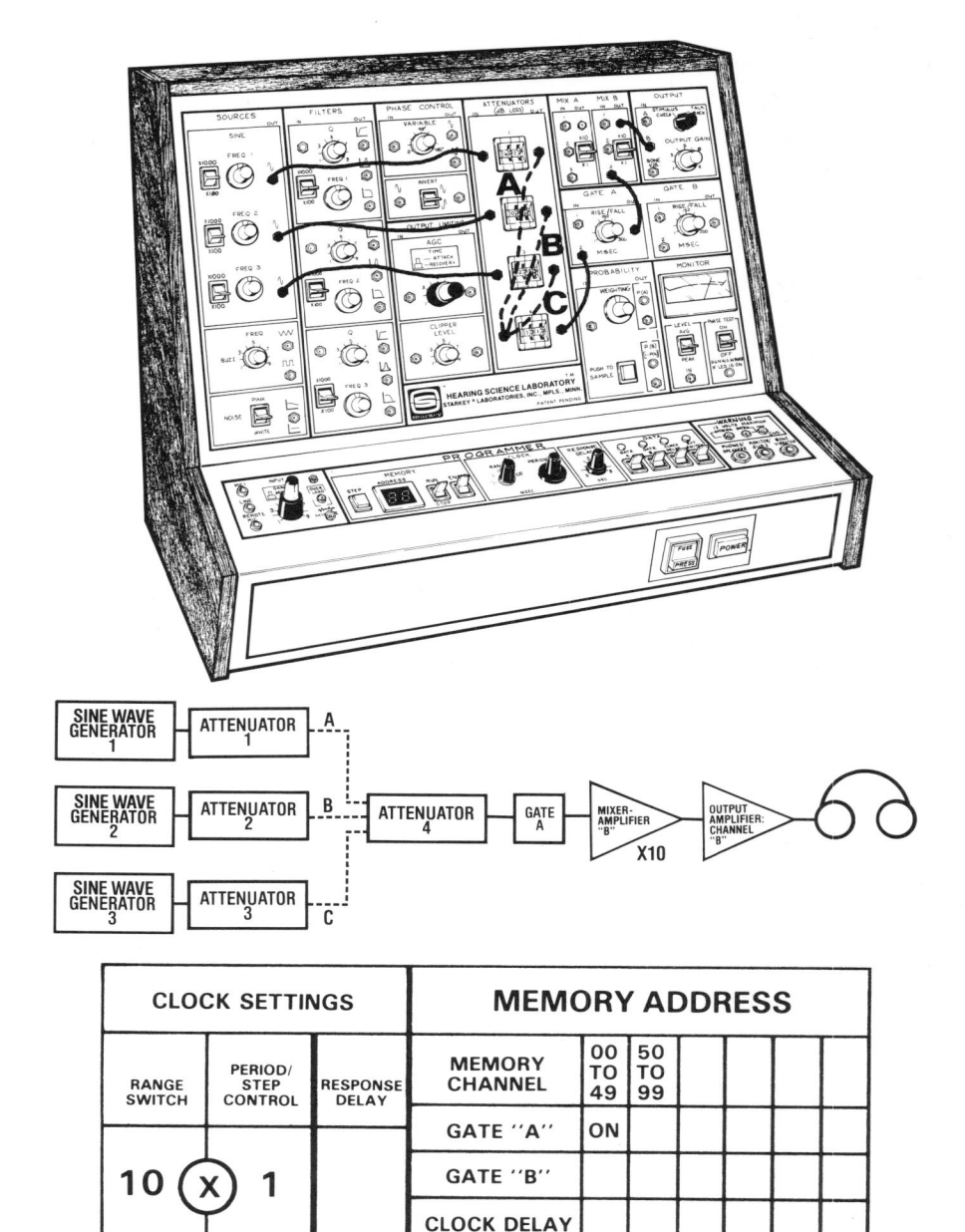

Purpose:
To examine clinical standards for the threshold of audibility.

Background Principle:
The Science of Audiology is vitally concerned with measurements of abnormal, as well as normal, phenomena of hearing. Over the past fifty years, clinical and laboratory researchers have shared in the development of meaningful standards for normal hearing threshold levels. Without such uniform guidelines, descriptions of the exact nature and extent of a listener's hearing impairment might vary substantially from one testing facility to the next. A great many experiments and test surveys with otologically healthy young adults have contributed to the evolution of the currently accepted standards for "normal" hearing levels. The results from these studies have been statistically pooled to form the standard sound pressure levels shown in Table I, below. These values, specified by the *American National Standards Institute (ANSI)* in 1969, serve as landmarks to which every *pure tone audiometer* must be calibrated. A pure tone audiometer is an electroacoustic device which generates the tonal stimuli used in the clinical determination of a listener's *hearing threshold levels* or *hearing levels.* The graph which shows the minimal sound requirements for detection, as a function of test tone frequency, is known as an *audiogram*. The audiogram portrayed in Figure "A" was derived from the ANSI (1969) standard values. Notice that at threshold levels, human listeners require more sound pressure level at the extremes of the frequency range than in the mid frequencies between 1000-4000 Hz. To facilitate the classification of deviations from the normal threshold of audibility, the ANSI dB SPL values themselves have been "normalized", or transformed, into the zero dB reference standard for *decibels Hearing Level (dB HL)*, a system universally used in clinical audiology. Figure "B" shows that the

Test Frequency (in Hz)	ANSI 1969 Level (in dB SPL)
125	45.0
250	25.5
500	11.5
750*	8.6*
1000	7.0
1500	6.5
2000	9.0
3000	10.0
4000	9.5
6000	15.5
8000	13.0

TABLE I: "Normal" hearing threshold levels (i.e., 0dB HL) standardized by ANSI, 1969 for TDH-39 earphones.
*Note: There is no ANSI level for 750 Hz. The value shown is taken from *International Standards Organization (ISO)* recommendation R389, 1964, as corrected for TDH-39 phones by Cox and Bilger, 1960.

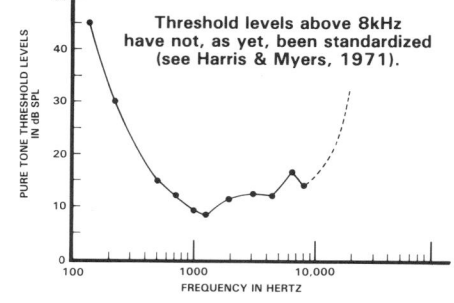

FIGURE A: This audiogram shows the "normal" pure tone threshold of audibility curve based upon the ANSI 1969 standard sound pressure level values. Threshold levels above 8kHz have not, as yet, been standardized (see Harris & Myers, 1971).

FIGURE B: A straight line is formed by the threshold data when they are normalized to 0 dB HL values on this "clinical" audiogram. Note that "normal" hearing is considered to lie within a range of values below 25 dB HL.

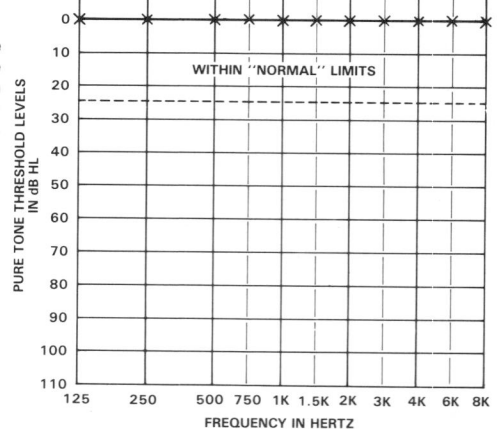

ANSI levels form a straight line at the top of a "clinical audiogram." A properly calibrated pure tone audiometer will produce the ANSI specified dB SPL levels at each test frequency when the audiometer attenuator is fixed at 0 dB HL.

Procedure:

The performance of a three-frequency pure tone audiometer may be simulated by routing the outputs from the three Sine Wave Generators to separate "calibration" Attenuators. Attenuator #4 will serve as the dB HL level control for the demonstration and should be set to an initial level of 50 dB which is analogous to the zero dB HL reference point. Connect dashed wires "A", "B", and "C", in turn, to the Input Jack of the fourth Attenuator. Adjust Attenuators 1, 2, and 3, respectively, to determine the threshold of audibility for a group of normal hearing subjects at three selected pure tone frequencies (e.g., 250 Hz, 500 Hz, 1 kHz). The average settings obtained for Attenuators 1, 2, and 3 will form the "standardized" reference levels for the audiometer. Decreasing the setting of Attenuator #4 indicates a deviation from the standard. Note, however, from Figure "B" that "normal" hearing lies within a range of threshold levels rather than at a single value. The output from Attenuator #4 is sent through an Electronic Gate which has been programmed to switch the signal on and off every half second. Twenty decibels of gain is provided for this demonstration by sending the output of the Gate through a Mixer-Amplifier (set to the X 10 position) before routing the stimulus through an Output Amplifier and headphone.

Exercises:

(1) Obtain a 3-frequency "clinical" audiogram for a subject before and after he or she wears an earplug. Note the threshold shifts produced by this kind of induced *conductive hearing loss*.

(2) Recalibrate the audiometer, as outlined in the Procedure section above, for such high frequencies as 4, 6, and 8 KHz. Repeat exercise #1 and note if the conductive loss produces the same degree of threshold shift you obtained in exercise #1. Can you explain the differences in your data?

NOTES:

Selected References:

American National Standards Institute [ANSI] (1969). Specifications for audiometers. S3.6.

Cox, J.R., Jr. and Bilger, R.D. (1960). Suggestion relative to the standardization of loudness-balance data for the telephonics TDH-39 earphone. *J. Acoust. Soc. Am.*, **32,** 1080-1082.

Dadson, R.S. and King, J.H. (1952). A determination of the normal threshold of hearing and its relation to the standardization of audiometers. *J. Laryngol. Otol.*, **66,** 366-378.

Davis, H. (1965). Guide for the classification and evaluation of hearing handicap in relation to the international audiometric zero. *Trans. Am. Acad. Opthal. Otolar.*, **69,** 710-751.

Davis, H. (1970). Hearing handicap, standards for hearing, and medicolegal rules. In H. Davis and S.R. Silverman (Eds.) *Hearing and deafness*. Third ed. Holt, Rinehart and Winston, New York.

Davis, H. and Kranz. F.W. (1964a). International audiometric zero. *J. Acoust. Soc. Am.*, **36,** 1450-1454.

Davis, H. and Kranz, F.W. (1964b). The international standard reference zero for pure-tone audiometers and its relations to the evaluation of impairment of hearing. *J. Speech Hear. Res.*, **7,** 7-16.

Davis, H. and Usher, J.R. (1957). What is zero hearing loss? *J. Speech Hear. Dis.*, **22,** 662-690.

Harris, J.D. (1954). Normal hearing and its relation to audiometry. *Laryngoscope*, **64,** 928-957.

Harris, J.D. and Myers, C.K. (1971). Tentative audiometric threshold-level standards from 8 through 18 kHz. *J. Acoust. Soc. Am.*, **49,** 600-601.

Jerger, J.F., Carhart, R., Tillman, T.W., and Peterson, J.L. (1959). Some relations between normal hearing for pure tones and for speech. *J. Speech Hear. Res.*, **2,** 126-140.

Northern, J.L., Downs, M.P., Rudmose, W., Glorig. A., and Fletcher, J.L. (1972). Recommended high-frequency audiometric threshold levels (8000-18000 Hz). *J. Acoust. Soc. Am.*, **52,** 585-595.

Watson, C.S., Franks, J.R., and Hood, D.C. (1972). Detection of tones in the absence of external masking noise. I. Effects of signal intensity and signal frequency. *J. Acoust. Soc. Am.*, **52,** 633-643.

Weissler, G. (1968). International standard reference zero for audiometers. *J. Acoust. Soc. Am.*, **44,** 264-275.

Yeowart, N.S. and Evans, M.J. (1974). Thresholds of audibility for very low-frequency pure tones. *J. Acoust. Soc. Am.*, **55,** 814-818.

EXPERIMENT II-7: THE OCCLUSION EFFECT

Purpose:
To note the influence of the external ear canal on bone conduction thresholds.

Background Principle:
We normally hear our own voices through two main "channels": air and bone conduction. Sound traveling via the air conduction route passes through the ear canal, or *external auditory meatus,* and vibrates our *tympanic membrane* (i.e., the eardrum) to which the three bones of the middle ear *ossicular-chain* are connected. The movement of these structures disturbs the fluid filled inner ear chamber which contains the sense organ of hearing. It is here that the transduction from physical vibration into electrical nerve impulses originates before traveling up the neural pathways to the brain. It is far more difficult, however, to describe the complex multiple pathways which are involved in the process of bone conduction. Tonndorf (1964, 1968 and 1972) discusses the details of this mechanism and points out that the outer, middle, and inner ear structures all influence and contribute to the bone conduction process. One phenomenon associated with the external ear component is known as the *occlusion effect.* In this instance, the detection of a pure tone signal that has been coupled to the skull bones by means of a bone vibrator will be enhanced in an ear that is covered. If, instead, the opposite ear is occluded, then the tone will appear to move, or *lateralize,* to that ear. The effect is more pronounced for very low frequencies (e.g., below 500 Hz) and becomes negligible above about 1000 Hz. In an explanation of the occlusion effect, Tonndorf (1968) points out that bone conducted signals vibrate the walls of the ear canal thereby producing sound within the meatus. Some of this sound energy will disturb the tympanic membrane and be propagated through the entire hearing mechanism. Occluding the ear alters the resonance, or filtering characteristics, of the external canal from its normal high-pass configuration shown in Figure "A". The covered ear behaves, instead, more like a low-pass filter which enhances the transmission and perception of low frequency signals.

Procedure:
A pure tone signal is routed through an Attenuator and into the Bone Vibrator Amplifier Input Jack (see Figure I-41E). The amplified signal is then delivered to the transducer from the Bone Vibrator Output Jack (Figure I-42C). (Note: most clinical bone vibrators are designed to operate between approximately 250 Hz to 4000 Hz.)

Exercises:
(1) Obtain a listener's bone conduction 50% threshold for a frequency near 300 Hz by using the adaptive test procedure described in Experiment II-4.

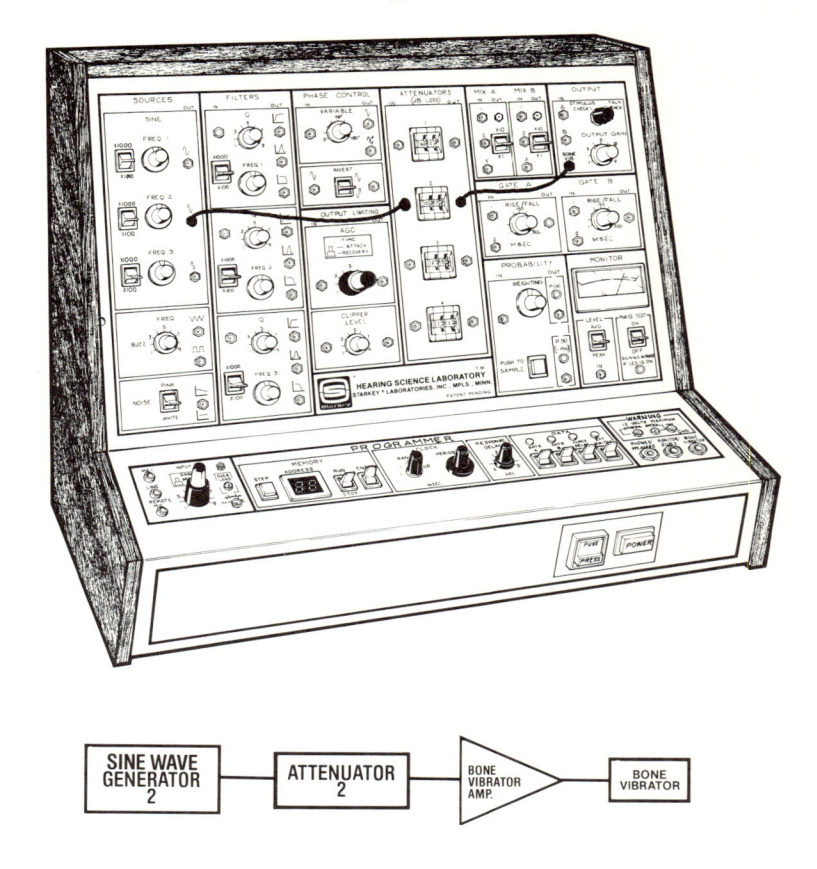

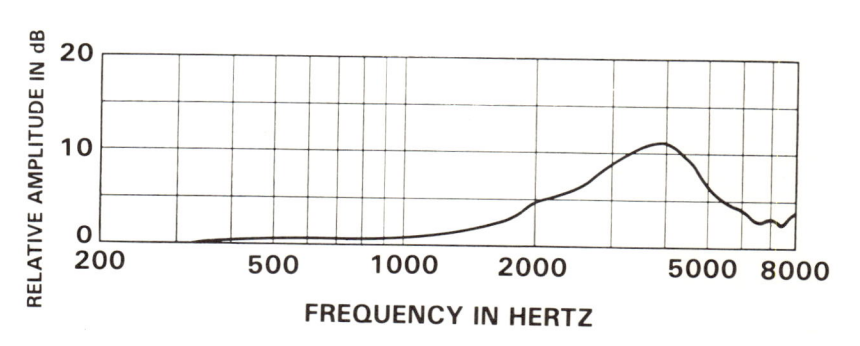

FIGURE A: The resonant characteristics of the external auditory meatus. The ratios between the sound pressures at the eardrum and the entrance to the canal are expressed in decibels. Note the presence of a resonant "peak" between 3000 and 5000 Hz. (After Wiener, 1947).

When this has been achieved, have the subject cover first one ear and then the other. Note the lateralization of the tone. Increase the Attenuator setting and determine the subject's new threshold level when the ear is occluded.

(2) Repeat exercise #1 for frequencies of 500, 700, 1000, 2000, and 4000 Hz for several subjects and note the variability of the effect from one frequency and listener to another.

(3) Repeat exercise #1 for speech and white noise signals. Note any changes in the quality of the stimulus when the ear is covered. How do you account for these changes?

NOTES:

Selected References:

Elpern, B.S. and Naunton, R.F. (1963). The stability of the occlusion effect. *Archs Otolar.*, **77**, 376-384.

Goldstein, D. and Hayes, C. (1965). The occlusion effect in bone conduction hearing. *J. Speech Hear. Res.*, **8**, 137-148.

Huizing, E.H. (1960). Bone conduction. *Acta Oto-Lar., Suppl.*, 155.

Naunton, R.F. (1957). Clinical bone-conduction audiometry: the use of a frontally applied bone-conduction receiver and the importance of the occlusion effect in clinical bone-conduction audiometry. *Archs Otolar.*, **66**, 281-298.

Sullivan, J.A., Gotleib, C.C., and Hodges, W.E. (1947). Shift of bone conduction threshold on occlusion of the external ear canal. *Laryngoscope*, **57**, 690-703.

Tonndorf, J. (1964). Animal experiments in bone conduction: clinical conclusions. *Ann. Otol. Rhinol. Lar.*, **73**, 659-678.

Tonndorf, J. (1968). A new concept of bone conduction. *Archs Otolar.*, **87**, 595-600.

Tonndorf, J. (1972). Bone conduction. In J.V. Tobias (Ed.) *Foundations of modern auditory theory*. Vol. 2. Academic Press, New York.

Tonndorf, J., Greenfield, E.C., and Kaufman, R.S. (1966). The occlusion of the external ear canal: its effect upon bone conduction in cats. *Acta Oto-Lar., Suppl.*, **213**, 80-104

Watson, N.A. and Gales, R.S. (1943). Bone conduction threshold measurements: effects of occlusion, enclosures, and masking devices. *J. Acoust. Soc. Am.*, **14**, 207-215.

Wiener, F.M. (1947). On the diffraction of a progressive sound wave by the human head. *J. Acoust. Soc. Am.*, **19**, 143-146.

EXPERIMENT II-8: CANCELLATION OF BONE CONDUCTED SOUND BY AIR CONDUCTION SIGNALS

Purpose:
To demonstrate that air and bone conducted signals share a common mechanical or acoustical pathway.

Background Principle:
The complex pathways by which air and bone conducted sounds stimulate our auditory system were once thought to be wholly independent from each other. Bone conducted signals were originally believed to reach the auditory nerves without the involvement of the cochlea "way station." Von Békésy (1932), however, demonstrated that air and bone conducted sounds must share a mutual transmission route since the two signals could be made to cancel each other by introducing an appropriate phase shift between them (see Laboratory Experiment I-1). Since a bone conducted signal stimulates both cochleae simultaneously, a broad-band masking noise will be delivered to one ear, effectively removing it from the listening task. The listener varies the phase relationship between the air conducted signal in the unmasked ear and an identical bone conducted sound.

Procedure:
The test tone from Sine Wave Generator #1 is sent to the Variable Phase Shifter whose Reference and Variable Phase outputs are passed through separate Attenuators and Electronic Gates. The output from Gate "A" is delivered to the Bone Vibrator Output Amplifier and Bone Vibrator while Gate "B" passes the signal to one Output Amplifier channel and headphone. By appropriate switching of one or both Gates, the subject may compare the air and bone conducted signals independently or simultaneously. The white noise masking signal is sent through its own Attenuator, Output Amplifier channel and the second headphone. The noise may be set to any comfortable level, such as 50 or 60 dB above threshold.

Exercises:
(1) Select an initial tone frequency of 4000 Hz. The subject should listen to the air and bone conduction signals one at a time and adjust their respective levels until the loudness of each signal is the same. With both stimuli on, the listener should vary the variable phase control and note if a "null" in the strength of the combined signal can be obtained.

(2) Exercise #1 should be repeated for a variety of signal frequencies and sensation levels to determine if the cancellation effect is influenced by these variables.

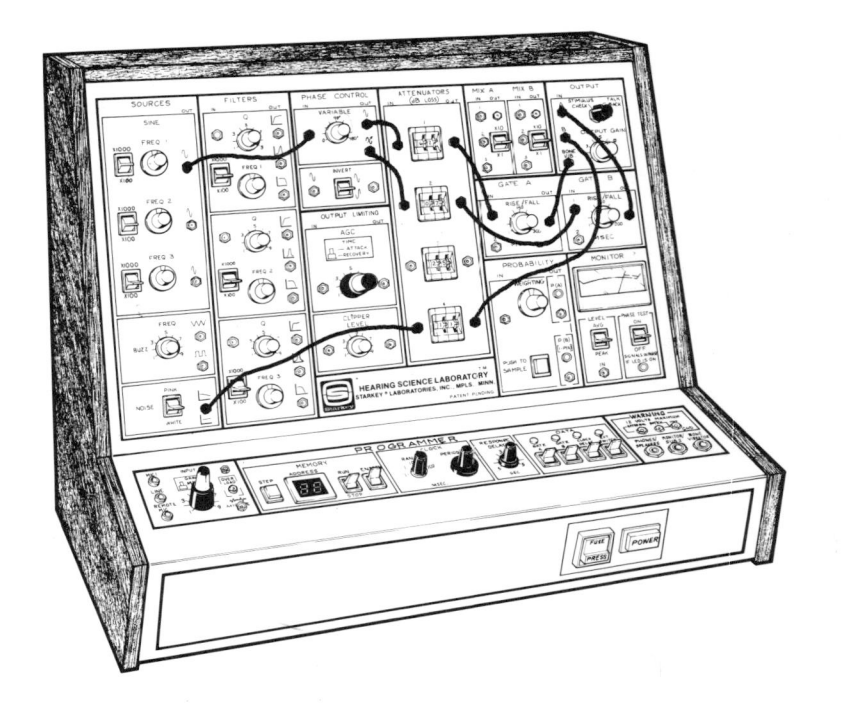

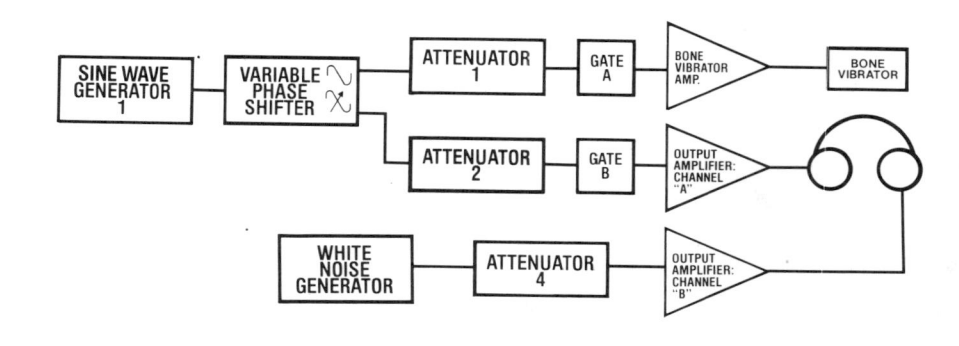

CLOCK SETTINGS			MEMORY ADDRESS		
RANGE SWITCH	PERIOD/ STEP CONTROL	RESPONSE DELAY	MEMORY CHANNEL	AIR CONDUCTION ONLY	BONE CONDUCTION ONLY	AIR & BONE CONDUCTION
CLOCK STOPPED			GATE "A"		ON	ON
			GATE "B"	ON		ON
			CLOCK DELAY			
MILLISECONDS	SECONDS		EXT. SWITCH			

(3) Exercises #1 and #2 should be repeated for several different bone vibrator placements including: the *mastoid process of the temporal bone* (i.e., the bony prominence behind the pinna); the forehead; and even contact with the teeth. Does placement of the vibrator affect cancellation of the signals?

NOTES:

Selected References:

von Békésy, G. (1932). Zur Theorie des Hörens bei der Schallaufnahme durch Knochenleitung. *Poggendorff's Annln Phys. Chem.*, **13**, ser. **5**, 111-136.

von Békésy, G. (1960). *Experiments in hearing.* pp. 207-238. McGraw-Hill, New York.

Khanna, S.M., Tonndorf, J., and Queller, J.E. (1976). Mechanical parameters of hearing by bone conduction. *J. Acoust. Soc. Am.*, **60**, 139-154.

Lowy, K. (1942). Cancellation of the electrical cochlear response with air- and bone-conducted sound. *J. Acoust. Soc. Am.*, **14**, 156-158.

Tonndorf, J. (1972). Bone conduction. In J.V. Tobias (Ed.) *Foundations of modern auditory theory.* Vol. 2. Academic Press, New York.

Tyszka, F.A. and Goldstein, D.P. (1975). Interaural phase and amplitude relationships of bone-conduction signals. *J. Acoust. Soc. Am.*, **57**, 200-206.

Intensity and Loudness

III

EXPERIMENT III-1: THE DIFFERENTIAL THRESHOLD FOR INTENSITY

Purpose:
To determine the smallest intensity increment that a listener can detect.

Background Principle:
An individual who whispers to his neighbor in a library reading room would probably be reproached for disturbing the quiet. In the midst of a noisy cocktail party, however, the same whisper would surely go unnoticed. The smallest detectable change in a physical stimulus, such as intensity, is known as a *just noticeable difference (JND)* or *difference limen (DL)*. It should be clear from the two listening situations mentioned above that the size of the differential threshold for intensity is dependent, to some degree, upon the intensity of the sound to which the increment is added. A psychoacoustic measure which takes this fact into account is called the *Weber Fraction*, in honor of Psychologist E.H. Weber (1795-1878). The measure is formed by the ratio of the intensity increment (ΔI) and the original stimulus level (I):

$$\text{Weber Fraction} = \frac{\Delta I}{I} \simeq \text{constant}$$

The difference in decibels between two compared sounds may be used as a convenient and legitimate metric for difference limen experiments (the decibel itself having been derived from an intensity ratio). The smallest JND's for intensity range between about 0.4 dB to 1 dB, depending upon the particular experimental procedure employed (see also Laboratory Experiment III-2). For this exercise, we shall require the listener to compare two alternating tones which have identical frequencies and different intensities. The subject's responsibility is to report whether the stimuli are the same or different in intensity while the experimenter gradually brings the level of one signal closer to that of its counterpart.

Procedure:
The output from one Sine Wave Generator is sent to two Attenuators and two Electronic Gates. Both gated signals are combined within a Mixer-Amplifier and delivered to one Output Amplifier channel and headphone. The suggested programming instructions will alternate the two signals every half second.

Exercises:
The JND for intensity may be influenced by such factors as the test frequency employed and the signal level of the tones themselves.

(1) Obtain JND values for a variety of low, mid, and high frequencies (e.g., 200 Hz, 1000 Hz and 6000 Hz). Is the size of the JND the same for each frequency?

(2) Determine if there is any difference in the size of the JND when relatively soft (e.g., near threshold) or loud tones are used.

(3) Use the Programmer Delay Channel to create a period of silence between the two tones. This can be accomplished with a single delay command at Memory Address 50. Vary the duration of this pause from 0.5 second to 5 seconds and note if the size of the JND is affected by the listener's ability to remember the loudness of the first signal.

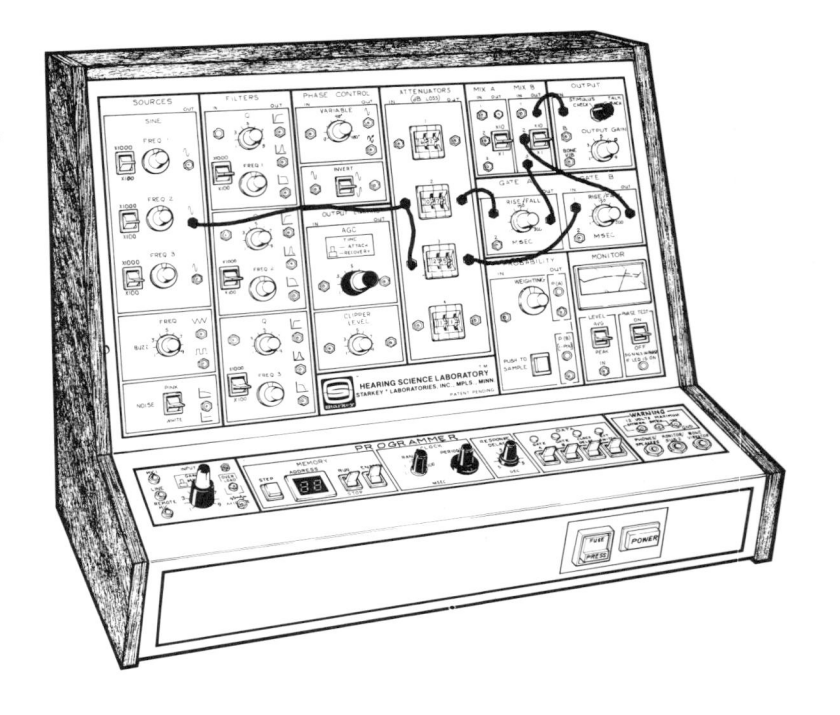

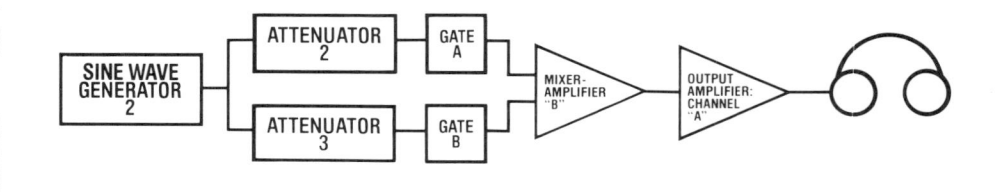

CLOCK SETTINGS			MEMORY ADDRESS	
RANGE SWITCH	PERIOD/STEP CONTROL	RESPONSE DELAY	MEMORY CHANNEL	00 TO 49 / 50 TO 99
10	X	1	GATE "A"	ON
			GATE "B"		ON
MILLISECONDS		SECONDS	CLOCK DELAY	
			EXT. SWITCH	

NOTES:

Selected References:

Ekman, G. (1959). Weber's law and related functions. *J. Psychol.*, **47**, 343-352.

Garner, W.R. and Miller, G.A. (1944). Differential sensitivity to intensity as a function of the duration of the comparison tone. *J. Exp. Psychol.*, **34**, 450-463.

Harris, J.D. (1963). Loudness discrimination. *J. Speech Hear. Dis. Mon. Suppl.*, **11**, 1-63.

Jesteadt, W. and Wier, C.C. (1977). Comparison of monaural and binaural discrimination of intensity and frequency. *J. Acoust. Soc. Am.*, **61**, 1599-1603.

Jesteadt, W., Wier, C.C., and Green, D.M. (1977). Intensity discrimination as a function of frequency and sensation level. *J. Acoust. Soc. Am.*, **61**, 169-177.

Luce, R.D. and Green, D.M. (1972). A neural timing theory for response times and the psychophysics of intensity. *Psychol. Rev.*, **79**, 14-57.

Moray, N. (1970). Introductory experiments in auditory time sharing: detection of intensity and frequency increments. *J. Acoust. Soc. Am.*, **47**, 1071-1073.

Moore, B.C.J. and Raab, D.H. (1974). Pure-tone intensity discrimination: some experiments relating to the "near-miss" to Weber's law. *J. Acoust. Soc. Am.*, **55**, 1049-1054.

Rowland, R.C. and Tobias, J.V. (1967). Interaural intensity difference limens. *J. Speech Hear. Res.*, **10**, 745-756.

Penner, M.J. and Viemeister, N.F. (1973). Intensity discrimination of clicks: the effects of click bandwidth and background noise. *J. Acoust. Soc. Am.*, **54**, 1184-1188.

Schacknow, P.N. and Raab, D.H. (1973). Intensity discrimination of tone bursts and the form of the Weber function. *Percept. Psychophys.*, **14**, 449-450.

Viemeister, N.F. (1972). Intensity discrimination of pulsed sinusoids: the effects of filtered noise. *J. Acoust. Soc. Am.*, **51**, 1265-1269.

Yost, W.A. (1972). Weber's fraction for the intensity of pure tones presented binaurally. *Percept. Psychophys.*, **11**, 61-64.

EXPERIMENT III-2: PEDESTAL EXPERIMENTS (THE SISI TEST)

Purpose:
To examine the size of the JND for intensity, using a *pedestal experiment* (i.e., one in which there is a brief increase in level for an ongoing pedestal, or "carrier," signal).

Background Principle:
Early research findings (Lüscher and Zwislocki, 1949; Jerger, 1952) tended to indicate that individuals with an inner ear type of hearing loss displayed a smaller size JND for intensity than did normal listeners. These initial conclusions have, however, been contraindicated by more recent investigations. A clinical test procedure known as the *Short Increment Sensitivity Index (SISI)* was a once familiar part of the clinical Audiology test battery which explored the intensity JND for hearing impaired subjects. The stimulus for this test was composed of a continuously-on tone set to 20 dB above a listener's threshold for a particular frequency. Every five seconds the magnitude of the tone is momentarily increased. The subject's responsibility is to report the presence of any abrupt intensity change in the ongoing tone (the *pedestal*). After several practice trials (with noticeably large dB increments, such as 4 or 5 dB), the experimenter decreases the size of the stimulus increment down to one decibel changes. A total of twenty such increments are presented to the subject who receives five percentage points for each correct identification. It was originally suggested that SISI scores above 70% often accompany cochlear pathology. A great many normal hearing listeners, however, also yield "positive" SISI scores, and thus the test is no longer considered an accurate indicator of inner ear impairment. Recent investigations, however, reveal that when the SISI test is performed at high levels, such as 75 dB HL, individuals with retrocochlear hearing impairment are unable to hear the intensity increment while normal hearing subjects obtain a high percentage of increment detections (see, for example, Cooper and Owen, 1976).

Procedure:
A single pure tone is passed through two Attenuators, one of whose outputs is sent to an Electronic Gate while the other is routed directly to a Mixer-Amplifier. The output of the Gate is also sent to the Mixer-Amplifier. This wiring configuration permits the tone to remain continuously on with periodic intensity increments provided by the Gated signal. The combined stimulus from the Mixer Output Jack is delivered to one Output Amplifier channel and headphone. The suggested programming instructions will create a 200 millisecond intensity increment every 5 seconds.

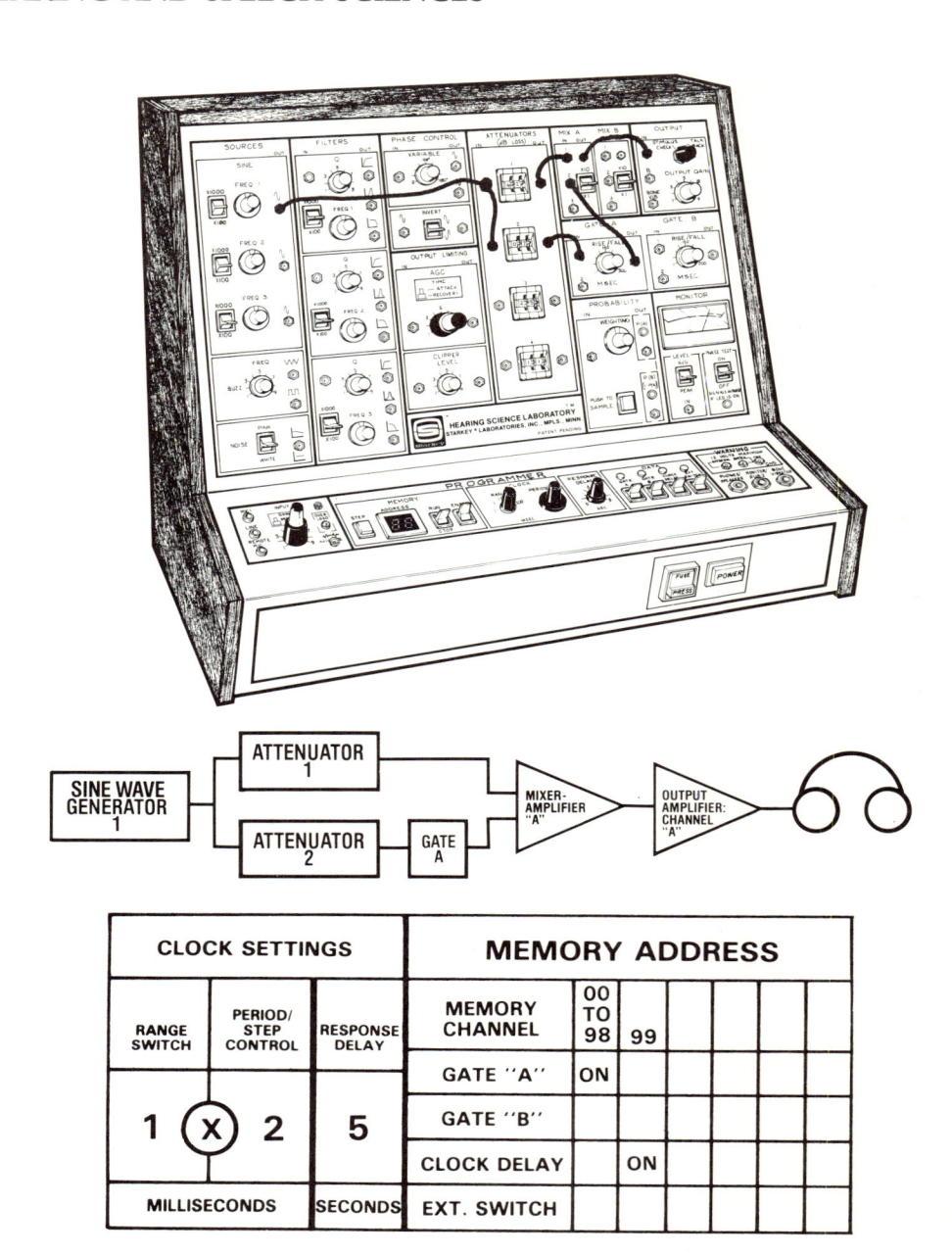

Exercises:
Differences between such factors as the rise/fall characteristics and duration of the tonal increments may have contributed to the disparate research findings that have been gathered on the efficacy of the SISI test.

(1) Examine a listener's SISI score for various rise/fall time settings of the two Electronic Gates. Does the SISI score increase when the tonal increment is switched on and off more abruptly?

(2) Perform the SISI task at several different stimulus levels. Are the increments more easily detected near or far above the subject's threshold?

(3) Repeat exercise #1 with several different test tone frequencies. Do the increments become easier to detect at very low or high frequencies?

(4) Reprogram Electronic Gate "A" so that the intensity increments remain on for several different durations. How does this variable affect the detectability of the stimulus increments?

NOTES:

Selected References:

Cooper, J.C., Jr. and Owen, J.H. (1976). In defence of SISIs. The short increment sensitivity index. *Archs Otolar.*, **102**, 396-399.

Hanley, C.N. and Utting, J. F. (1965). An examination of the normal hearer's response to the SISI. *J. Speech Hear. Dis.*, **30**, 58-65.

Hirsh, K.J., Palva, T., and Goodman, A. (1954). Difference limen and recruitment. *Archs Otolar,* (Chicago), **60**, 525-540.

Jerger, J. (1952). A difference limen recruitment test and its diagnostic significance. *Laryngoscope*, **62**, 1316-1332.

Jerger, J., Shedd, J.L., and Harford, E. (1959). On the detection of extremely small changes in sound intensity. *Archs Otolar.*, **69**, 200-211.

Lüscher, E. and Zwislocki, J. (1949). A simple method for indirect monaural determination of the recruitment phenomenon (difference limen in intensity in different types of deafness). *Acta Otolaryng. (Stockholm)*, **78**, 156-168.

Martin, F.N. (1972). The short increment sensitivity index (SISI). In J. Katz (Ed.) *Handbook of Clinical Audiology.* The Williams and Wilkins Co., Baltimore, Maryland.

Owens, E. (1965). The SISI test and VIIIth nerve versus cochlear involvement. *J. Speech Hear. Dis.*, **30**, 252-262.

Sanders, J. (1966). The effect of increment size on the short increment sensitivity index scores. *J. Speech Hear. Res.*, **9**, 297-304.

Swisher, L.P. (1966). Response to intensity change in cochlear pathology. *Laryngoscope*, **10**, 1706-1713.

Swisher, L.P., Stephens, M.M., and Doehring, D.G. (1966). The effects of hearing level and normal variability on sensitivity to intensive change. *J. Aud. Res.*, **6**, 249-259.

Thompson, G. (1963). A modified SISI technique for selected cases with suspected acoustic neurinoma. *J. Speech Hear. Dis.*, **28**, 299-302.

Yantis, P.A., and Decker, R.L. (1964). On the short increment sensitivity index (SISI test). *J. Speech Hear. Dis.*, **29**, 231-246.

Young, I.M. and Harbert, F. (1967). Significance of the SISI test. *J. Aud. Res.*, **7**, 303-311.

EXPERIMENT III-3: EQUAL LOUDNESS CONTOURS

Purpose:
To match the loudness of two tones which differ in frequency.

Background Principle:
In addition to detecting minimal changes in physical magnitudes, most observers display the ability to judge when two stimuli produce identical sensations. It is, for example, commonplace for individuals to match paint colors or heft objects in each hand to equate their weights. A less familiar, and often more difficult, psychophysical task is to equate the loudness of two different sounds. In one procedure, a listener is required to match the loudness of different frequency test tones to that of a 1000 Hz reference tone fixed at a specific sound pressure level. For equally loud tones, the number of *loudness level* units, or *phons,* is equal to the dB SPL value of the 1000 Hz reference tone (e.g., 40 dB SPL at 1 KHz = 40 Phons). Any sound which is judged equal in loudness to a 40 dB SPL 1000 Hz tone would also possess a loudness level of 40 phons. Results from this type of experiment reveal that different test tone frequencies require different sound pressure levels to be equal in loudness to the 1000 Hz reference tone. The curve that connects these various decibel levels is known as an *equal loudness contour,* or *phon line.* Several phon lines, like those shown in Figure "A", can be obtained by repeating the basic experiment with a number of different reference tone levels. Note that the phon lines flatten slightly at higher signal levels and appear to converge at both extremes of the frequency range. How would you account for the fact that the Threshold of Audibility, obtained in an earlier experiment, is also regarded as one member of the family of phon lines?

Procedure:
The test and reference pure tone signals are passed through separate Attenuators and Electronic Gates. The outputs from the Gates are combined within a Mixer-Amplifier and then sent into one Output Amplifier channel and headphone. The suggested programming instructions may be used to present alternating 0.5 second tones to the listener's ear.

Exercises:
(1) Adjust Sine Wave Generator #1 to provide the reference tone frequency of 1000 Hz. The Attenuator for this signal should be set to a value that delivers 40 dB more sound pressure level than the subject requires at his or her threshold (i.e., 40 dB less attenuation). Present each test tone from Sine Wave Generator #2 well above the listener's threshold for that frequency. Employ a series of test tones which span a large frequency range (e.g., 100 Hz, 400 Hz, 700 Hz, 2000 Hz, 4000 Hz, and 6000 Hz). The listener or the

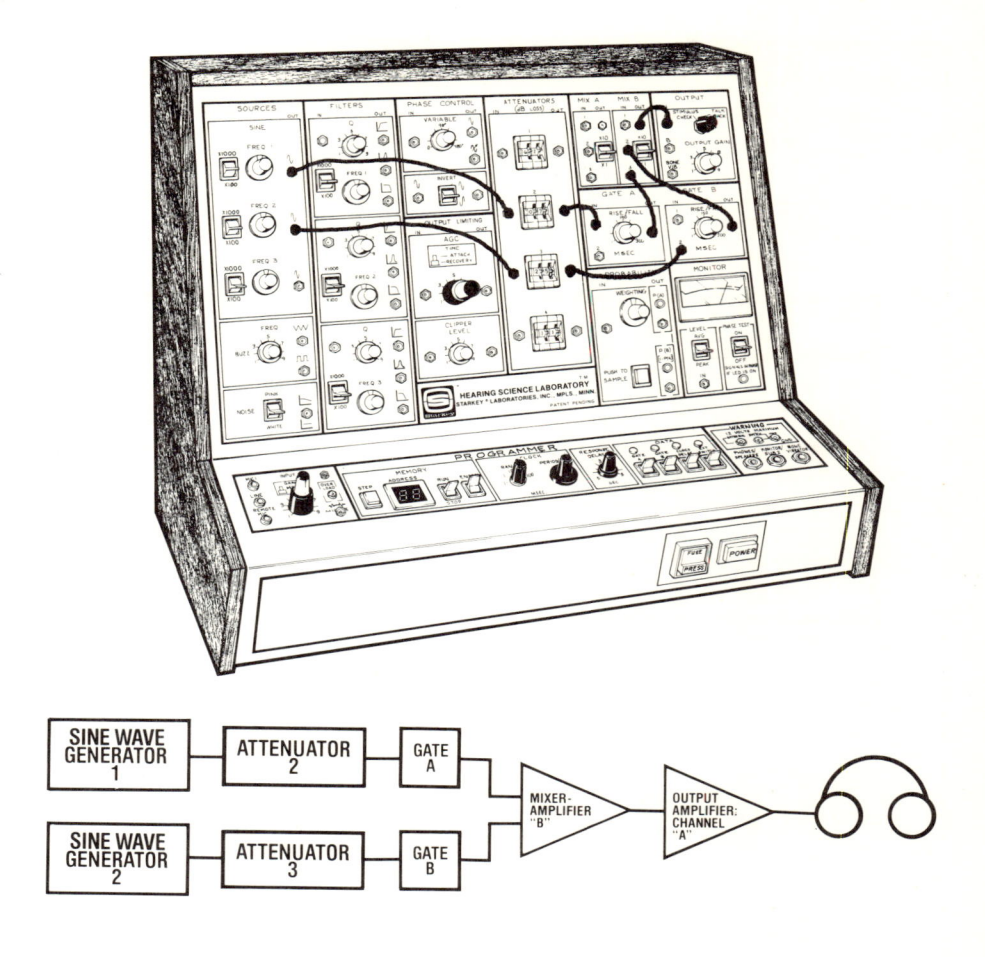

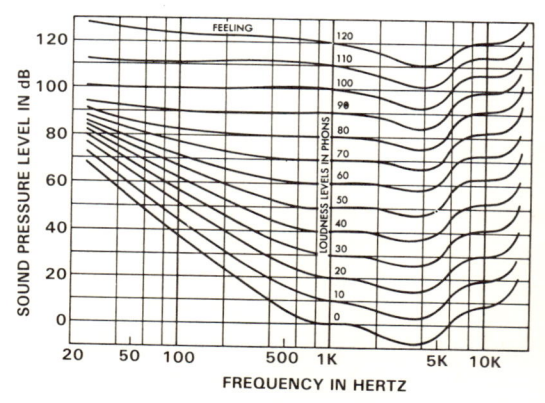

FIGURE A: These phon lines reveal that different frequency tones require differing sound magnitudes in order to have the same loudness level as a 1000 Hz reference signal. Note that the number of phons equals the decibel level of the 1000 Hz reference tone. (After Fletcher and Munson, 1933. From *The Speech Chain* by P.B. Denes and E.N. Pinson. © 1963 by Bell Telephone Laboratories, Inc. Reproduced by permission of Doubleday & Company, Inc.)

experimenter may vary the test tone's magnitude until the subject reports that both stimuli are equal in loudness. Record both Attenuator settings for each test frequency and plot a smooth equal loudness level contour on Figures "B" and "C", respectively.

(2) Repeat exercise #1 for different reference tone levels (e.g., 30 dB above and below the reference tone level setting used in exercise #1). How do the phon lines you obtained compare with those to be found in the cited literature?

NOTES:

1000 Hz REFERENCE		TEST TONE FREQUENCY IN HERTZ (RECORD ATTENUATOR #3 SETTINGS IN dB)					
IN dB SL (i.e. dB ABOVE THRESHOLD)	ATTENUATOR #2 SETTING (IN dB)	100	400	700	2000	4000	6000
40							
10							
70							

FIGURE B: Sample Data Chart.

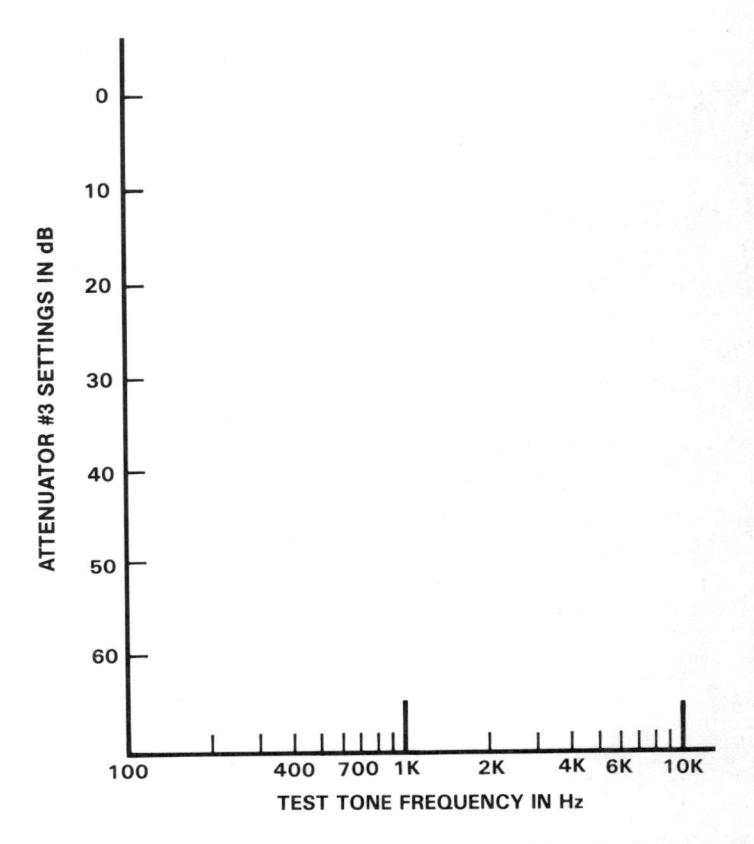

FIGURE C: Sample Data Graph. Attenuator #2 reference tone settings should be entered at 1000 Hz on the graph.

Selected References:

Carver, W.F. (1972). Loudness balance procedures. In J. Katz (Ed.) *Handbook of clinical audiology.* The Williams and Wilkins Co., Baltimore, Maryland.

Churcher, B.G. and King. A.J. (1937). The performance of noise meters in terms of the primary standard. *J. Inst. Elect. Engrs.,* **81,** 57-90.

Fletcher, H. and Munson, W.A. (1933). Loudness, its definition, measurement and calculation. *J. Acoust. Soc. Am.,* **5,** 82-108.

Molino, J.A. (1973). Pure-tone equal-loudness contours for standard tones of different frequencies. *Percept. Psychophys.,* **14,** 1-4.

Robinson, D.W. and Dadson, R.S. (1956). A redetermination of the equal loudness relations for pure tones. *Brit. J. App. Phy.,* **7,** 166-181.

Robinson, D.W. and Dadson, R.S. (1957). Threshold of hearing and equal-loudness relations for pure tones, and the loudness function. *J. Acoust. Soc. Am.,* **29,** 1284-1288.

Ross, S. (1967). Matching functions and equal-sensation contours for loudness. *J. Acoust. Soc. Am.,* **42,** 778-793.

Schneider, B., Wright, A.A., Edelheit, W., Hock, P., and Humphrey, C. (1972). Equal loudness contours derived from sensory magnitude judgments. *J. Acoust. Soc. Am.,* **51,** 1951-1959.

Stevens, S.S. (1959). On the validity of the loudness scale. *J. Acoust. Soc. Am.,* **31,** 995-1003.

EXPERIMENT III-4: THE SONE SCALE

Purpose:
To examine the abilities of a listener to estimate the loudness differences between sounds.

Background Principle:
The Equal Loudness Contours obtained in Laboratory Experiment III-3 indicate that a sound such as 80 phons is subjectively louder than one at 40 phons loudness level. But is 80 phons twice as loud as 40 phons? In order to answer this kind of question, one must perform an experiment in which a subject actually tells us by **how much** one sound is louder than another. In one class of experiments called *ratio estimation* procedures, a listener is presented with two alternating tones, of differing level, and is required to report the loudness ratio that is perceived to exist between the stimuli. The subject could also be asked to actually adjust the level of a *comparison stimulus* with respect to some *standard stimulus* until the comparison signal is either some multiple (commonly twice) or fraction (typically one-half) of the standard. Both the *method of multiple stimuli* and the *method of fractionation* come under the general heading of *ratio production* scaling techniques. The levels at which these loudness doublings or halvings take place become the starting values for the next experimental trial. By continuing in this manner, a loudness, or *sone scale*, can be established. Researchers have adopted the convention that one sone is equal to a loudness level of 40 phons (i.e., 40 dB SPL at 1000 Hz). Experiments have shown that there is no simple, one to one relationship between the perceived loudness, the loudness level, and the physical intensity of a sound. It has been determined, for example, that a four-fold increase in loudness may result from a doubling of the loudness level of a sound. That is, a change from 1 sone to 4 sones requires that a 20 phon 1000 Hz tone be raised to a value of 40 phons. Since the number of phons equals the number of decibels at 1000 Hz, this should be recognized as a 20 dB, or 100 fold, increase in physical intensity. As might be expected, studies that employ differing procedures often yield somewhat different findings. With this in mind, it is not surprising that the precise nature of the loudness phenomenon remains unresolved and controversial.

Procedure:
The same pure tone signal is sent to two separate Attenuators whose outputs are delivered to two separate Electronic Gates. The suggested programming instructions permit the reference and test signals to alternate in the listener's ear. A 50 millisecond silent interval separates the two 450 millisecond tones. The outputs from both Electronic Gates are combined within a Mixer-Amplifier and then routed to one Output Amplifier channel and headphone.

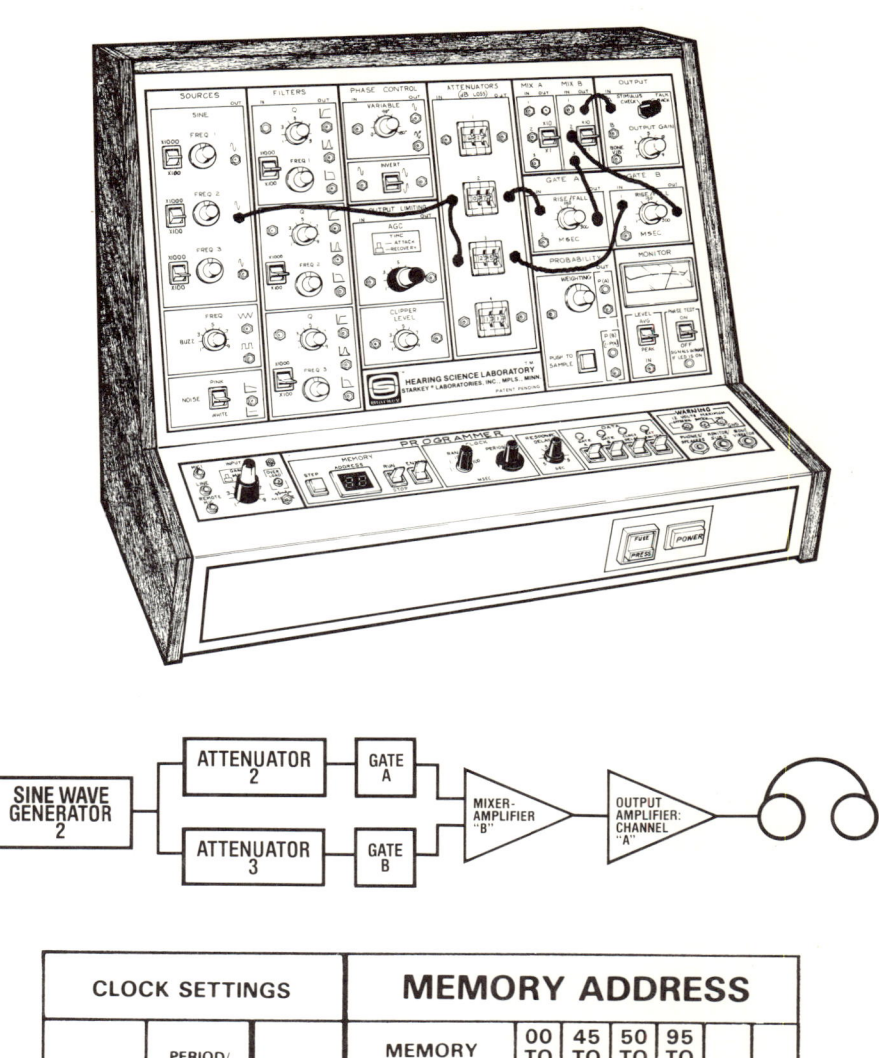

Exercises:
(1) Adjust the pure tone frequency to a value near 1000 Hz. Choose one Attenuator as the reference and set its level to provide the subject with a signal that is roughly 40 dB greater in magnitude than was required at threshold (i.e., 40 dB less attenuation than at threshold). For our purposes, this signal may be considered to have a reference loudness of one sone. While both tones alternate, the subject varies the level of the test signal Attenuator until it is roughly twice as loud as the reference stimulus. Record this Attenuator setting as two sones. Repeat this procedure with the two-sone level setting as the new starting value. Continue in this fashion and plot each doubling in sones as a function of the corresponding Attenuator settings on the axes of Figure "A." Other loudness ratios, such as

halvings or triplings, may be used if desired. Does the shape of your sone curve match those shown in the literature cited? If not, try to identify differences between the procedures and variables you employed and those of the other investigators.

(2) Use the method of *ratio estimation* to obtain a scale of subjective loudness. In this case, the subject reports how many fold louder one sound is than another. The reference Attenuator may be reset to the same initial value that was used for exercise #1 (i.e., 40 dB above the listener's threshold, or roughly one sone). The experimenter varies the non-reference Attenuator and asks, after each change in level, how many times louder the non-reference tone is than the reference tone. Plot the relative loudness estimates on the ordinate of Figure "B" which shows corresponding Attenuator settings on the abscissa. Contrast this sone scale with the one obtained for exercise #1.

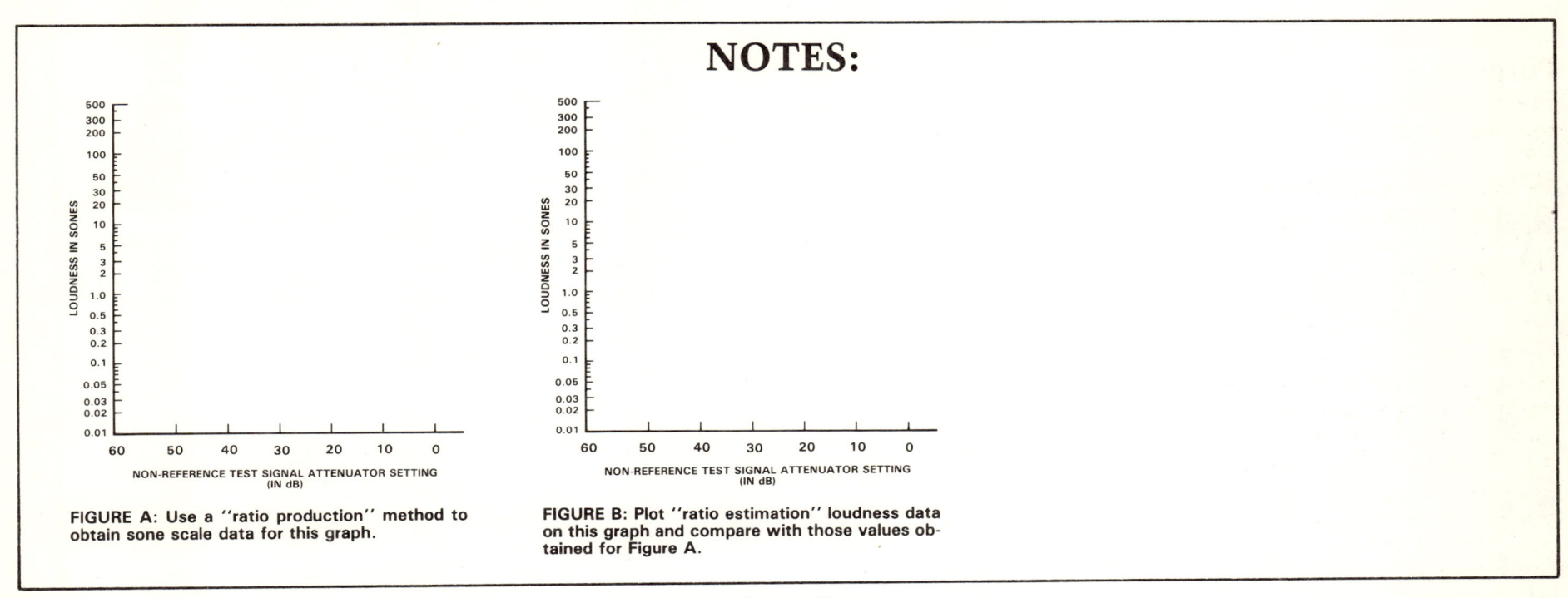

NOTES:

FIGURE A: Use a "ratio production" method to obtain sone scale data for this graph.

FIGURE B: Plot "ratio estimation" loudness data on this graph and compare with those values obtained for Figure A.

Selected References:

de Barbenza, C.M., Bryan, M.E., McRobert, H., and Tempest, W. (1970). Individual loudness susceptibility. *Sound*, **4**, 75-79.

Garner, W.R. (1954). Technique and a scale for loudness measurement. *J. Acoust. Soc. Am.*, **26**, 73-88.

Hellman, R.P. and Zwislocki, J.J. (1961). Some factors affecting the estimation of loudness. *J. Acoust. Soc. Am.*, **33**, 687-694.

Howes, W.L. (1971). Loudness determined by power summation. *Acustica*, **25**, 343-349.

McRoberts, H., Bryan, M.E., and Tempest, W. (1965). Magnitude estimation of loudness. *J. Sound Vib.*, **2**, 391-401.

Poulton, E.C. and Stevens, S.S. (1955). On the halving and doubling of the loudness of white noise. *J. Acoust. Soc. Am.*, **27**, 329-331.

Richards, A.M. (1974). Non-metric scaling of loudness. I. 1000-Hz tones. *J. Acoust. Soc. Am.*, **56**, 582-588.

Robinson, D.W. (1953). The relation between the sone and the phon scales of loudness. *Acustica*, **3**, 344-358.

Robinson, D.W. (1957). The subjective loudness scale. *Acustica*, **7**, 217-233.

Stevens, S.S. (1936). A scale for the measurement of a psychological magnitude: loudness. *Psychol. Rev.*, **43**, 405-416.

Stevens, S.S. (1955). The measurement of loudness. *J. Acoust. Soc. Am.*, **27**, 815-820.

Stevens, S.S. (1956). The direct estimation of sensory magnitude — loudness. *Am. J. Psychol.*, **69**, 1-25.

Stevens, S.S. (1957a). Concerning the form of the loudness function. *J. Acoust. Soc. Am.*, **29**, 603-606.

Stevens, S.S. (1957b). Calculating loudness. *Noise Control*, **3**, 11-22.

Stevens, S.S. (1957c). On the psychophysical law. *Psychol. Rev.*, **64**, 153-181.

Stevens, S.S. (1959). On the validity of the loudness scale. *J. Acoust. Soc. Am.*, **31**, 995-1003.

Stevens, S.S. (1972). 1971 Rayleigh gold medal address: calculating the perceived level of light and sound. *J. Sound Vib.*, **23**, 297-306.

Stevens, S.S. (1975). In G. Stevens (Ed.) *Psychophysics*, Wiley, New York.

Stevens, S.S. and Poulton, E.C. (1956). The estimation of loudness by unpracticed observers *J. Exp. Psychol.*, **51**, 71-78.

Ward, L.M. (1972). Category judgments of loudness in the absence of an experimenter-induced identification function: sequential effects and power-function fit. *J. Exp. Psychol.*, **94**, 179-184.

Ward, L.M. (1973). Repeated magnitude estimations with a variable standard: sequential effects and other properties. *Percept. Psychophys.*, **13**, 193-200.

Warren, R.M. (1970). Elimination of biases in loudness judgments for tones. *J. Acoust. Soc. Am.*, **48**, 1397-1403.

Warren, R.M. (1973). Anomalous loudness function for speech. *J. Acoust. Soc. Am.*, **54**, 390-396.

EXPERIMENT III-5: THE PSYCHOPHYSICAL POWER LAW

Purpose:
To use a *method of magnitude estimation* to determine the relationship between the physical intensity of a sound stimulus and the sensation of loudness it produces.

Background Principle:
In addition to the ratio scaling procedures mentioned in Laboratory Experiment III-4, it is also common to require a subject to provide a *magnitude estimation* of the stimulus loudness. In this instance, the listener assigns some numerical value to the magnitude of the loudness percept. The standard tone is fixed at some level (e.g., 60 dB SPL) and is usually assigned an arbitrary loudness value, or *modulus,* such as 100. The comparison stimuli would then be presented to the subject in a random sequence of levels (e.g., at 60, 30, 50, 70, 20 dB SPL, etc.). The results of Stevens (1956), shown in Figure "A", display the relationship between the loudness estimations of listeners and various sound pressure levels. The relationship between the magnitude of a subject's sensation (Ψ) for a given stimulus magnitude (S) may be expressed in mathematical terms as follows:

$$\Psi = kS^n$$

The values for the constants k and n will depend upon the particular sense modality under consideration. Note that a straight line, or *linear function,* is formed by the two variables when a logarithmic scale is used on the

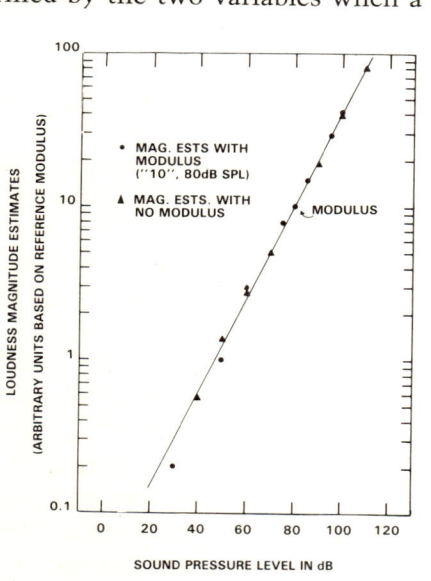

FIGURE A: The relationship between a subject's loudness magnitude estimations for various sound pressure levels appears as a "linear function" when plotted on log-log coordinates. (After Stevens, 1956).

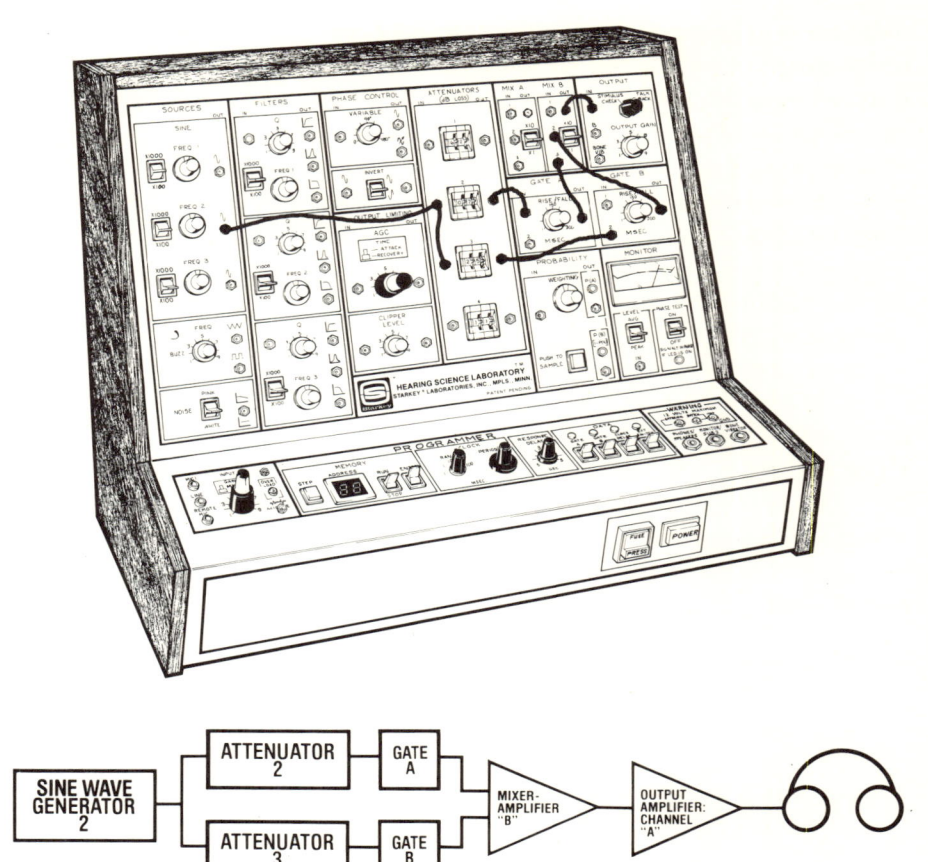

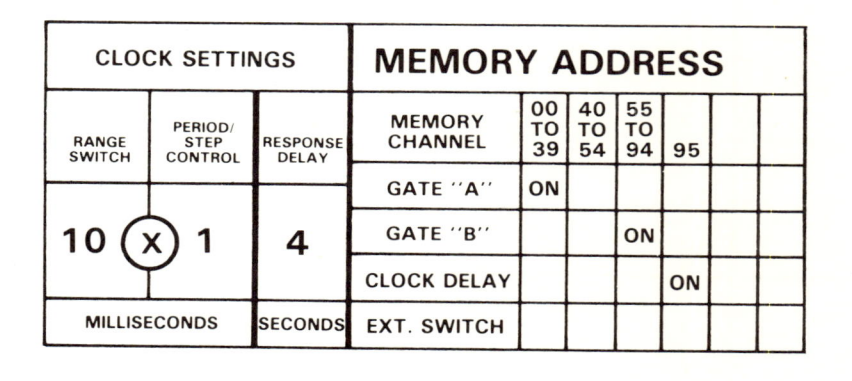

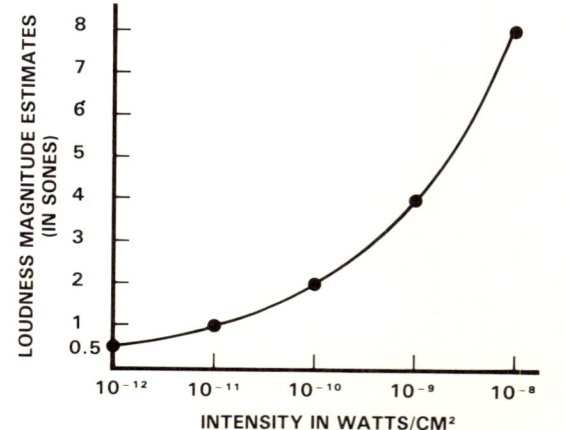

FIGURE B: A doubling in sound loudness roughly corresponds to a ten-fold increase in the physical intensity of the stimulus. This is seen as a "power function" when plotted on a graph with linear scale rulings on both axes.

ordinate and a logarithmic unit (i.e., the decibel) appears on the x-axis. A linear function on "double logarithmic," or *log-log coordinates,* indicates that perceived loudness appears as a *power function* when plotted against an equally ruled scale of physical stimulus intensity (see Figure "B"). It can be seen from these graphic representations that every doubling or halving in loudness is linked to an approximate 10 dB change in the physical stimulus. This power function for loudness has a slope, or exponent, of 0.3 for sound intensity and 0.6 for sound pressure units. Other sensory modalities involving brightness, taste, heaviness, et al. have been shown to have different exponents for their power functions (see Stevens, 1957, for more details about his general *Psychophysical Law*).

Procedure:

As in the preceding experiment, a pair of tones are produced by routing one sinusoid through two Attenuators and Electronic Gates. The Gates are programmed to present the signals in sequence followed by a 4 second pause for the subject's response and the experimenter's changing of the Attenuator. Both stimuli are combined within a Mixer-Amplifier and delivered to one Output Amplifier channel and headphone.

Exercises:

(1) Select a pure tone frequency near 1000 Hz. Attenuator #2 and Gate "A" will control the standard tone, whereas Attenuator #3 and Gate "B" will control the comparison (i.e., variable) stimulus. Set Attenuator #2 to provide a standard tone level 40 dB above the subject's threshold for 1000 Hz. Assign a numerical modulus of 100 to this value. The comparison stimuli may be Attenuator increments between 0 and 60 in steps of 10 dB presented in a random order. The listener must compare both stimuli and assign some numerical value to each level increment based upon the reference loudness value of 100. Plot your data points on the axes provided in Figure "C."

(2) Repeat exercise #1 for several different frequencies and standard tone level settings. Does the slope of your loudness scale change for the different test conditions?

(3) Repeat exercise #1 for several different arbitrary magnitude references. Does the slope of the power function change?

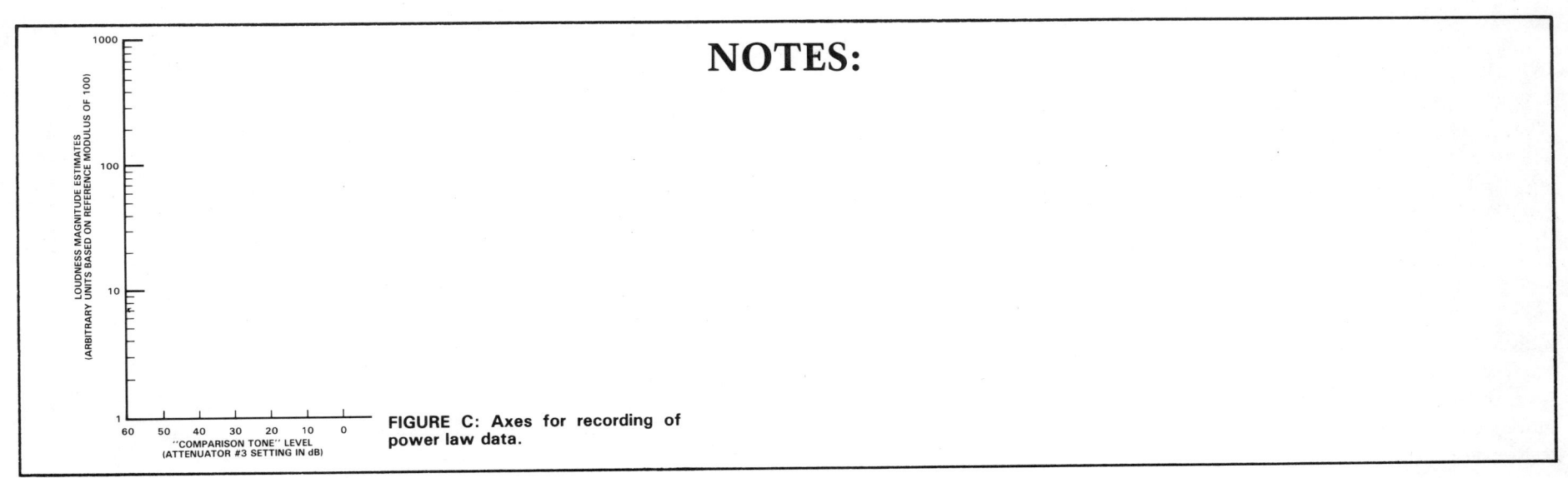

FIGURE C: Axes for recording of power law data.

NOTES:

Selected References:

Hellman, R.P. (1976). Growth of loudness at 1000 and 3000 Hz. *J. Acoust. Soc. Am.,* **60,** 672-679.

Hellman, W.S., and Hellman, R.P. (1975). Relation of the loudness function to the intensity characteristic of the ear. *J. Acoust. Soc. Am.,* **57,** 188-192.

MacKay, D.M. (1963). Psychophysics of perceived intensity: a theoretical basis for Fechner's and Stevens' laws. *Science,* **139,** 1213-1216.

Stevens, S.S. (1955). The measurement of loudness. *J. Acoust. Soc. Am.,* **27,** 815-829.

Stevens, S.S. (1956). The direct estimation of sensory magnitude — loudness. *Am. J. Psychol.,* **69,** 1-25.

Stevens, S.S. (1957). Concerning the form of the loudness function. *J. Acoust. Soc. Am.,* **29,** 603-606.

Stevens, S.S. (1961a). To honor Fechner and repeal his law. *Science.* **133,** 80-86.

Stevens, S.S. (1961b). The psychophysics of sensory function. In W.A. Rosenblith (Ed.) *Sensory communication.* pp. 1-33. M.I.T. Press & John Wiley and Sons, Inc., New York.

Stevens, S.S. (1962). The surprising simplicity of sensory metrics. *Am. Psychol.,* **17,** 29-39.

Stevens, S.S. (1964). Concerning the psychophysical power law. *Q. J. Exp. Psychol.,* **16,** (Part IV), 383-385.

Teghtsoonian, R. (1971). On the exponents in Stevens' law and the constant in Ekman's law. *Psychol. Rev.,* **78,** 71-80.

Treisman, M. (1964). Sensory scaling and the psychophysical law. *Q. J. Exp. Psychol.,* **16,** 11-22.

Yilmaz, H. (1967). Perceptual invariance and the psychophysical law. *Percept. and Psychophys.,* **2,** 533-538.

Zwislocki, J.J. (1973). On intensity characteristics of sensory receptors: a generalized function. *Kybernetik,* **12,** 169-183.

Zwislocki, J.J. (1974). A power function for sensory receptors. In H.R. Moskowitz, B. Scharf, and J.C. Stevens (Eds.) *Sensation and measurement.* Reidel, Dordrecht, Holland.

EXPERIMENT III-6: ALTERNATE BINAURAL LOUDNESS BALANCING

Purpose:
To match the loudness of tones switched between the two ears.

Background Principle:
Individuals who have a hearing loss due to cochlea pathology may suffer from an abnormally rapid growth of the loudness of sounds. This condition, known as *loudness recruitment,* is portrayed graphically in Figure "A". Curve "A" depicts a normal loudness curve. A given dB increase in a reference tone results in an equal loudness increase in a comparison tone. Curve "B" shows the manner in which an individual with recruitment might respond to various stimuli levels. Notice that below 50 dB, this hypothetical subject cannot detect the presence of the comparison tone because of his hearing loss. Above this threshold level, however, sounds are judged as substantially louder for a relatively smaller change in the physical intensity of the tone than we would expect. At the highest intensity levels, an individual with recruitment may respond in the same fashion as a normal listener. In one commonly used clinical test for recruitment, a tone at a given frequency is presented alternately to the two ears, and the listener is asked to adjust one until it is equally loud with the other (reference) tone. This so-called *alternate binaural loudness balance (ABLB)* procedure requires that the subject have one normal ear for the reference to which the damaged side is compared. Electronic techniques are available to provide a hearing impaired listener who has recruitment with amplified sound that is automatically kept at levels above his threshold of audibility, but below his threshold of discomfort. (See section on Output Limitation in Part I of this text.)

Procedure:
A 1000 Hz pure tone is delivered to two separate Attenuators whose outputs enter separate Electronic Gates. Each gated signal is then sent to a different Output Amplifier channel and headphone. The suggested programming instructions will permit the two signals to switch on and off, alternately, for 0.5 second each.

Exercises:
(1) Select one of the subject's ears as the reference side. Adjust the sound magnitude delivered to that ear to be ten decibels greater than the level of sound required at threshold for the particular test frequency employed. Vary the Attenuator setting for the opposite test ear until the listener is satisfied that both tones are equal in loudness level. Repeat this procedure with several different reference tone levels and plot the data values on the

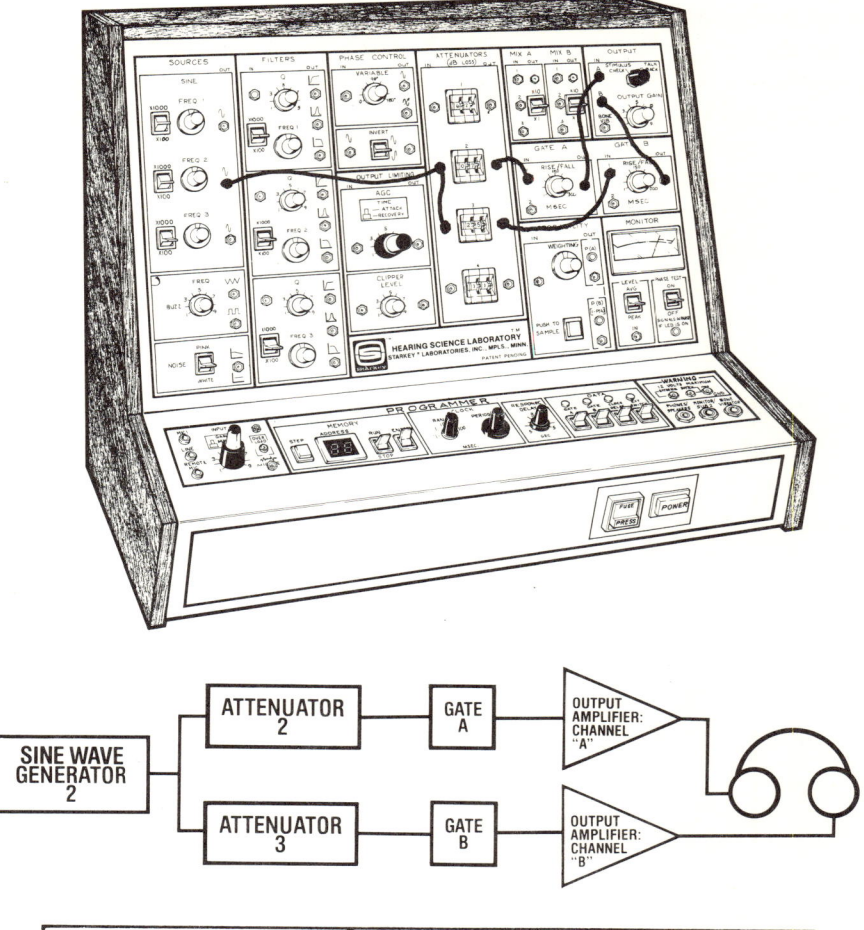

CLOCK SETTINGS			MEMORY ADDRESS					
RANGE SWITCH	PERIOD/ STEP CONTROL	RESPONSE DELAY	MEMORY CHANNEL	00 TO 49	50 TO 99			
10	X 1		GATE "A"	ON				
			GATE "B"		ON			
			CLOCK DELAY					
MILLISECONDS		SECONDS	EXT. SWITCH					

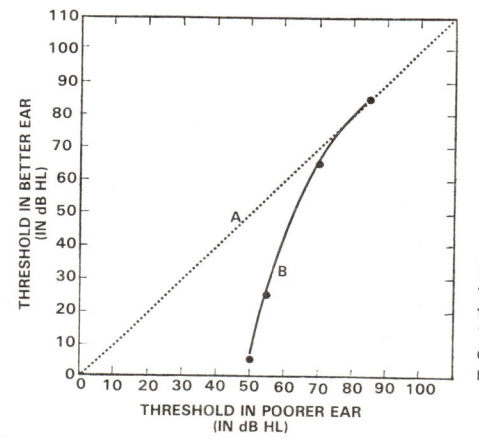

FIGURE A: The "growth" of loudness for two normal ears is represented by the dotted diagonal line, "A." Curve "B" indicates how an individual with one normal and one recruiting ear might respond. (After Carver, 1972).

so-called "laddergram" in Figure "B." What variables might affect the accuracy of the subject's ability to match loudness between the two ears?
(2) Repeat exercise #1 for tones of differing frequency. Is the listening task more difficult to perform at high or low frequencies?

(3) Occlude one of the listener's ears with an earplug and repeat exercises #1 and #2. Contrast the laddergram you obtain for this simulated conductive hearing loss with the normal pattern obtained for the preceding exercises.

NOTES:

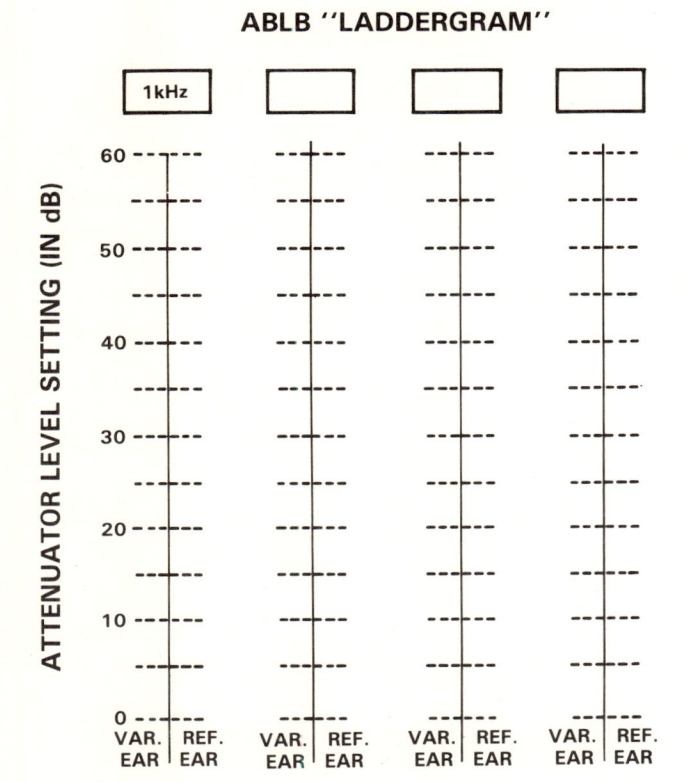

ABLB "LADDERGRAM"

FIGURE B: For each test tone frequency, plot the reference and variable ear Attenuator settings at which equal loudness is obtained. Use "O" and "X" respectively, to indicate the right and left ear levels. Connect data points of equal loudness with straight lines.

Selected References:

Carver, W.F. (1970). The reliability and precision of a modification of the ABLB test. *Ann. Otolar.*, **79**, 398-412.

Carver, W.F. (1972). Loudness balance procedures. In J. Katz (Ed.) *Handbook of clinical audiology*. Williams and Wilkins Co., Baltimore.

Dix, M.R. (1965). Observations upon the nerve fibre deafness of multiple sclerosis. With particular reference to the phenomenon of loudness recruitment. *J. Laryn.*, **79**, 695-706.

Fowler, E.P. (1950). The recruitment of loudness phenomenon. *Laryngoscope*, **60**, 680-695.

Graham, A.B. (Ed.) (1967). Alternate loudness balance techniques. *Sensorineural hearing processes and disorders.* pp. 245-257. Little, Brown and Company, Boston.

Harris, J.D. (1953). A brief critical review of loudness recruitment. *Psychol. Bull.*, **50**, 190-203.

Jerger, J.F., and Harford, E.R. (1960). The alternate and simultaneous balancing of pure tones. *J. Speech Hear. Res.*, **3**, 17-30.

Miskolczy-Fodor, F. (1964). Automatically recorded loudness balance testing. *Arch. Otolar.*, **79**, 355-365. Chicago.

Palva, T. (1957). Recruitment testing. *Archs. Otolar.*, **66**, 93-98.

Simmons, F.B., and Dixon, R.F. (1966). Clinical implications of loudness balancing. *Archs. Otolar.*, **83**, 449-454.

Stokinger, T.E., Cooper, W.A., Jr., and Lankford, J.E. (1970). Effect of interval durations on interaural loudness balancing. *J. Aud. Res.*, **10**, 35-44.

Tillman, T.W. (1969). Special hearing tests in otoneurologic diagnosis. *Archs. Otolar.*, **89**, 25-30.

EXPERIMENT III-7: "RECRUITMENT" IN NORMAL EARS

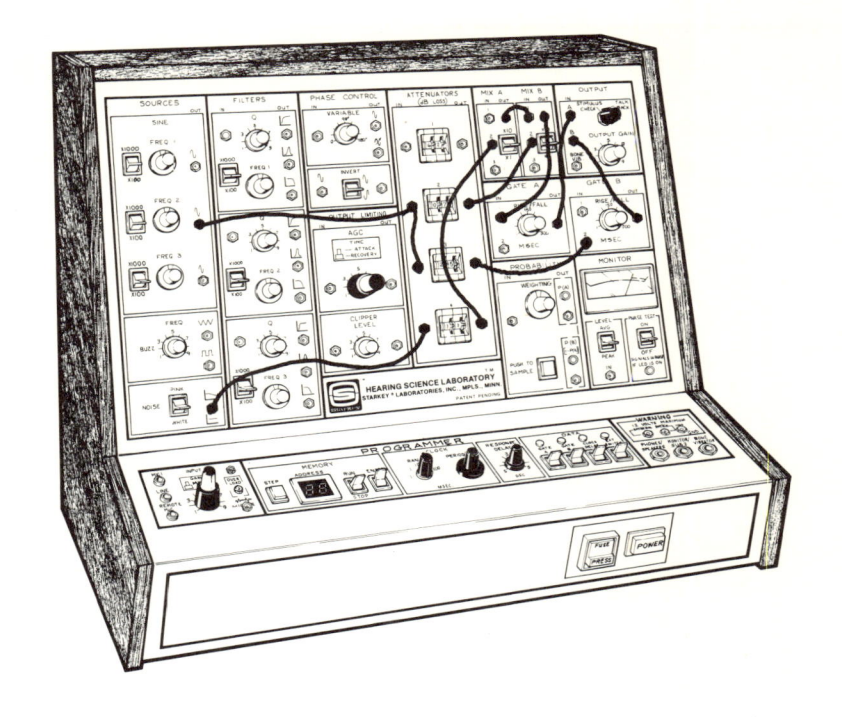

Purpose:
To examine the growth of loudness for a tone in a background of white noise.

Background Principle:
In Laboratory Experiment III-6, the topic of loudness recruitment was introduced. Under certain conditions, an abnormally rapid growth of loudness can be seen in normal hearing listeners. In one demonstration of *simulated recruitment*, a 1000 Hz pure tone of moderate intensity is presented to one of a subject's ears. A fixed level of wide band noise is then introduced to the same ear. The subject is required to vary the level of a 1000 Hz tone-in-quiet in the opposite ear until it is the same loudness as the tone-in-noise. This task is repeated for several of the tone-in-noise levels, and the results are plotted on axes labeled as in Figure "A". A display similar to Figure "A" in the preceding experiment should be obtained. It is believed that the masking stimulus raises the normal exponent of the psychophysical relationship between the physical intensity and the loudness of the signal (see Laboratory Experiment III-5 and Stevens, 1966, for more details).

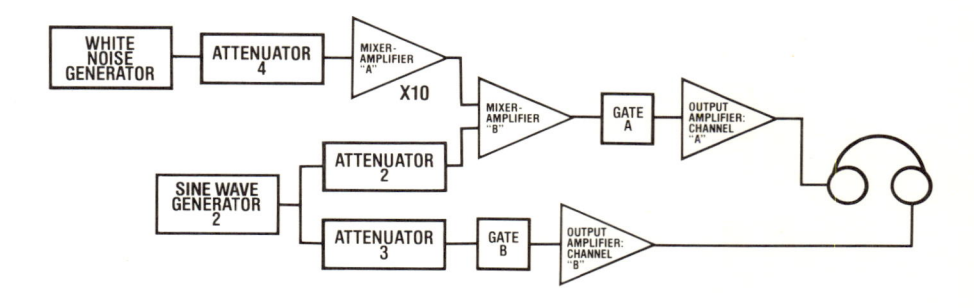

Procedure:
The pure tone signal from Sine Wave Generator #2 is passed through Attenuators #2 and #3. The stimulus from Attenuator #3 is sent through Electronic Gate "B" and one Output Amplifier channel and headphone. The tone emerging from Attenuator #2 is combined with a continuous high level white noise within Mixer-Amplifier "B" before being sent to Electronic Gate "A" and the second Output Amplifier and headphone. Be sure to set Mixer-Amplifier "A" to the *X* 10, 20 dB gain switch position in order to produce the high level of masking noise required for the listening task. The suggested programming instructions will result in the tone and tone-in-noise stimuli alternating on and off every half-second.

Exercises:
(1) Select an initial test tone frequency near 1000 Hz. Set the tone-in-noise level (i.e., Attenuators 2 and 4) to values that permit the signal to remain clearly audible slightly above its masked threshold. Vary Attenuator #3 (i.e., the tone-in-quiet level) until the subject reports that the signals in each headphone are equally loud. Repeat this procedure for a series of increasing tone-in-noise levels (e.g., decreasing Attenuator #2 in steps of 10 dB). Record your data values on Figure "A" and compare the results with the curves shown in the selected references cited below.

(2) Repeat exercise #1 for tones of 250 Hz and 4000 Hz and a variety of noise levels. Describe the differences in the test results you obtain for these listening conditions.

NOTES:

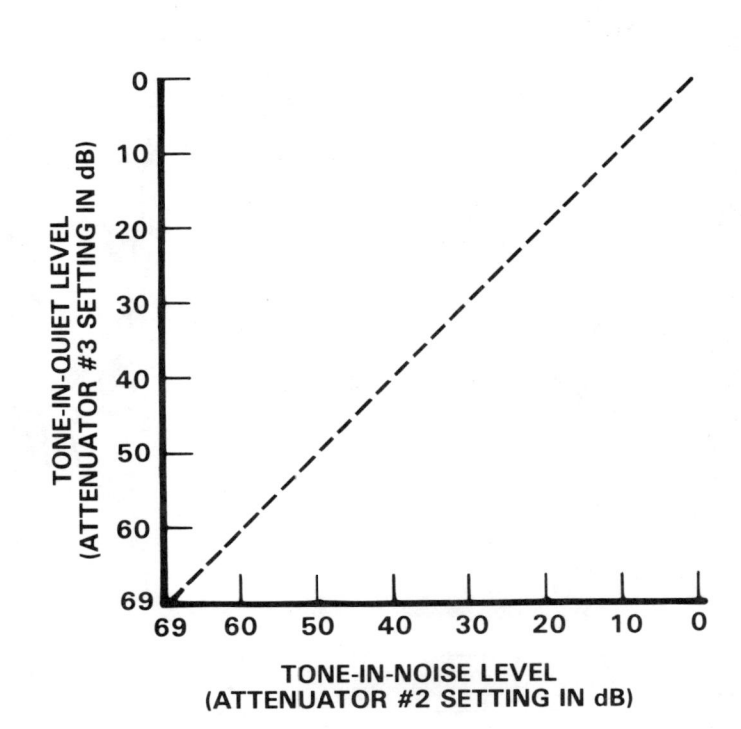

FIGURE A: Plot the data points for exercise #1 on these axes. The dashed diagonal line represents an equal loudness response for equal attenuation levels at the two ears.

Selected References:

Hellman, R.P. (1970). Effect of noise bandwidth on the loudness of a 1000-Hz tone. *J. Acoust. Soc. Am.*, **48**, 500-504.

Hellman, R.P., and Zwislocki, J. (1963). Monaural loudness function at 1000 cps and interaural summation. *J. Acoust. Soc. Am.*, **35**, 856-865.

Hellman, R.P., and Zwislocki, J. (1964). Loudness function of a 1000-cps tone in the presence of a masking noise. *J. Acoust. Soc. Am.*, **9**, 1618-1627.

Hellman, R.P. and Zwislocki, J. (1968). Loudness determination at low sound frequencies. *J. Acoust. Soc. Am.*, **43**, 60-64.

Lochner, J.P.A., and Burger, J.F. (1961). Form of the loudness functions in the presence of masking noise. *J. Acoust. Soc. Am.*, **33**, 1705-1707.

Richards, A.M. (1968). Monaural loudness functions under masking. *J. Acoust. Soc. Am.*, **44**, 599-605.

Stevens, S.S. (1966). Power-group transformations under glare, masking and recruitment. *J. Acoust. Soc. Am.*, **39**, 725-735.

Stevens, S.S. and Guirao, M. (1967). Loudness functions under inhibition. *Percept. Psychophys.*, **2**, 459-465.

EXPERIMENT III-8: THE RELATIONSHIP BETWEEN INTENSITY AND PITCH

Purpose:
To demonstrate the effects of signal intensity upon the pitch of a tone.

Background Principle:
The manner in which the ear responds to sound is most unlike that of a laboratory measurement device. We have already observed that the perception of loudness varies in a complex fashion with the level of a signal; a machine would have faithfully displayed any change in a stimulus in a simple manner. We shall now investigate the phenomenon of one acoustic characteristic of a signal influencing the perception of another. Musicians have long been aware of the fact that the intensity of a sound may slightly alter the pitch that is perceived. The direction and extent of this pitch change seems to vary with the frequency, complexity, and intensity of the stimulus employed. The results of one early study which used pure tone signals (Stevens, 1935) indicated that as intensity was increased, low frequency tones dropped in pitch; mid frequencies remained about the same; and high frequencies increased in their perceived pitch (see Figure "A"). A more recent study (Cohen, 1961) showed that the basic effect may not be as pronounced as originally thought.

Procedure:
A single pure tone is passed through two Attenuators, each of whose outputs is sent to a different Electronic Gate. The suggested programming instructions will permit both signals to be switched on and off sequentially. The Programmer Delay Channel provides a 0.5 second pause after each stimulus presentation to facilitate the comparison task. The two stimuli are combined within a Mixer-Amplifier and then routed to one Output Amplifier channel and headphone.

Exercises:
(1) Begin the demonstration with a low frequency tone near 200 Hz, where the effect is most likely to be noticed. Adjust the two Attenuator settings to initial values that are only 10 dB apart (e.g., 50 dB and 40 dB). The Output Amplifier Gain Control should be set to a position that permits both signals to be clearly audible. If more signal level is needed, set the Mixer-Amplifier Gain Switch to the X 10 (i.e., 20 dB) position. Before each test trial, increase the difference between the two level settings by 10 additional decibels (e.g., 50-30 dB, 50-20 dB, etc.). How many decibels of level separation are needed before any pitch change is detected?

(2) Repeat exercise #1 with a variety of test frequencies. Are your perceptions in agreement with the early results reported by Stevens (1935)?

(3) Use different stimuli, such as a squarewave or filtered noise, as your test signals. Does the pitch of such complex sounds alter with intensity? Is the effect more or less noticeable with complex rather than pure tone sounds?

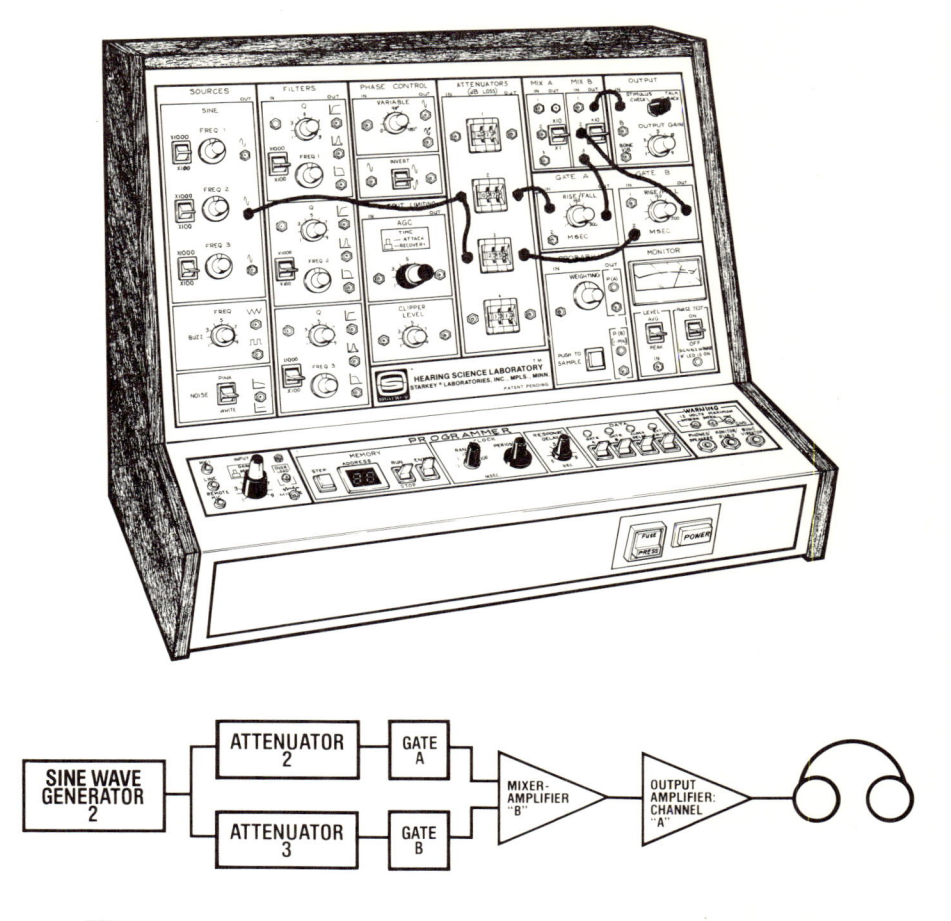

CLOCK SETTINGS			MEMORY ADDRESS			
RANGE SWITCH	PERIOD/ STEP CONTROL	RESPONSE DELAY	MEMORY CHANNEL	00 TO 48	49	50 TO 98	99
10	X 1	0.5	GATE "A"	ON			
			GATE "B"			ON	
			CLOCK DELAY		ON		ON
MILLISECONDS		SECONDS	EXT. SWITCH				

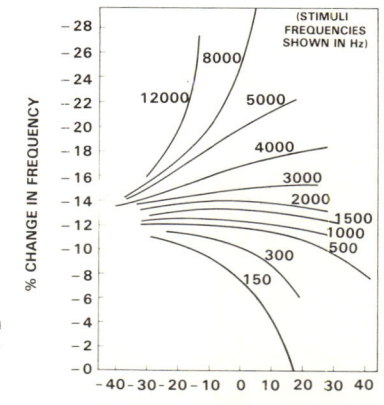

FIGURE A: The change of pitch as a function of the intensity of the signal. (After Stevens, 1935).

NOTES:

Selected References:

Cohen, A. (1961). Further investigation of the effects of intensity upon the pitch of pure tones. *J. Acoust. Soc. Am.*, **33**, 1363-1376.

Jauhiainen, T., Häkkinen, V., Lindroos, R., and Raij, K. (1967). On pitch and loudness interaction. *J. Aud. Res.*, **7**, 41-46.

Lewis, D., and Cowan, M. (1936). The influence of intensity on the pitch of violin and cello tones. *J. Acoust. Soc. Am.*, **8**, 20-22.

Morgan, C.T., Garner, W.R., and Galambos, R. (1951). Pitch and intensity. *J. Acoust. Soc. Am.*, **23**, 658-663.

Snow, W.B. (1936). Change of pitch with loudness at low frequencies. *J. Acoust. Soc. Am.*, **8**, 14-19.

Stevens, S.S. (1935). The relation of pitch to intensity. *J. Acoust. Soc. Am.*, **6**, 150-154.

Stevens, S.S. (1975). *Psychophysics*. Chapters 3 and 4. Wiley, New York.

Thurlow, W.R. (1943). Binaural interaction and the perception of pitch. *J. Exp. Psychol.*, **32**, 13-36.

Frequency and Pitch

IV

EXPERIMENT IV-1: OHM'S ACOUSTIC LAW

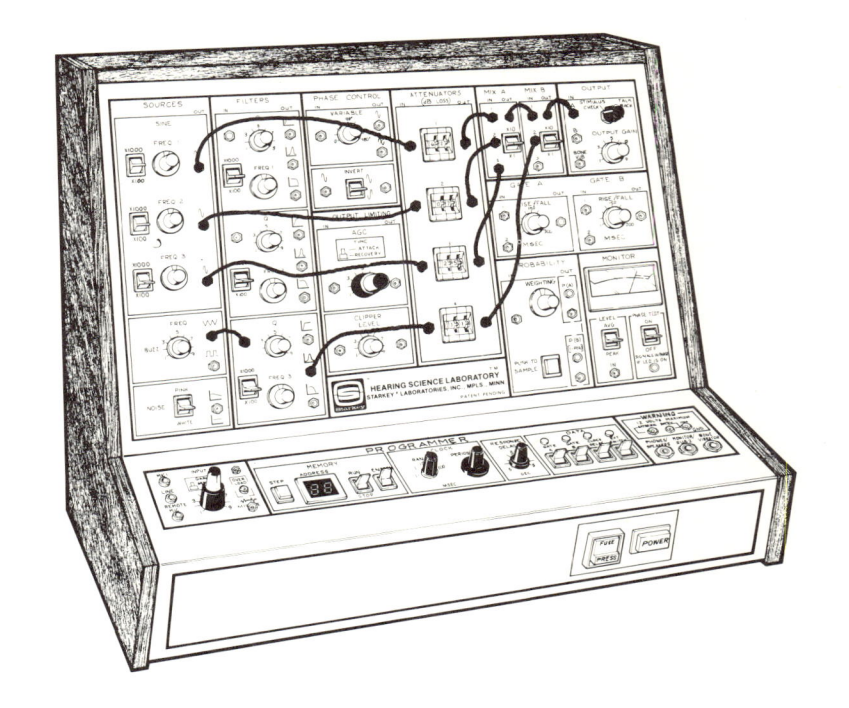

Purpose:
To explore the ear's ability to detect the pure tone components in a complex sound.

Background Principle:
In 1843, Georg S. Ohm (1789-1854) postulated that the ear was capable of analyzing a complex sound into a series of sinusoidal components after the fashion of Fourier's Theorem (see experiment I-2). Ohm's so-called "Acoustic Law" stimulated extensive research and controversy on a number of experimental and theoretical issues that remain unresolved to this day. Does a listener have the ability to perceive the individual components that make up a complex sound? A good musician will surely identify the several notes in a musical chord. Each of these sounds, however, is itself complex in nature and, therefore, comprised of a combination of tones. In the present experiment, a complex sound will be synthesized from four tones, and a subject will be asked to hum or sing each pitch he discerns. The fact that some musically inclined listeners might easily accomplish this task should not, however, be taken as conclusive proof of Ohm's notion. We shall find in upcoming experiments that two tones may create only a single pitch percept that fluctuates in magnitude or varies in subjective quality. Some two-tone combinations may actually produce more than one pitch, while still other tonal groupings create the illusion of non-existent sound percepts. In addition to these phenomena, we shall explore how one sound may "mask" or render another sound inaudible.

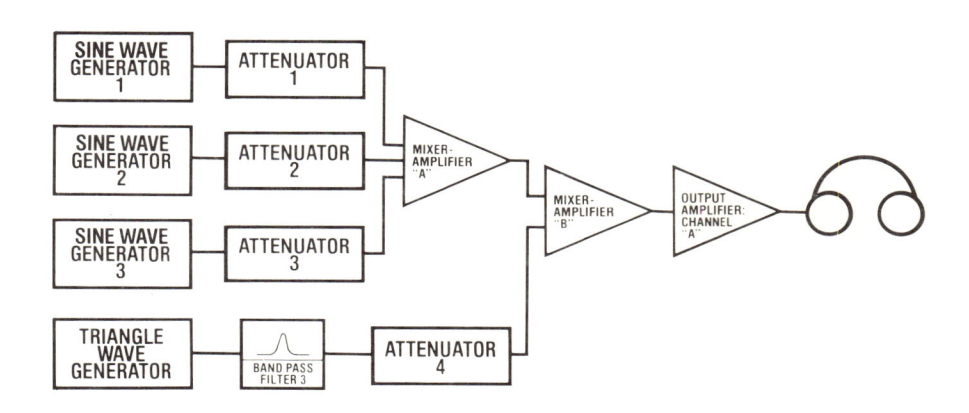

Procedure:
In addition to the signals from Sine Wave Generators 1, 2, and 3, a fourth pure tone may be produced by passing a triangle waveform through a narrow band filter. The maximum pure tone signal output will emerge from the filter when its center frequency is adjusted to be the same as that for the triangle waveform (i.e., at the triangle waveform fundamental frequency). This maximum amplitude may be monitored with the Level Meter, an oscilloscope, or by listening for the loudest sound output. Rotate the Filter "Q" control to the fully clockwise position for maximum Filter selectivity. Each of the four sinusoidal waveforms are sent to separate Attenuators whose outputs are mixed together within Mixer-Amplifiers "A" and "B". This combined signal is then sent to one Output Amplifier channel and headphone.

Exercises:
(1) Select four different signal frequencies (e.g., 200, 300, 400, and 800 Hz) and adjust their Attenuator settings so that each tone is clearly audible by itself. Listen to the combined signal in the headphone and try to sing or hum the lowest tone in the series (i.e., 200 Hz). By alternately unplugging and replacing the 200 Hz signal wire, the tone should become easier to identify so that the accuracy of the listener's response may be verified. In the same manner, try to individually reproduce each of the other tones in the series. Is one tone more easily identified than another? Can you account for why this may or may not be the case?

(2) Repeat exercise #1 with all four tones set near the subject's threshold or well above threshold for each frequency. Are the tones easier to recognize when soft or quite loud?

(3) Repeat exercise #1 with the signal frequencies more widely spaced apart (e.g., 200 Hz, 1000 Hz, 3000 Hz, and 7000 Hz). Is identification made easier in this case?

NOTES:

Selected References:

von Helmholtz, H. (1863). *On the sensation of tone as a physiological basis for the theory of music.* (First American ed. of the second English ed. of the fourth German ed.) Dover, New York, 1954.

Licklider, J.C.R., (1956). Auditory frequency analysis. In C. Cherry (Ed.) *Information theory, fourth symposium.* Butterworth & Co., Ltd., London.

Plomp, R. (1964). The ear as a frequency analyzer. *J. Acoust. Soc. Am.,* **36,** 1628-1636.

Pollack, I. (1964). Ohm's acoustical law and short-term auditory memory. *J. Acoust. Soc. Am.,* **36,** 2340-2345.

Schouten, J.F. (1940). The residue, a new concept in subjective sound analysis. Proc. Kon. Ned. Akad. v. Wetensch. Amsterdam, **43,** 356-365. (In J.D. Harris. *Forty germinal papers in human hearing,* J. Audit. Res., Groton, Connecticut, 1969).

Schouten, J.F., Ritsma, R.J., and Cardozo, B.L. (1962). Pitch of the residue. *J. Acoust. Soc. Am.,* **34,** 1418-1424.

Small, A.M. (1955). Some parameters influencing the pitch of amplitude modulated signals. *J. Acoust. Soc. Am.,* **27,** 751-760.

Wever, E.G. (1949). *Theory of hearing.* Wiley, New York.

Wightman, F.L. and Green, D.M. (1974). The perception of pitch. *American Scientist,* **62,** 208-215.

EXPERIMENT IV-2: OBJECTIVE BEATS

Purpose:
To listen for the resultant produced by two pure tones that have dissimilar frequencies.

Background Principle:
When two tones of different frequency are added together, they alternately reinforce and cancel one another and yield a resultant that fluctuates in magnitude with the passage of time. The fluttering sound sometimes heard from a combination of tones is known as a *beat*. The number of amplitude fluctuations per second is called the *beat frequency* and is equal to the difference in hertz between the two components making up the complex. Tone pairs of either 504 and 500 Hz or 496 and 500 Hz would, therefore, yield four beats per second (see Figure "A"). If the magnitudes of both tones are identical, complete cancellation (i.e., silence) or complete reinforcement (i.e., double the resultant amplitude) would occur at those instants when the phase relationship between the tones is 180° and 0°, respectively. This condition is known as *best beats*.

Procedure:
The outputs from the two Sine Wave Generators are delivered to separate Attenuators so that the magnitude of each pure tone component may be independently adjusted. Both Attenuator outputs are combined within a Mixer-Amplifier and routed to one Output Amplifier channel and headphone. The listener may easily compare the single versus the double tone conditions by alternately unplugging and replacing either of the signal generator wires.

Exercises:
(1) Select an initial pair of tones near 500 Hz and, as you listen to the beating, slowly vary the frequency of one of the signal generators. Note the effect upon the number of beats per second that are produced. What seems to be the maximum number of beats per second that can be distinguished before the individual fluctuations become blurred and indistinct?

(2) Create beats with pairs of very low and high as well as mid frequency tones (e.g., pairs of tones near 200 Hz, 1000 Hz, and 6000 Hz). Is it easier to detect the phenomenon of beats at particular frequencies?

(3) Adjust both signal Attenuators until they are set to the identical levels. Are you able to obtain best beats? How could you confirm best beats with the Level Meter or an oscilloscope?

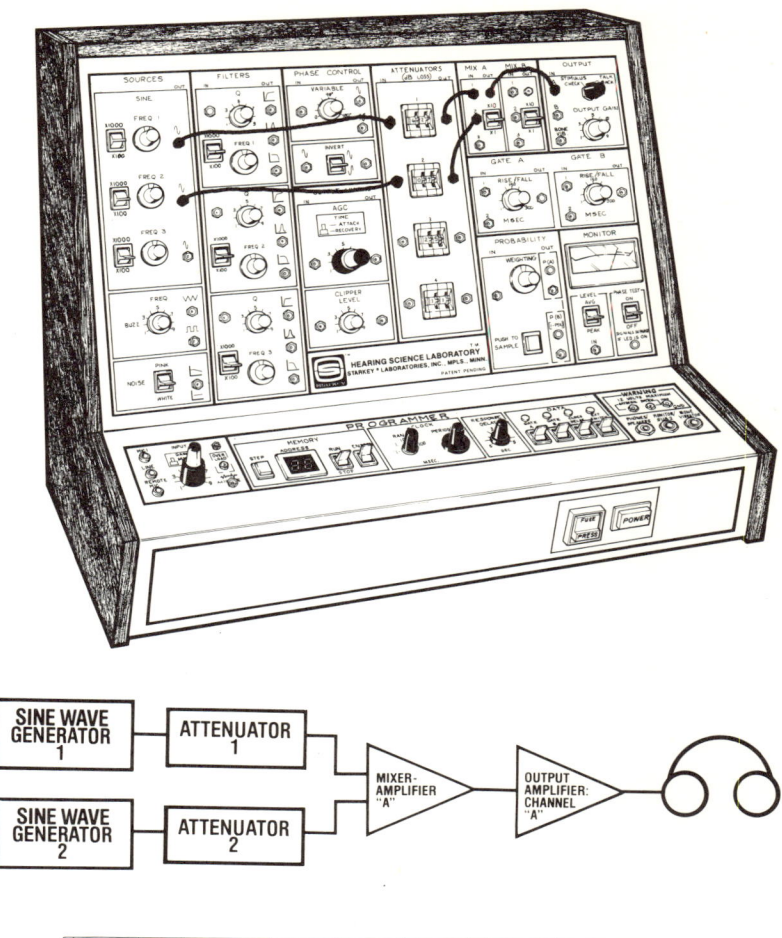

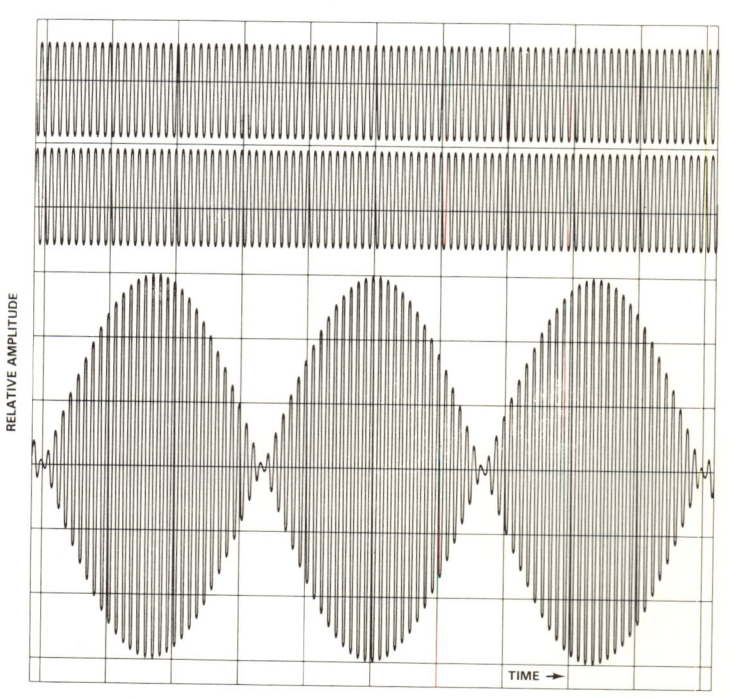

FIGURE A: The instantaneous phase relationship between two different frequency sine waves will vary from one moment to the next. The resultant wave will fluctuate in amplitude, or "beat," as the two component signals alternately cancel and reinforce one another. (After Oster, 1973).

NOTES:

Selected References:

Egan, J.P. and Klumpp, R.G. (1951). The error due to masking in the measurement of aural harmonics by the method of best beats. *J. Acoust. Soc. Am.*, **23**, 275-286.

von Helmholtz, H. (1863). *On the sensation of tone as a physiological basis for the theory of music.* (First American ed. of the second English ed. of the fourth German ed.) Dover, New York, 1954.

Oster, G. (1973). Auditory beats in the brain. *Scientific Am.*, **229 (10)**, 76-84.

Plomp, R. (1967). Beats of mistuned consonances. *J. Acoust. Soc. Am.*, **42**, 462-474.

Tonndorf, J. (1959). Beats in cochlear models. *J. Acoustic Soc. Am.*, **31**, 608-619.

EXPERIMENT IV-3: CONSONANCE, DISSONANCE, AND MUSICAL INVERVALS

Purpose:
To explore the subjective quality of selected tone pairs.

Background Principle:
As beat frequencies greater than about seven hertz are produced, the percept of a fluttering tone gives way to a series of sounds that listeners report display either a disturbing roughness (i.e., *dissonance*) or decidedly pleasant, or *consonant*, character. Figure "A" portrays the relative consonance of two tones as their frequency ratio is altered. Note that certain frequency ratios (e.g., 5/4, 4/3, 3/2, and 2/1) yield particularly consonant sound percepts, at least to Western ears. Exactly why these frequency combinations, known as musical *intervals*, affect us the way they do is not fully understood. There is evidence to suggest some form of synchronous impulse pattern is established in our nervous systems in response to these intervals, but precisely where in the system this takes place remains a point of speculation.

Procedure:
The outputs from the two Sine Wave Generators are delivered to separate Attenuators so that the magnitude of each pure tone component may be independently adjusted. Both Attenuator outputs are combined within a Mixer-Amplifier and routed to one Output Amplifier channel and headphone.

Exercises:
(1) Select an initial pair of tones which are near 500 Hz. Slowly adjust one Sine Wave Generator until the frequency separation of the signals reaches a point of maximum unpleasantness or dissonance. For most listeners, this occurs at frequency separations of roughly thirty hertz.

(2) Adjust the frequency controls of the two Sine Wave Generators in accordance with the following chart of tone pair combinations. Rank order the relative consonance or dissonance for each of the intervals created.

F2 in Hz	F1 in Hz	F2/F1	Name of Musical Interval
100	100	1/1	Unison
200	100	2/1	Octave
300	200	3/2	Fifth
400	300	4/3	Fourth
500	400	5/4	Major Third
600	500	6/5	Minor Third
500	300	5/3	Major Sixth
800	500	8/5	Minor Sixth
900	800	9/8	Major Second

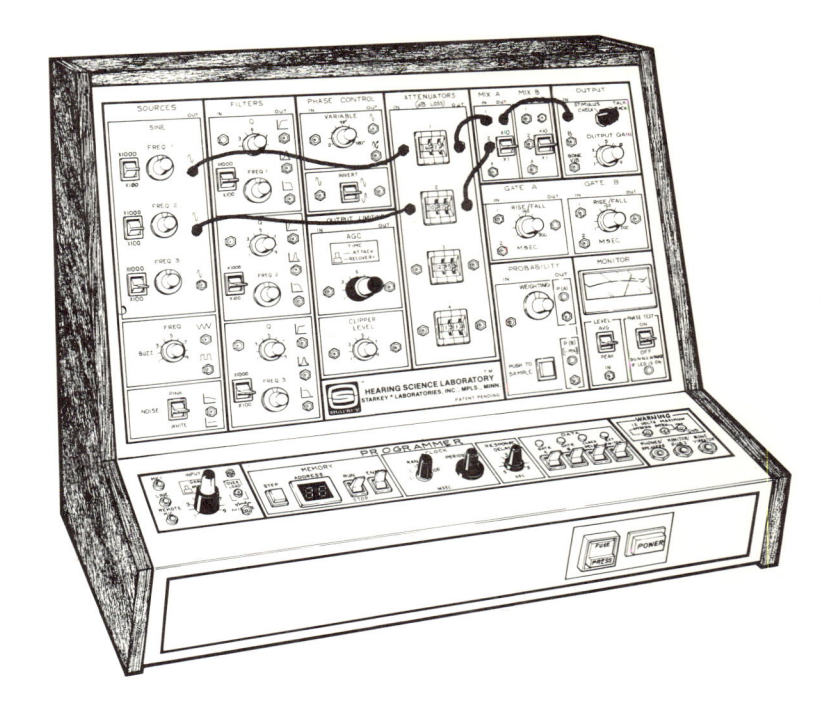

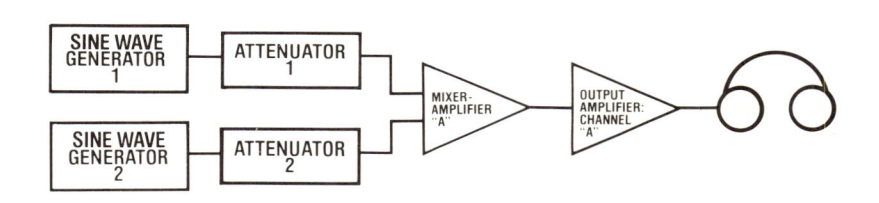

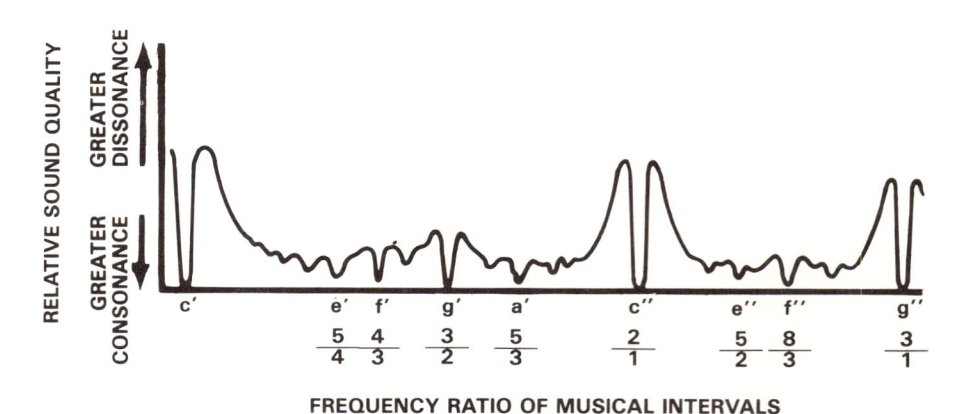

FIGURE A: The relative consonance and dissonance of musical intervals. The lowest tone (c') remains on while the second note is gradually increased in frequency. (After Helmholtz, 1863).

NOTES:

Selected References:

Backus, J. (1969). *The acoustical foundations of music.* W.W. Norton and Company, Inc., New York.

Cazden, N. (1959). Musical intervals and simple number ratios. *J. Res. Music Educ.,* **7,** 197-220.

Cazden, N. (1962). Sensory theories of musical consonance. *J. Aesth. Art Criticism,* **20,** 301-319.

Corso, J.F. (1957). Absolute judgments of musical tonality. *J. Acoust. Soc. Am.,* **29,** 138-144.

Culver, C.A. (1956). *Musical acoustics.* McGraw-Hill Book Company, New York.

van de Geer, J.P., Levelt, W.J.M., and Plomp, R. (1962). The connotation of musical consonance. *Acta Psychol.,* **20,** 308-319.

von Helmholtz, H. (1863). *On the sensation of tone as a physiological basis for the theory of music.* (First American ed. of the second English ed. of the fourth German ed.) Dover, New York, 1954.

Houtsma, A.J.M. and Goldstein, J. (1972). The central origin of the pitch of complex tones: evidence from musical interval recognition. *J. Acoust. Soc. Am.,* **51,** 520-529.

Plomp, R. and Levelt, W.J.M. (1965). Tonal consonance and critical bandwidth. *J. Acoust. Soc. Am.,* **38,** 548-560.

Plomp, R., Wagenaar, W.A., and Mimpen, A.M. (1973). Musical interval recognition with simultaneous tones. *Acustica,* **29,** 101-109.

Rigden, J.S. (1974). Variations of sound intensity for mistuned consonances. *J. Acoust. Soc. Am.,* **55,** 1095-1097.

Sundberg, J.E.F. and Lindqvist, J. (1973). Musical octaves and pitch. *J. Acoust. Soc. Am.,* **54,** 922-929.

Terhardt, E. (1974). Pitch, consonance, and harmony. *J. Acoust. Soc. Am.,* **55,** 1061-1069.

Ward, W.D. (1970). Musical perception. In J.V. Tobias (Ed.) *Foundations of modern auditory theory.* Vol. I. Academic Press, New York.

Winckel, F. (1967). *Music, sound and sensation: a modern exposition.* Dover, New York.

Wood, A. (1950). *The physics of music.* (5th ed.). Methuen & Co., London.

EXPERIMENT IV-4: COMBINATION TONES

Purpose:
To examine one type of frequency distortion in the hearing mechanism.

Background Principle:
If the magnitudes of either or both of the pure tones used in the previous experiment are increased beyond roughly 60 dB SPL, most listeners will perceive the presence of a sound (or sounds) which was not actually delivered to their ears. The pitch of this so-called *combination tone* is usually associated with a frequency that is equal to the numerical sum, or difference, in Hz of the two original pure tone components (e.g., tones of $F_1 = 700$ Hz and $F_2 = 1200$ Hz, if sufficiently intense, will produce summation and difference tones of $F_1 + F_2 = 1900$ Hz and $F_2 - F_1 = 500$ Hz, respectively). At still greater tone levels (e.g., 80 dB above threshold), a myriad of combination tones, including $3F_1$, $3F_2$, $2F_1 + 2F_2$, $2F_1 - 2F_2$, et al. may be perceived. A vibrating system, such as our hearing mechanism which produces such spurious responses, is said to contain *distortion*. One way the frequency associated with summation, or difference, tones may be determined is to introduce a low intensity *exploring tone*, or *probe tone*, into the subject's ear and adjust its frequency until it produces simple beats with the combination tone. The exploring tone frequency at which the beats slow to 3 beats/sec. is often used to reveal the frequency of the sum, or difference, tone. A probe tone may also be used to cancel out a combination tone when presented at 180° out of phase at the same frequency and amplitude.

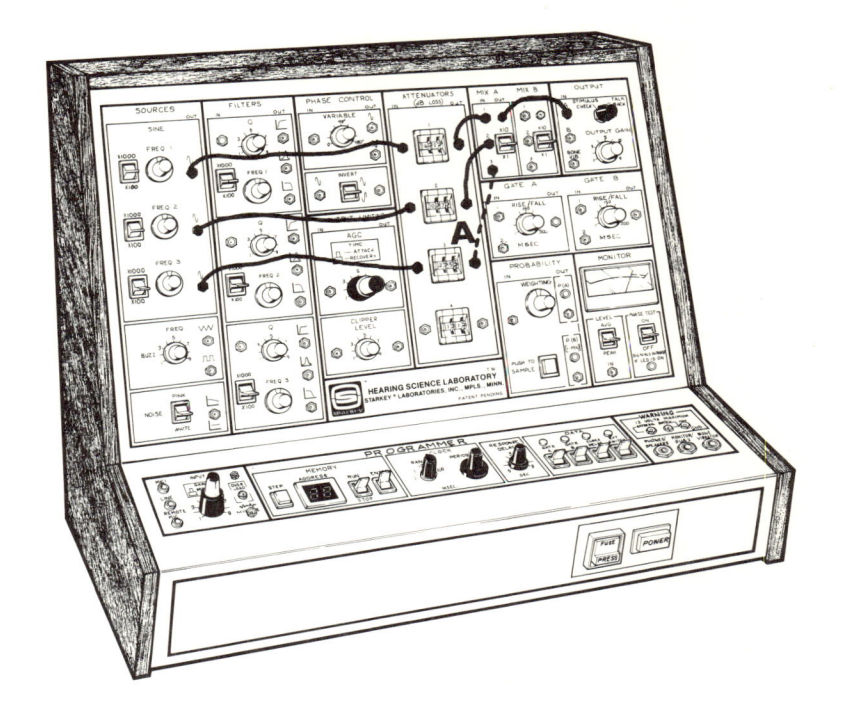

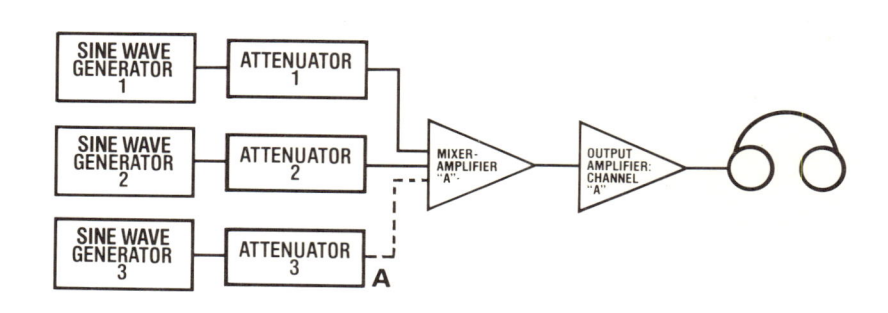

Procedure:
The stimuli from three Sine Wave Generators are routed to separate Attenuators and combined within Mixer-Amplifier "A". This combined signal is then sent to one Output Amplifier channel and headphone. By alternately unplugging and replacing the dashed circuit wire "A", the exploring tone can be contrasted with the combinational tone.

Exercises:
(1) Adjust Sine Wave Generators 1 and 2 to have frequencies near 700 Hz and 1200 Hz, respectively. The levels for these tones should be set to a value that is roughly 50 dB more intense than their threshold levels for the listener. The third, exploring tone signal should be set near 1900 Hz or 500 Hz. When a summation, or difference, tone is noticed, add the exploring tone to the complex sound and try to beat this signal with the combinational tone. If no beats can be perceived, it may be necessary to increase the stimuli levels by an additional 20 to 30 dB. CAUTION: Do not listen to any sound that is **uncomfortably** loud as this may fatigue the ear!

(2) Repeat exercise #1 for a variety of two-tone component frequencies and rank order the relative loudness of the combination tones you discover. (e.g., $F_1 = 1000$ Hz and $F_2 = 1300$ Hz should provide good test results.)

NOTES:

Selected References:

Crane, H.D. and Bell, D.W. (1976). Phase effect of an input f_2-f_1 tone on the level of the $2f_1$-f_2 combination tone. *J. Acoust. Soc. Am.*, **59**, 123-128.

Goldstein, J.L. (1967). Auditory non-linearity. *J. Acoust. Soc. Am.*, **41**, 676-689.

Goldstein, J.L. (1970). Aural combination tones. In R. Plomp and G. Smoorenburg (Eds.) *Frequency analysis and periodicity detection in hearing.* A.W. Sijthoff, Leiden.

Greenwood, D.D. (1971). Aural combination tones and auditory masking. *J. Acoust. Soc. Am.*, **50**, 502-543.

Greenwood, D.D. (1972a). Masking by narrow bands of noise in proximity to more intense pure tones of higher frequency: application to measurement of combination band levels and some comparisons with masking by combination noise. *J. Acoust. Soc. Am.*, **52**, 1137-1143.

Greenwood, D.D. (1972b). Masking by combination bands: estimation of the levels of the combination bands $(n + 1) f_1$-nf_h. *J. Acoust. Soc. Am.*, **52**, 1144-1154.

Greenwood, D.D. (1972c). Combination bands of even order: masking effects and estimation of level of the difference bands $(f_h$-$f_1)$ and $2 (f_h$-$f_1)$. *J. Acoust. Soc. Am.*, **52**, 1155-1167.

Hall, J.L. (1972a). Auditory distortion products f_2-f_1 and $2f_1$-f_2. *J. Acoust. Soc. Am.*, **51**, 1863-1871.

Hall, J.L. (1972b). Monaural phase effect: cancellation and reinforcement of distortion products f_2-f_1 and $2f_1$-f_2. *J. Acoust. Soc. Am.*, **51**, 1872-1881.

Houtsma, A.J.M. and Goldstein, J.L. (1972). The central origin of the pitch of complex tones: evidence from musical interval recognition. *J. Acoust. Soc. Am.*, **51**, 520-529.

Plomp, R. (1965). Detectability threshold for combination tones. *J. Acoust. Soc. Am.*, **37**, 1110-1123.

Plomp, R. (1967). Pitch of complex tones. *J. Acoust. Soc. Am.*, **41**, 1526-1533.

Plomp, R. (1970). Timbre as a multidimensional attribute of complex tones. In R. Plomp and F.G. Smoorenburg (Eds.) *Frequency analysis and periodicity detection in hearing.* A.W. Suithoff, Leiden.

Ritsma. R.J. (1967). Frequencies dominant in the perception of pitch of complex sounds, *J. Acoust. Soc. Am.*, **42**, 191-198.

Schodder, G.R. and David, E.E., Jr. (1960). Pitch discrimination of two-tone frequency complexes. *J. Acoust. Soc. Am.*, **32**, 1426-1435.

Smoorenburg, G.F. (1970). Pitch perception of two-frequency stimuli. *J. Acoust. Soc. Am.*, **48**, 924-942.

Smoorenburg, G.F. (1972a). Audibility region of combination tones. *J. Acoust. Soc. Am.*, **52**, 603-614.

Smoorenberg, G.F. (1972b). Combination tones and their origin. *J. Acoust. Soc. Am.*, **52**, 615-632.

Sutton, R.A. and Williams, R.P. (1970). Residue pitches from two-tone complexes. *J. Sound Vib.*, **13**, 195-199.

Zurek, P.M. and Leshowitz, B.H. (1976). Measurement of the combination tones f_2-f_1 and $2f_1$-f_2. *J. Acoust. Soc. Am.*, **60**, 155-168.

EXPERIMENT IV-5: PITCH OF COMPLEX TONES ("THE CASE OF THE MISSING FUNDAMENTAL")

Purpose:
To examine the pitch of a complex waveform.

Background Principle:
Most listeners will report hearing a pitch corresponding to 100 Hz when they are presented with a complex tone having components of 1000, 900, 800, and 700 hertz. Since 100 Hz corresponds to the fundamental frequency, or greatest common divisor, in this series of tones, and because no energy was actually delivered at 100 Hz, this mysterious phenomenon has been called the "Case of the Missing Fundamental." Could this low frequency percept be some form of difference tone and, therefore, due to distortion within the ear? Such an explanation is unlikely, for, among other reasons, the missing fundamental emerges even when the levels of the component signals lie well below the magnitudes required for the creation of difference tones. While the ear's pitch extraction mechanism remains open to question, recent studies suggest that the brain may actually perform a type of Fourier analysis on the incoming waveform and "project" the existence of the missing fundamental.

Procedure:
In addition to the signals from Sine Wave Generators 1, 2, and 3, a fourth pure tone may be produced by passing a triangle waveform through a narrow band filter. The frequency of this fourth tone will be equal to the center frequency of the bandpass filter when a maximum output is obtained from the filter. Be sure to rotate the Filter "Q" control to the fully clockwise position for maximum filter selectivity. Each of the four sinusoidal waveforms are sent to separate Attenuators (set to identical levels) whose outputs are mixed together within Mixer-Amplifiers "A" and "B". This combined signal is then sent to one Output Amplifier channel and headphone.

Exercises:
(1) Search for the missing fundamental in each of the following tone combinations. You will surely hear the pure tone components, but listen for a low frequency overall pitch. It is being created in your own auditory system!

	FREQUENCY IN HERTZ			
	F_1	F_2	F_3	F_4
I.	1000	900	800	700
II.	1000	800	600	400
III.	1400	1200	1000	800
IV.	4000	3000	2000	1000

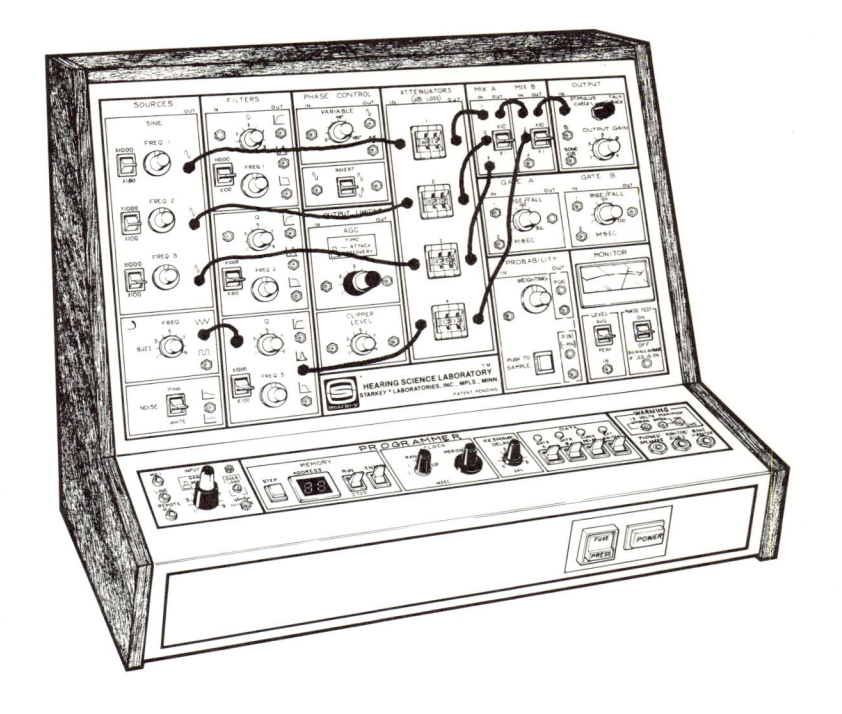

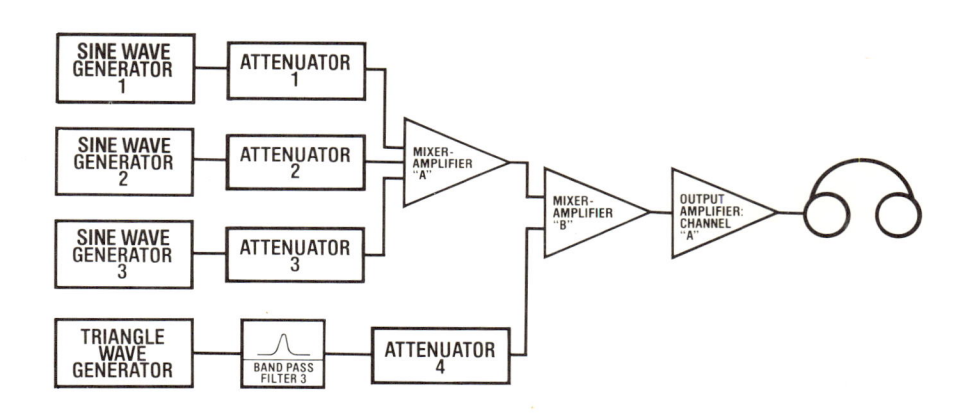

Is the effect more or less noticeable when large frequency differences exist between tones? Is the effect most obvious within a certain frequency "region"?

(2) Disconnect any one of the four signal sources and note if the missing fundamental remains or disappears. Remove any two signals and note the effect. Is the phenomenon more readily observed when more tonal ingredients are present?

(3) Instead of unplugging a signal, simply shift its frequency slightly up or down. Is the low-pitch percept influenced in any way?

(4) Reduce all four signal levels by 15 dB for those tone mixtures that produce a distinct missing fundamental and note if the effect disappears or persists.

NOTES:

Selected References:

von Békésy, G. (1972). The missing fundamental and periodicity detection in hearing. *J. Acoust. Soc. Am.*, **51**, 631-637.

Bilsen, F.A. (1973). On the influence of the number and phase of harmonics on the perceptibility of the pitch of complex signals. *Acustica*, **28**, 60-65.

Buunen, T.J.F., Festen, J.M., Bilsen, F.A., and van den Brink, G. (1974). Phase effects in a three-component signal. *J. Acoust. Soc. Am.*, **55**, 297-303.

Heffner, H. and Whitfield, I.C. (1976). Perception of the missing fundamental by cats. *J. Acoust. Soc. Am.*, **59**, 915-919.

Moore, B.C.J. (1973). Some experiments relating to the perception of complex tones. *Q. J. Exp. Psychol.*, **25**, 451-475.

Patterson, R. (1973). Physical variables determining residue pitch. *J. Acoust. Soc. Am.*, **53**, 1565-1572.

Patterson, R.D. and Wightman, F.L. (1976). Residue pitch as a function of component spacing. *J. Acoust. Soc. Am.*, **59**, 1450-1459.

Plomp, R. (1967). Pitch of complex tones. *J. Acoust. Soc. Am.*, **41**, 1526-1533.

Ritsma, R. (1963). Existence region of the tonal residue. II. *J. Acoust. Soc. Am.*, **35**, 1241-1245.

Ritsma, R. (1967). Frequencies dominant in the perception of the pitch of complex sounds. *J. Acoust. Soc. Am.*, **42**, 191-198.

Schouten, J.F. (1940). The residue, a new concept in subjective sound analysis Proc. Kon. Ned. Akad. v. Wetensch. Amsterdam, **43**, 356-365. (In J.D. Harris, *Forty germinal papers in human hearing*. J. Aud. Res., Groton, Connecticut, 1969).

Schouten, J.F., Ritsma, R.J., and Cardozo, B.L. (1962). Pitch of the residue. *J. Acoust. Soc. Am.*, **34**, 1418-1424.

Small, A. (1970). Periodicity pitch. In J.V. Tobias (Ed.) *Foundations of modern auditory theory*. Vol. 1. Academic Press Inc., New York.

Wightman, F.L. (1973). The pattern transformation model of pitch. *J. Acoust. Soc. Am.*, **54**, 407-416.

Wightman, F.L. and Green, D.M. (1974). The perception of pitch. *American Scientist*, **62**, 208-215.

EXPERIMENT IV-6: THE RELATIONSHIP BETWEEN FREQUENCY AND PITCH

Purpose:
To examine a listener's pitch perception for different tone frequencies.

Background Principle:
We have already observed that a listener can assign numerical values to the perceived loudness of different sounds. This ability to scale sensations also exists for the perception of pitch. Most subjects who are presented with two alternating tones of equal loudness level can usually report when one signal is twice (or half) as high in pitch as the other. By convention, a 1000 Hz tone has been assigned a value of 1000 subjective pitch units called *mels*. Tones half (or twice) as high as this reference value would possess subjective pitch levels of 500 and 2000 mels, respectively. As in the case of the loudness (i.e., sone) scale, however, the relationship between perceived pitch and physical frequency is complex rather than simply proportional. Experiments have shown, for example, that a pure tone of 4000 Hz may be judged to have only twice the pitch of a 1000 Hz signal, while 400 Hz is perceived to be half as high in pitch as 1000 Hz (see Figure "A"). This relationship becomes even more complicated with multi-tone complex signals.

Procedure:
The outputs from two Sine Wave Generators are sent to separate Attenuators and Electronic Gates. Both signals are combined within a Mixer-Amplifier whose output is delivered to one Output Amplifier channel and headphone. The Programmer instructions will switch the two Gates and their signals on and off, alternately.

Exercises:
(1) Set both Attenuators to identical levels such that the two pure tones are clearly audible to the listener. Adjust the frequency control of one Sine Wave Generator to produce an initial reference tone near 1000 Hz. The listener or experimenter must adjust the Frequency Control of the second generator until its tone is perceived to be half as high in pitch as the reference signal. Repeat this procedure with each of the following frequencies serving as new reference tones: 250, 500, 2000, and 5000 Hz. Record the approximate frequency dial settings for the non-reference test tone signal. For more accurate frequency determinations, a calibrated oscilloscope, or frequency counter, should be employed. Plot your data values on Figure "B."

(2) Repeat exercise #1, but require the listener to judge doublings in perceived pitch rather than halvings. Plot the data values on Figure "B." Account for any differences you obtain from the two sets of mel scale data.

(3) If you try this experiment on a musically trained listener, you may obtain a one-to-one correspondence between frequency and perceived pitch. How would you account for this phenomenon?

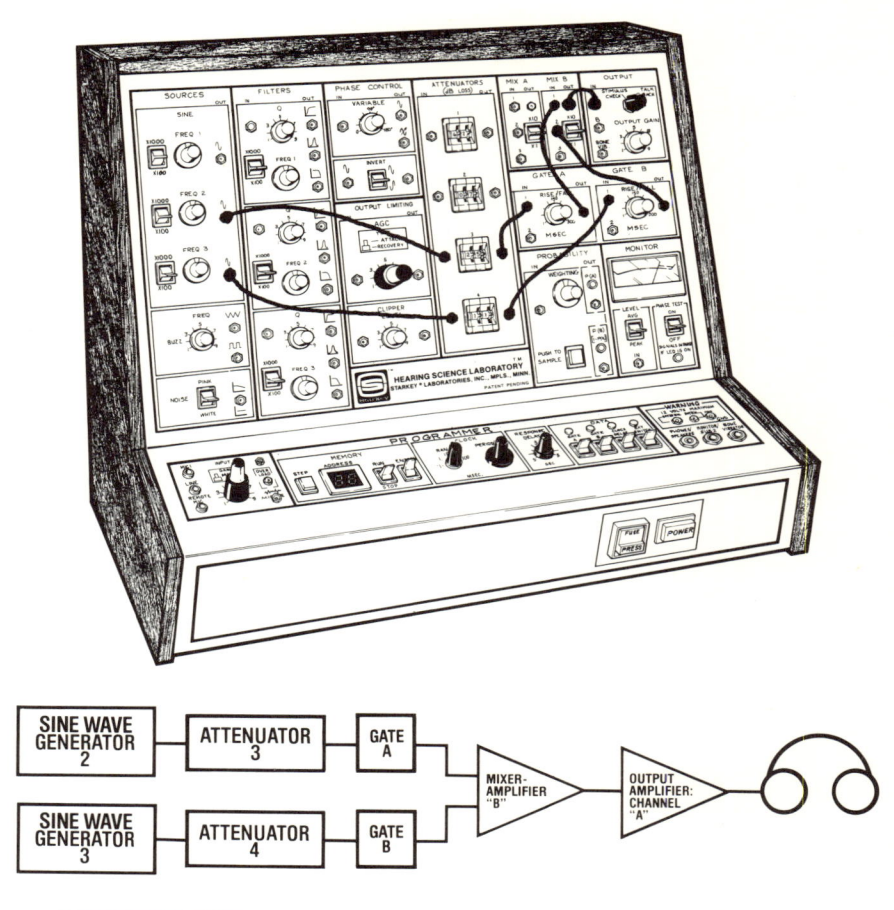

FIGURE A: The Mel scale displays the relationship between frequency and pitch. Note that 1000 Hz is assigned a value of 1000 mels. (After Stevens and Volkmann, 1940).

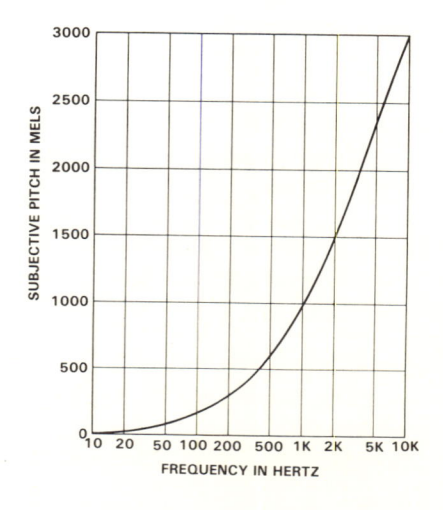

NOTES:

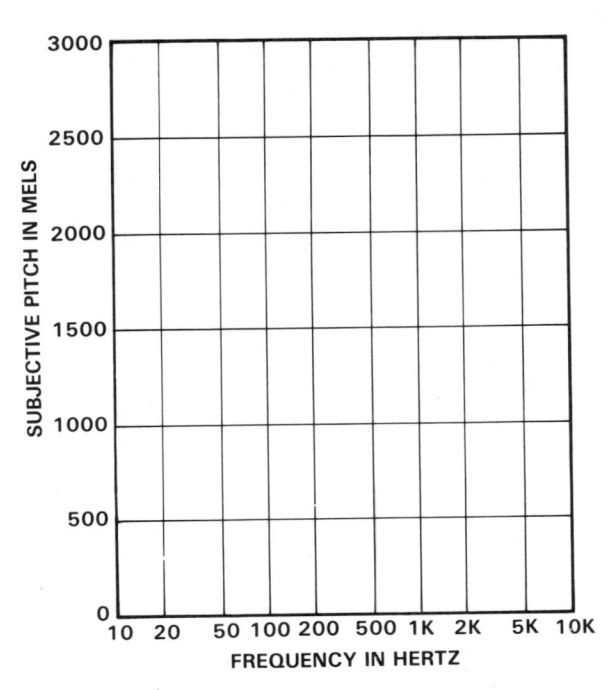

FIGURE B: Mel scale data graph.

Selected References:

Beck, J. and Shaw, W.A. (1963). Single estimates of pitch magnitude. *J. Acoust. Soc. Am.*, **35**, 1722-1724.

Elfner, L. (1964). Systematic shifts in the judgment of octaves of high frequencies. *J. Acoust. Soc. Am.*, **36**, 270-276.

Harris, J.D. (1960) Scaling of pitch intervals. *J. Acoust. Soc. Am.*, **22**, 1575-1581.

Shepard, R.N. (1964). Circularity in judgments of relative pitch. *J. Acoust. Soc. Am.*, **36**, 2346-2353.

Siegel, R.J. (1964). A reproduction of the mel scale for pitch. *Am. J. Psychol.*, **78**, 615-620.

Stevens, S.S. (1954). Pitch discrimination, mels, and Koch's contention. *J. Acoust. Soc. Am.*, **26**, 1075-1077.

Stevens, S.S. (1975). *Psychophysics.* Chapters 3 and 4. Wiley, New York.

Stevens, S.S. and Volkmann, J. (1940). The relation of pitch to frequency: a revised scale. *Am. J. Psychol.*, **53**, 329-353.

Stevens, S.S., Volkmann, J., and Newman, E.B. (1937). A scale for the measurement of the psychological magnitude pitch. *J. Acoust. Soc. Am.*, **8**, 185-190.

Ward, W.D. (1954). Subjective musical pitch. *J. Acoust. Soc. Am.*, **26**, 369-380.

Ward, W.D. (1970). Musical perception. In J.V. Tobias (Ed.) *Foundations of auditory theory.* Vol. 1. Academic Press, New York.

EXPERIMENT IV-7: THE JND FOR FREQUENCY

Purpose:
To examine the frequency discrimination abilities of the ear.

Background Principle:
How far apart must the frequencies of two tones be in order for a listener to just notice a difference between them? Several aspects of this seemingly straightforward research question remain controversial, even after more than a century of investigation. As in the case of just noticeable intensity changes (see Laboratory Experiment III-1), it is important to keep the distinction clear between the differential threshold (also called the just noticeable difference, "JND", or difference limen, "DL") and the *differential sensitivity*, or Weber fraction (i.e., the JND/Absolute Stimulus Value). The JND is that minimum physical change in a stimulus parameter that is required for the observer to notice a change exists. The Weber fraction relates the JND to the absolute physical value of the stimulus prior to any increment. In Figure "A", it can be seen that a greater frequency separation between two tones is needed to notice a difference at higher, rather than lower, frequencies. When, however, we plot this same data on a graph whose ordinate relates the JND to the absolute frequency of the stimulus (i.e., the Weber fraction), we find that frequency discrimination remains relatively constant above 1000 Hz (see Figure "B"). The performance of the listener has not changed; only the graphic representation of the test results. Along with a scrutiny of how research findings are displayed, the careful student must also consider the various experimental procedures that have been employed to gather the data. Differences between methods and equipment have yielded conflicting test results as to the exact measure of frequency discrimination.

Procedure:
Both the reference and variable test tone stimuli are passed through separate Attenuators whose outputs are sent to two locations. Each tone is sent to Mixer-Amplifier "A" as well as to separate Electronic Gates. The signals that emerge from the Gates are combined within Mixer-Amplifier "B" and are routed to one Output Amplifier channel and headphone. The suggested programming instructions will switch the two tones on and off, alternately. The duration for each tone is approximately 0.5 second. The Programmer Delay channel will provide a 0.5 second pause after each tone presentation to facilitate the comparison task. The dashed circuit wire "A", shown in the wiring guide and block diagram, allows us to make use of the phenomenon of beats to accurately monitor the frequency difference between the two signals. Note that the combined tones which leave Mixer-Amplifier "A" are sent directly to an additional Attenuator and into the Level Meter. The rate of fluctuation of the meter needle will reflect the approximate number of beats per second and hence the frequency difference, in hertz, that exists between the two tones. Attenuator #4 should be

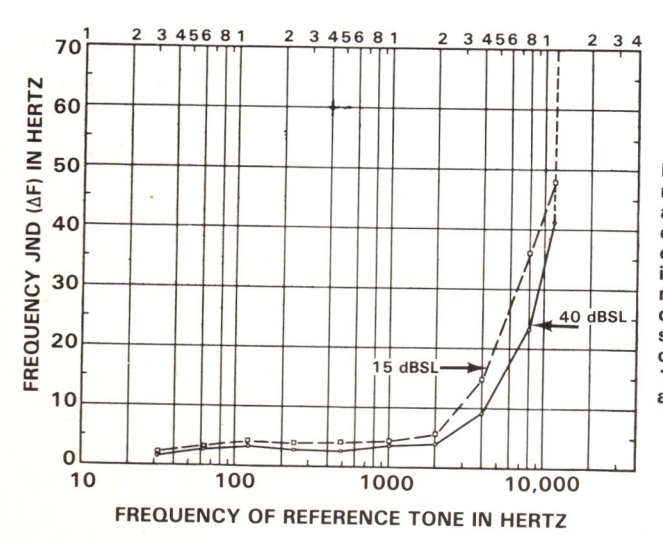

FIGURE A: The JND is one measure of a listener's ability to discriminate a change in the frequency of a tone. Note that larger increments (in Hz) are needed at high frequencies in order for the subject to discern a pitch change. (After Wever, 1949; Data from Shower and Biddulph, 1931).

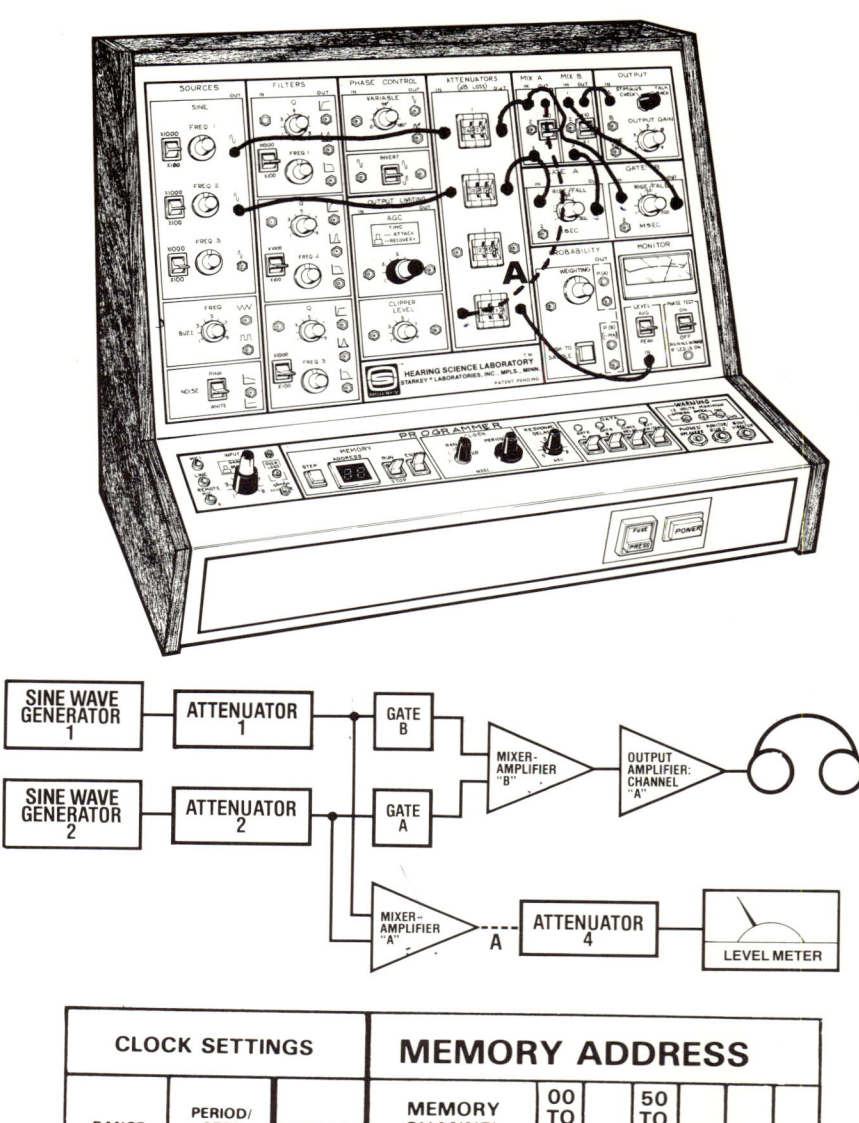

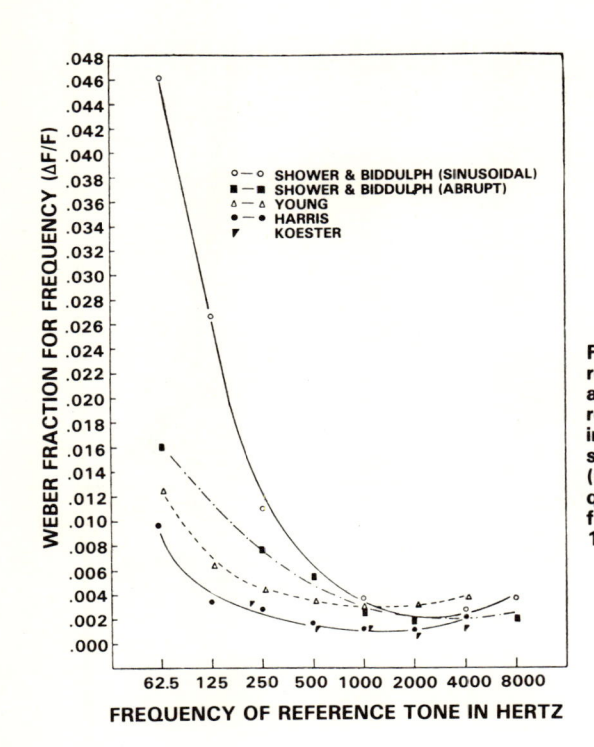

FIGURE B: The Weber Fraction relates the frequency JND to the absolute frequency of the reference tone. When displayed in this manner, the differential sensitivity is seen to "improve" (i.e., decrease) at higher frequencies. (Harris, 1952; Data from Shower and Biddulph, 1931 and others).

adjusted to a level that provides a satisfactory Meter scale reading. A frequency counter may, of course, also be used to determine the component frequencies.

Exercises:

(1) Let Sine Wave Generator #1 provide the reference tone and set its Frequency Control to an initial value near 1000 hertz. Find the subject's threshold for the stimulus and adjust both tone Attenuators to provide the same suprathreshold level (e.g., 40 dB greater than the threshold value). Sine Wave Generator #2 should be adjusted to a frequency that is roughly four or five Hz distant from the reference tone (as indicated by 4 or 5 fluctuations on the meter needle per second). The subject's responsibility is to report after each test sequence if the two tones were the same or different in pitch. The experimenter adjusts the test tone in the search for the smallest frequency difference (i.e., corresponding to the slowest beat rate) which the subject can detect. This value provides our estimate of the JND for frequency.

(2) There are a number of variables which affect, and may indeed confound, the measurement of the frequency JND. Repeat exercise #1 for very low and high frequencies as well as with different stimuli sound pressure levels. Are your estimates of the JND in general agreement with the findings of past researchers?

NOTES:

Selected References:

Butler, R.A. and Albrite, M.J.P. (1956). The pitch-discriminative function of the pathological ear. *Archs. Otolar.*, **63**, 411-418.

Daniloff, R.G., Glattke, T.J., Keith, R.W., and Small, A.M., Jr. (1964). Procedural variables influencing estimations of differential thresholds for frequency. *J. Acoust. Soc. Am.*, **36**, 1733-1734.

Harris, J.D. (1948). Discrimination of pitch: suggestions toward method and procedure. *Am. J. Psychol.*, **61**, 309-322.

Harris, J.D. (1952). Pitch discrimination. *J. Acoust. Soc. Am.*, **24**, 750-755.

Henning, G.B. (1966). Frequency discrimination of random-amplitude tones. *J. Acoust. Soc. Am.*, **39**, 336-339.

Henning, G.B. (1970). A comparison of the effects of signal duration on frequency and amplitude discrimination. In R. Plomp and G.F. Smoorenburg (Eds.) *Frequency analysis and periodicity detection in hearing.* Sijthoff, Lieden.

Jesteadt, W. and Bilger, R.C. (1974). Intensity and frequency discrimination in one- and two-interval paradigms. *J. Acoust. Soc. Am.*, **55**, 1266-1276.

Jesteadt, W. and Sims, S.L. (1975). Decision processes in frequency discrimination. *J. Acoust. Soc. Am.*, **57**, 1161-1168.

Jesteadt, W. and Wier, C.C. (1977). Comparison of monaural and binaural discrimination of intensity and frequency. *J. Acoust. Soc. Am.*, **61**, 1599-1603.

Moore, B.C.J. (1973). Frequency difference limens for short-duration tones. *J. Acoust. Soc. Am.*, **54**, 610-619.

Nordmark, J.O. (1968). Mechanisms of frequency discrimination. *J. Acoust. Soc. Am.*, **44**, 1533-1540.

Rosenblith, W. and Stevens, K.N. (1953). On the DL for frequency. *J. Acoust. Soc. Am.*, **25**, 980-985.

Shower, E.G. and Biddulph, R. (1931). Differential pitch sensitivity of the ear. *J. Acoust. Soc. Am.*, **3**, 275-287.

Stevens, S.S. (1954). Pitch discrimination, mels, and Kock's contention. *J. Acoust. Soc. Am.*, **26**, 1075-1077.

Tanner, W.P., Jr. and Rivette, C.L. (1964). Experimental study of "tone deafness." *J. Acoust. Soc. Am.*, **36**, 1465-1467.

Wever, E.G. (1949). *Theory of hearing.* Chapter 13. Wiley, New York.

EXPERIMENT IV-8: THE EFFECTS OF PHASE ON THE PITCH OF A COMPLEX SOUND

Purpose:
To see the effect of inverting a complex waveform upon its pitch.

Background Principle:
As mentioned in part I of this text, altering the phase relationship between the pure tone components in a complex wave can affect the resultant waveshape and sound quality. What effect, however, do phase changes exert upon the pitch associated with the complex sound? Several auditory theories have suggested that pitch is determined from such "fine-structure" details of the complex waveform as the time interval between the higher amplitude waveform peaks. Since these peaks are affected by the phase relationship between the components in the signal, it would follow that relative phase changes should also affect pitch. Wightman (1973), however, reports the results of several experiments which tend to refute the "fine-structure" model of pitch perception. We shall consider one of these demonstrations in this exercise. The waveforms shown in Figure "A" and "B" are 3-tone harmonic complex signals that were formed by amplitude modulating a 1000 Hz sinusoid with a 200 Hz sinusoid. Both waveforms are identical except for the fact that the signal in Figure "B" is an inverted version of the one Figure in "A" (i.e., the two stimuli are 180° out of phase with each other). Note that the various time periods between the waveform peaks are similar for both signals:

Waveform A		Waveform B
t_1	=	t_1 or t_2
t_2	=	t_4
t_3	=	t_3

Despite these similarities, however, a "fine-structure" theory would predict that the two waveforms will produce different pitches because of the differences in their waveshapes. A simple listening task will, however, reveal that the low pitch associated with each waveform is the same.

Procedure:
The 1000 Hz sinusoid for this demonstration is obtained from Sine Wave Generator 3 whose output is sent through an Attenuator and into Electronic Gate "A". The suggested programming instructions will turn the signal on for 2.5 milliseconds and off for the same duration. Thus the amplitude of the tone is being "modulated," or varied, at a rate of 200 times per second (i.e., with a period of 5 msec). Varying the rise/fall time of Gate "A" will change the "depth of modulation" between 0 and 100%. For the

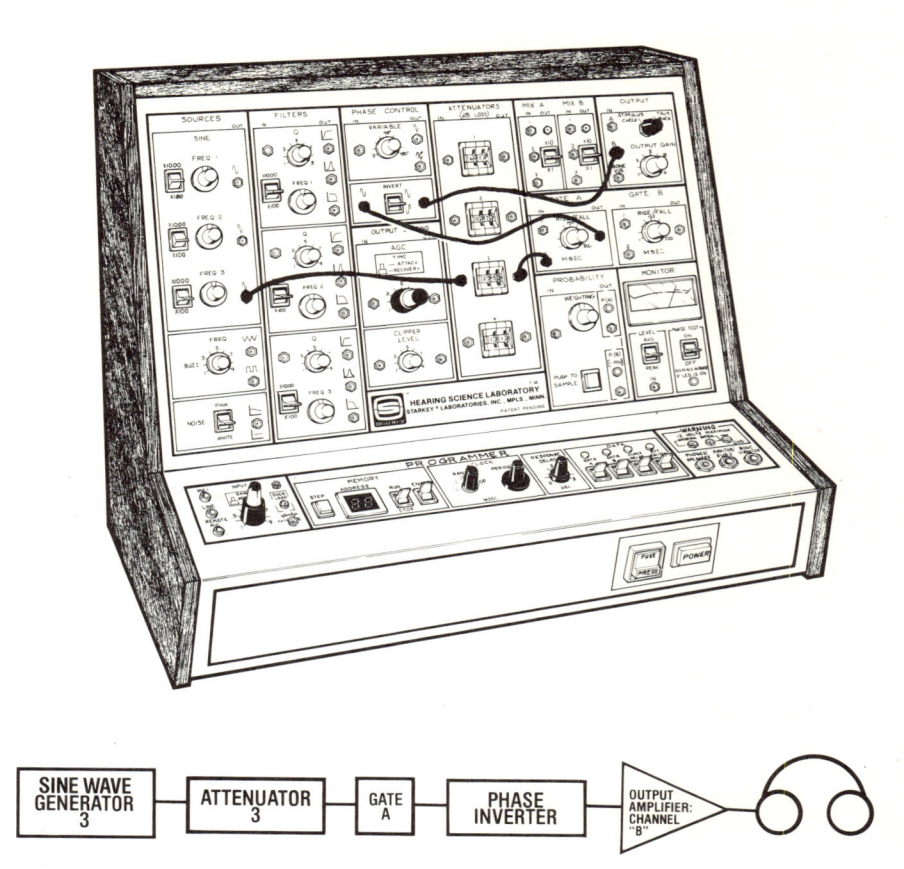

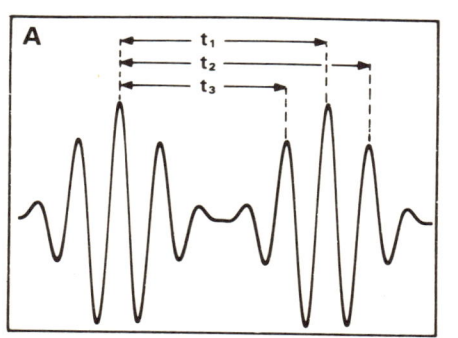

FIGURE A: Three component complex signal produced by amplitude modulating a 1000 Hz sinusoid with a 200 Hz sine wave.

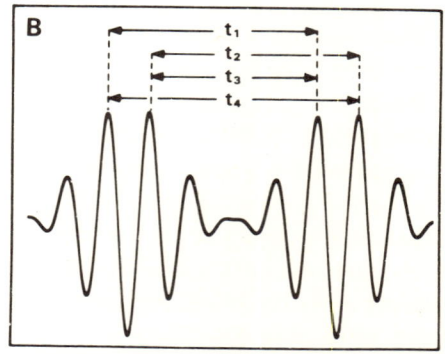

FIGURE B: Phase inverted version of waveform shown in Figure "A." Note similarities in the time periods between waveform peaks. (Wightman and Green, 1974).

present demonstration, gradually adjust the Rise/Fall Control of Gate "A" until the amplitude modulated signal shown in Figure "A" appears on a monitor oscilloscope display. This condition will be obtained near the extreme counterclockwise rotation of Rise/Fall Time Control. The output from the Electronic Gate is next sent to the Phase Inverter module and finally to one Output Amplifier channel and headphone (or loudspeaker). Note: since the rise/fall characteristics of the Gate are somewhat "triangular" rather than sinusoidal, the quasi-A.M. signal produced will have some additional energy at frequencies other than 800, 1000 and 1200 Hz.

Exercises:

(1) Listen to the A.M. signal at both soft and loud listening levels. Can you hear the low pitch (associated with a 200 Hz tone) that is formed from the interaction of the 800, 1000 Hz, and 1200 Hz components produced by the A.M. signal?

(2) Alternate the position of the Phase Inverter Switch and note if there is any change in the complex pitch from one listening condition to the next.

(3) Repeat exercises #1 and #2 with different carrier tone frequencies of 2000 Hz and 4000 Hz. Can you still perceive the presence of a low complex pitch? How do you account for what you do or do not hear in these instances?

(4) Repeat exercise #1 while slowly varying the modulation signal frequency. This may be achieved by altering the Programmer Clock settings. Describe the pitch changes that are created in this task.

NOTES:

Selected References:

Buunen, T.J.F., Festen, J.M., Bilsen, F.A., and van den Brink, G. (1974). Phase effects in a three-component signal. *J. Acoust. Soc. Am.,* **55,** 297-303.

Cabot, R.C., Mino, M.G., Dorans, D.A., Tackel, I.S., and Breed, H.E. (1976). Detection of phase shifts in harmonically related tones. *J. Audio Eng. Soc.,* **24,** 568-571.

Patterson, R. (1969). Noise masking of a change in residue pitch. *J. Acoust. Soc. Am.,* **45,** 1520-1524.

Raiford, C.A. and Schubert, E.D. (1971). Recognition of phase changes in octave complexes. *J. Acoust. Soc. Am.,* **50,** 559-567.

Ritsma, R. (1962). Existence region of the tonal residue, I. *J. Acoust. Soc. Am.,* **34,** 1224-1229.

Ritsma, R. (1967). Frequencies dominant in the perception of the pitch of complex sounds. *J. Acoust. Soc. Am.,* **42,** 191-198.

Ritsma, R. and Engel, F. (1964). Pitch of frequency-modulated signals. *J. Acoust. Soc. Am.,* **36,** 1637-1644.

Wightman, F.L. (1973a). Pitch and stimulus fine-structure. *J. Acoust. Soc. Am.,* **54,** 397-406.

Wightman, F.L. (1973b). The pattern-transformation model of pitch. *J. Acoust. Soc. Am.,* **54,** 407-416.

Wightman, F.L. and Green, D.M. (1974). The perception of pitch. *American Scientist,* **62,** 208-215.

Auditory Temporality V

EXPERIMENT V-1: WAVEFORM DURATION AND PERCEIVED TONALITY

Purpose:
To examine the influence of stimulus duration upon the quality of a sinusoid.

Background Principle:
It takes a certain amount of time for the mechanical vibrations of a sound wave to travel through the spiral tunnel of our inner ear and reach the appropriate point of stimulation on the basilar membrane that is associated with the test tone frequency. The minimal duration a tone must possess in order for it to be perceived as having a definite tonal, rather than click-like, quality has been found to range between 10 to 60 milliseconds, depending upon such variables as the stimulus frequency, intensity, and rise-fall time in addition to duration (see Figure "A").

Procedure:
The output of one Sine Wave Generator is passed through an Attenuator, into an Electronic Gate and one Output Amplifier channel and headphone. The suggested programming instructions will permit Electronic Gate "A" to switch on and off, sequentially. The duration that Gate "A" (and the test tone) remains on ranges from 10 to 80 milliseconds, with each succeeding test tone being 10 milliseconds longer than the previous one. The Programmer Delay Channel provides a one second pause between stimulus presentations. After some initial practice runs, the listener should be able to recognize which signal durations in the sequence produce a tonal sound quality.

Exercises:
(1) Select several different test tone frequencies ranging from 100 to 6000 Hz and determine the minimum duration required for tonality to be perceived. Plot these durations as a function of test tone frequency on Figure "B" and compare your graph with those shown in the references cited below.

(2) Repeat exercise #1 for different stimulus rise/fall times and signal levels. Can you account for the differences between test results?

(3) Reprogram the Memory to provide a series of ever-smaller durations instead of increasing ones and repeat exercises #1 and #2. Does this "descending" approach change any of your findings?

(4) Use the data shown in Figure "A" to compute the number of **cycles** required at each signal frequency for tonality to occur.

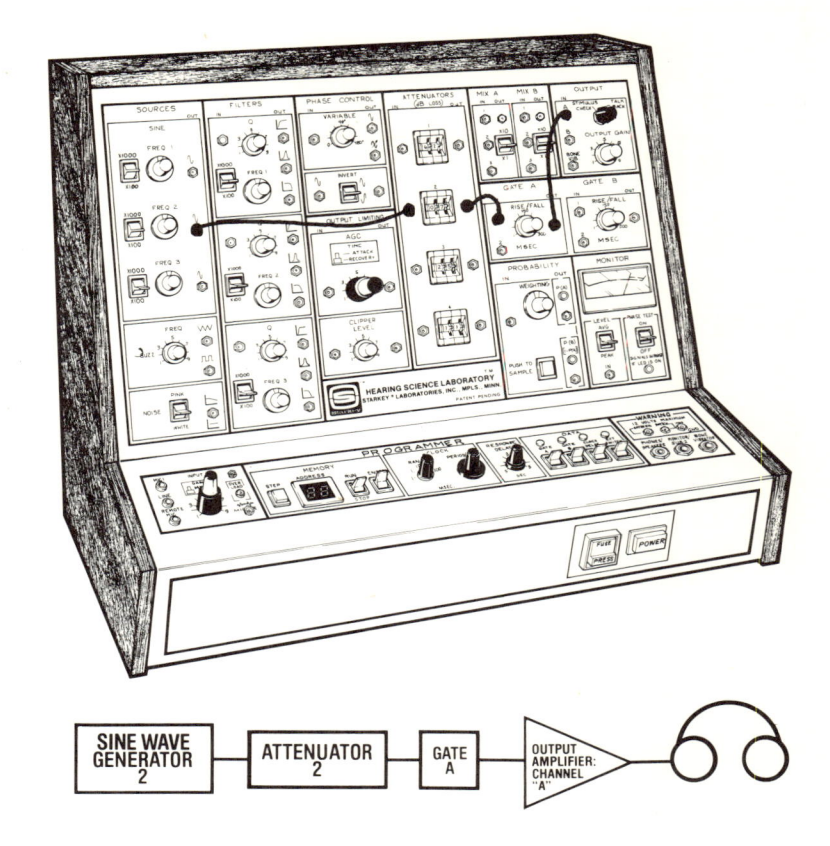

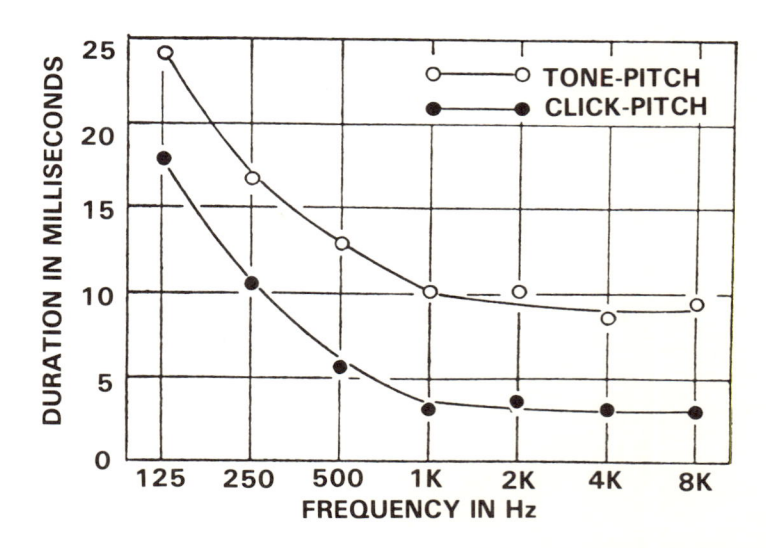

FIGURE A: Very brief sinusoidal signals (e.g., < 5 msec.) are perceived as clicks rather than tones. For signal durations ranging between 5 to 20 milliseconds, the click will assume a pitch-like quality depending upon the stimulus frequency. Additional increments in durations at each frequency produce a further increase in tonality. (Doughty and Garner, 1947).

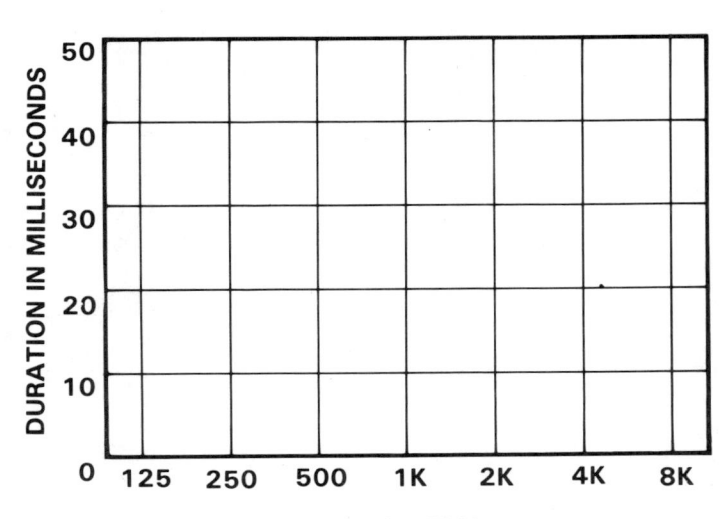

NOTES:

FIGURE B: Data graph for displaying the relationship between the required signal duration for tonality at a particular frequency.

Selected References:

Boomsliter, P.C., Creel, W., and Powers, S.R., Jr. (1964). Time requirements for the tonal function. *J. Acoust. Soc. Am.*, **36,** 1958-1959(A).

Doughty, J.M. and Garner, W.R. (1947). Pitch characteristics of short tones. I. Two kinds of pitch threshold. *J. Exp. Psychol.*, **37,** 351-365.

Doughty, J.M. and Garner, W.R. (1948). Pitch characteristics of short tones. II. Pitch as a function of tonal duration. *J. Exp. Psychol.*, **38,** 478-494.

Ward, W.D. (1970). Musical perception. In J.V. Tobias (Ed.) *Foundations of modern auditory theory.* Vol. 1. Academic, New York.

EXPERIMENT V-2: THE RISE AND FALL OF WAVEFORMS

Purpose:
To observe how the rise/fall time of a waveform influences the quality of a brief signal.

Background Principle:
The ideal pure tone would possess a single frequency of constant amplitude and would last for an infinite duration. In our everyday world, however, all sounds have a finite beginning and end. The notion of a perfectly pure tone must, therefore, remain as a hypothetical concept.

Consider the sinusoidal waveforms shown in Figure "A". Notice the abrupt onset and offset of waveform I (i.e., its almost instantaneous rise and fall to and from its maximum amplitude) and the more gradual rise/fall times of waveforms II-IV. The corresponding spectra for these signals, shown in Figure "B", reveal the presence of a wide spread of energy above and below the frequency of the basic pure tone signal for waveform I. These additional frequencies impart a click-like quality to the tone burst. For waveforms II-IV, however, the energy spread diminishes in amplitude and the click becomes less audible to the listener. Minimizing such transient energies is an important concern in experimental and clinical threshold testing; for the subject may respond to spurious spectral components, rather than to the desired test tone frequency.

We have already observed in Laboratory Experiment V-1 that brief duration tones also possess a click producing spread of energy above and below the stimulus frequency. A spectral analysis of **equal-energy,** different-duration *canonical signals* (i.e., stimuli which have received no envelope shaping or

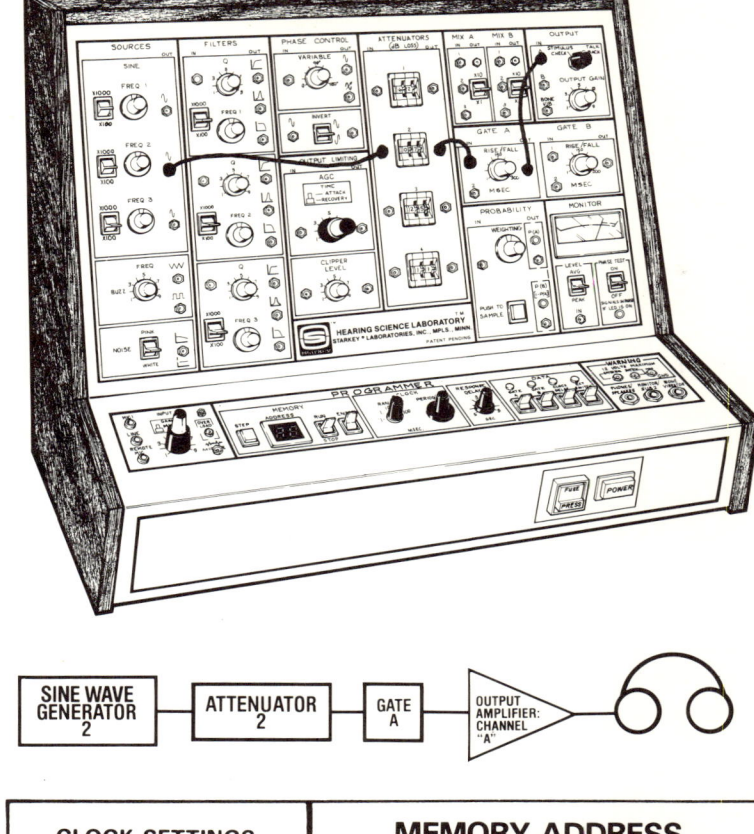

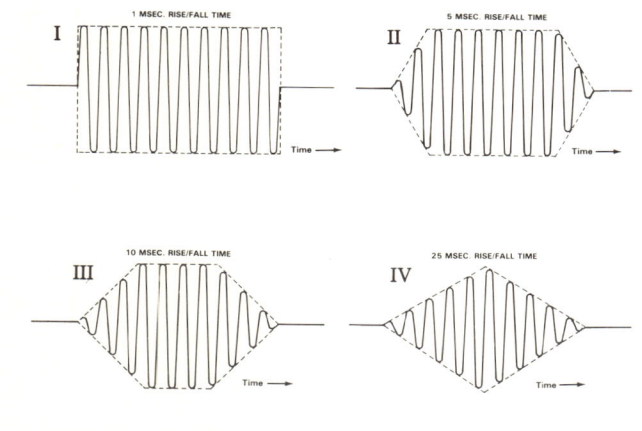

FIGURE A: Relative envelope and waveform shapes of sinusoids having different rise/fall times. Note rectangular envelope of tone burst with 1 millisecond rise/fall times.

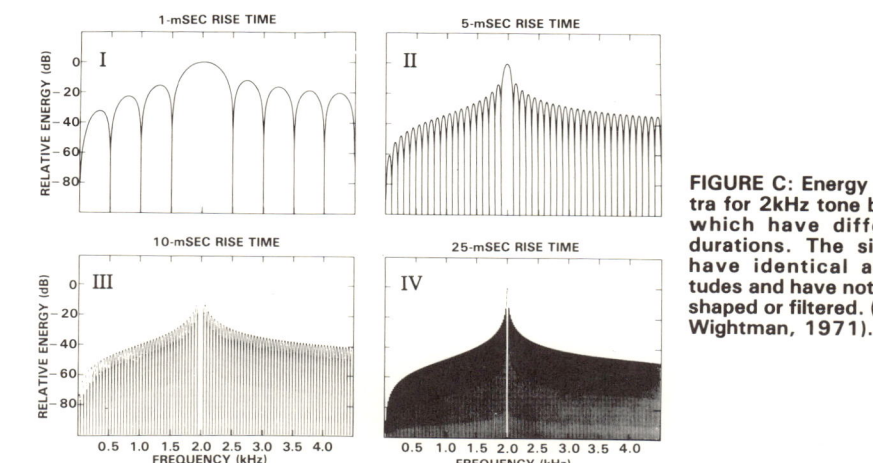

FIGURE B: Spectral distribution of energy for electronically switched sinusoids having different rise/fall times. Note increase of energy-spread amplitude for briefer rise/fall times. (Curves based upon transfer functions of filters which have equivalent spectral shaping characteristics to electronic switches with specified rise/fall times). (From Wightman 1971).

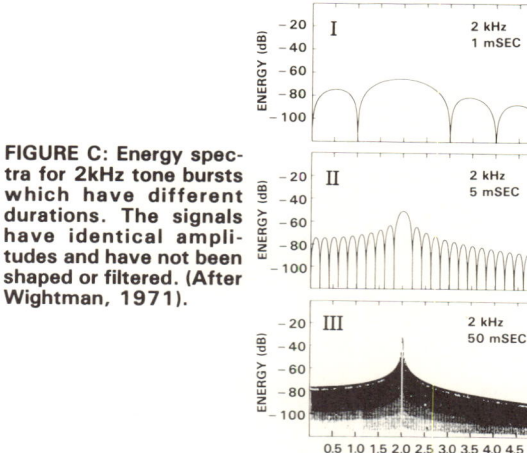

FIGURE C: Energy spectra for 2kHz tone bursts which have different durations. The signals have identical amplitudes and have not been shaped or filtered. (After Wightman, 1971).

filtering), reveals that there is a substantial spread of energy even for relatively long duration signals. Note, for example, that spectrum III in Figure "C" has essentially the same overall energy content as spectrum I despite being 50 times longer in duration! It should be clear from the graphs that the increased duration serves only to increase the energy near the original tone signal frequency.

One may describe the duration of a tone burst in terms of its exact moment of onset and offset or by its *equivalent duration* (after Dallos and Olsen, 1964). In this instance, the computed duration of the shaped sinusoid is the equivalent of a tone burst having a rectangular envelope (i.e., a signal with essentially instantaneous rise/fall times). One may use the following formula to calculate equivalent duration:

$$T = \frac{2R}{3} + P$$

where: T = Equivalent Duration
R = Rise/Fall Times (must be identical)
P = Duration for Peak Amplitude of Signal

Procedure:

The output of one Sine Wave Generator is passed through an Attenuator, into an Electronic Gate and one Output Amplifier channel and headphone. The suggested Programmer instructions permit the Electronic Gate to alternately switch the tone on and off for equal durations while the clock is running. Various attack and decay times can be imparted to the waveform by adjusting the Rise/Fall Control Knob on the Electronic Gate.

Exercises:

(1) Select several different pure tone frequencies and note the rise/fall time for each at which the presence of clicks first become audible. Are some frequencies more prone to the formation of clicks?

(2) Repeat exercise #1 for tones of differing signal level at each test frequency. Are the clicks more obvious well above or near threshold levels?

(3) Repeat exercise #1 for tone bursts of differing duration. Try a variety of Programmer Clock settings and note the effect of the rise/fall times on click perception.

NOTES:

Selected References:

Carter, N.L. (1972). Effects of rise time and repetition rate on the loudness of acoustic transients. *J. Sound Vib.*, **21**, 227-239.

Carter, N.L. and Dunlop, J.I. (1973). The effects of rise time and repetition rate on the thresholds for acoustic transients. *J. Sound Vib.*, **30**, 359-366.

Dallos, P.J. and Johnson, K.R. (1966). Influence of rise-fall time upon short-tone threshold. *J. Acoust. Soc. Am.*, **40**, 1160-1163.

Dallos, P.J. and Olsen, W.O. (1964). Integration of energy at threshold with gradual rise-fall tone pips. *J. Acoust. Soc. Am.*, **36**, 743-751.

Gjaevenes, K. and Rimstad, E.R. (1972). The influence of rise time on loudness. *J. Acoust. Soc. Am.*, **51**, 1233-1239.

Leshowitz, B.H. and Wightman, F.L. (1971). On-frequency masking with continuous sinusoids. *J. Acoust. Soc. Am.*, **49**, 1180-1190.

Wightman, F.L. (1971). Detection of binaural tones as a function of masker bandwidth. *J. Acoust. Soc. Am.*, **50**, 623-636.

Wright, H.N. (1958). Switching transients and threshold determination. *J. Speech and Hear. Res.*, **1**, 52-60.

EXPERIMENT V-3: TEMPORAL INTEGRATION

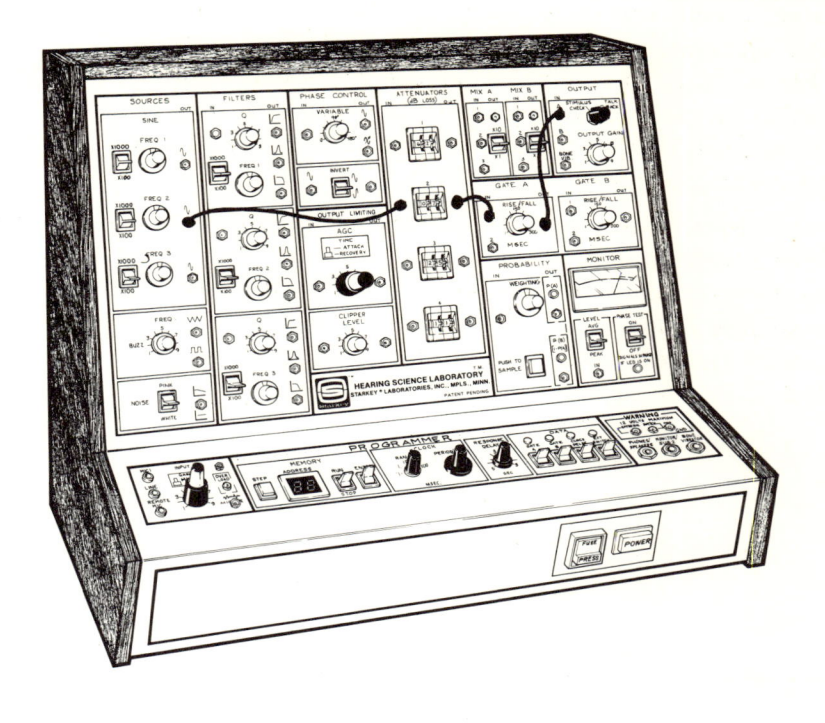

Purpose:
To examine the trading relationship that exists between the duration of a sound and its loudness.

Background Principle:
The threshold and loudness of a sound are closely linked to its duration. Researchers who have explored the ear's ability to analyze and *integrate* (i.e., summate) the energy in a sound have described a definite trading relationship between duration and loudness of a sound. Specifically, the loudness of sounds decreases as their duration decreases. It appears that for stimulus durations ranging between 10 to 200 milliseconds, any ten-fold reduction in the duration of a threshold level tone can be compensated for by a ten-fold increase in the energy of the sound (i.e., by 10 dB SPL). Increasing the duration of a signal beyond about 200 milliseconds does not enhance its detectability any further. For signals shorter than 10 milliseconds, the stimulus energy spreads above and below the test tone frequency, yielding clicks which confound the study of *temporal integration*. We have seen that the effects of such transients may be reduced through the use of a more gradual stimulus rise/fall time. Studies have attempted to show that individuals with different types of hearing loss do not respond to brief tones in the same manner, nor as normal hearing listeners do. The diagnostic usefulness of this effect is currently under investigation by clinical researchers (see, for example, Olsen et al., 1974).

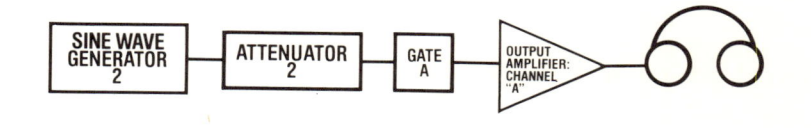

Procedure:
A pure tone is first sent through an Attenuator and then to an Electronic Gate that will switch the signal on and off in accordance with the suggested Programmer instructions. The pulsed tone that is created next enters an Output Amplifier channel and headphone. The Programmer Delay Channel will provide a one second pause before the delivery of each tone.

Exercises:
(1) Adjust the Sine Wave Generator to an initial frequency near 1000 Hz. Determine the subject's threshold for pulsed tones having the following durations: 2000, 200, 20, and 2 milliseconds. Each of these ten-fold reductions in pulse length may be easily obtained by rotating the Clock Range Switch counterclockwise, one step at a time. Do you find that roughly 10 dB more signal level must be added to the tone for it to remain audible at each ten-fold reduction in duration?

(2) Repeat exercise #1 for very low and high frequencies (e.g., 100 Hz and 10,000 Hz). Does the trading relationship remain the same at these different frequency regions?

(3) Repeat exercise #1 with a white noise as the test stimulus instead of a tone. This can be done by routing the Attenuator input wire to the White Noise Generator. Do you find that fewer decibels of noise are needed to compensate for each ten-fold reduction in stimulus duration than was the case for a tone?

NOTES:

Selected References:

Dallos, P.J. and Olsen, W.O. (1964). Integration of energy at threshold with gradual rise-fall tone pips. *J. Acoust. Soc. Am.*, **36**, 743-751.

Elliott, L.L. (1963). Tonal thresholds for short-duration stimuli as related to subject hearing level. *J. Acoust. Soc. Am.*, **35**, 578-580.

Evans, D.H. (1971). An experimental determination of the growth of auditory sensation for time periods greater than 125 ms. *J. Aud. Res.*, **11**, 374-384.

Garner, W.R. (1947). The effect of frequency spectrum on temporal integration of energy in the ear. *J. Acoust. Soc. Am.*, **19**, 808-815.

Gengel, R.W. (1972). Auditory temporal integration at relatively high masked-threshold levels. *J. Acoust. Soc. Am.*, **51**, 1849-1851.

Gengel, R.W. and Watson, C.S. (1971). Temporal integration: I. Clinical implications of a laboratory study: II. Additional data from hearing impaired subjects. *J. Speech Hear. Dis.*, **36**, 213-224.

Goldstein, R. and Kramer, J.C. (1960). Factors affecting thresholds for short tones. *J. Speech Hear. Res.*, **3**, 249-256.

Harris, J.D., Haines, H.L., and Myers, C.K. (1958). Brief tone audiometry. *Archs Otolar.*, **67**, 699-713.

Irwin, R.J. and Kemp. S. (1976). Temporal summation and decay in hearing. *J. Acoust. Soc. Am.*, **59**, 920-925.

Jerger, J.F. (1955). Influence of stimulus duration on the pure tone threshold during recovery from auditory fatigue. *J. Acoust. Soc. Am.*, **27**, 121-124.

Karlovich, R.S. et. al. (1971). Auditory threshold at 12.5 Hz as a function of signal duration and signal filtering. *J. Acoust. Soc. Am.* **49**, 1897-1899.

McFadden, D. (1975). Duration — intensity reciprocity for equal loudness. *J. Acoust. Soc. Am.*, **57**, 702-704.

Martin, F.N., and Wofford, M.J. (1970). Temporal summation of brief tones in normal and cochlear-impaired ears. *J. Aud. Res.*, **10**, 82-86.

Miller, G.A. (1948). The perception of short bursts of noise. *J. Acoust. Soc. Am.*, **20**, 160-170.

Miskolczy-Fodor, F. (1960). Relation between loudness and duration of tonal pulses: III. Response in cases of abnormal loudness function. *J. Acoust. Soc. Am.*, **32**, 486-492.

Olsen, W. and Carhart, R. (1966). Integration of acoustic power at threshold by normal hearers. *J. Acoust. Soc. Am.*, **40**, 591-599.

Olsen, W., Rose, D.E., and Noffsinger, D. (1974). Brief tone audiometry with normal, cochlear, and eighth nerve tumor patients. *Archs Otolar.*, **99**, 185-189.

Pedersen, C.B. and Elberling, C, (1972). Temporal integration of acoustic energy in normal hearing persons. *Acta Oto-Lar.*, **74**, 398-405.

Sanders, J.W. and Honig, E.A. (1967). Brief tone audiometry results in normal and impaired ears. *Archs Otolar.*, **85**, 640-647.

Stephens, S.D.G. (1973a). Auditory temporal integration as a function of intensity. *J. Sound Vib.*, **30**, 109-126.

Stephens, S.D.G. (1973b). Some experiments on the detection of short duration stimuli. *Brit. J. Audiol.*, **7**, 81-94.

Tempest, W. and Bryan, M.E. (1971). The auditory threshold for short-duration pulses. *J. Acoust. Soc. Am.*, **49**, 1901-1902.

Wright, H. (1958). Switching transients and threshold determination. *J. Speech Hear. Res.*, **1**, 52-60.

Wright, H. (1967). An artifact in the measurement of temporal summation at the threshold of audibility. *J. Speech Hear. Dis.*, **32**, 354-359.

Zwislocki, J. (1960). Theory of temporal auditory summation. *J. Acoust. Soc. Am.*, **32**, 1046-1060.

Zwislocki, J. (1969). Temporal summation of loudness: an analysis. *J. Acoust. Soc. Am.* **46**, 431-441.

EXPERIMENT V-4: FLUTTER FUSION

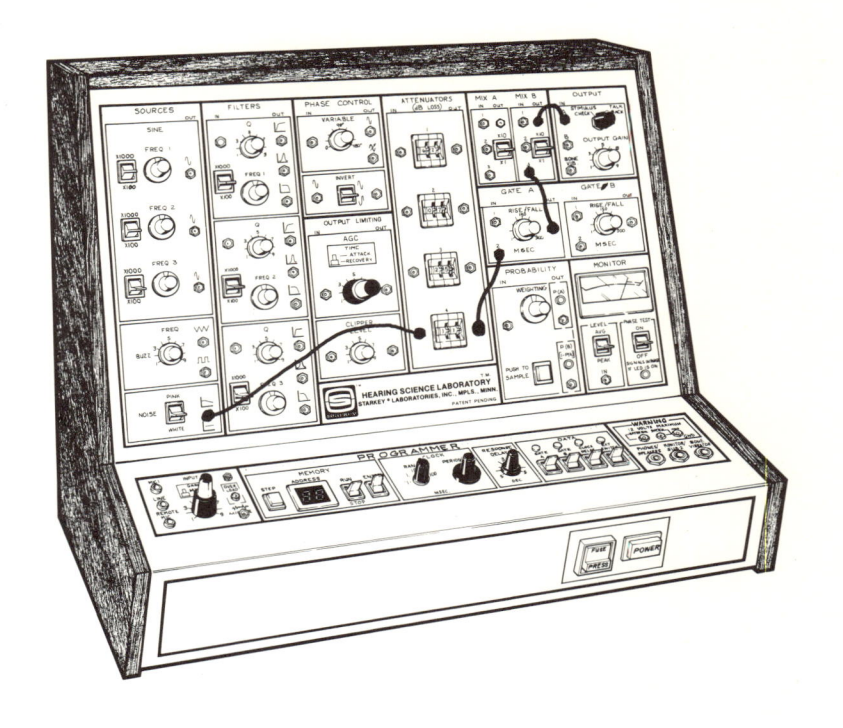

Purpose:
To explore the perception of a rapid series of acoustic events as a continuous-sounding phenomenon.

Background Principle:
When the bulbs on a movie-house marquee switch on and off in rapid succession, their individual flashing is perceived to fuse into continuous patterns of moving light. Similarly, the separate images on movie film fuse into the illusion of continuous motion when they pass before our eyes at the projection rate of sixteen images or more per second. An analogous version of this *flutter fusion* phenomenon exists in audition. Any sound will appear to flutter at slow interruption rates but will fuse into a continuous percept as faster repetition rates. Stimulus on-off time ratios, or *duty cycles,* can also affect the percept (see Laboratory Experiment VIII-11 for further details about duty cycle).

As we have already observed in Laboratory Experiment V-2, the frequency content of brief tone pulses will vary, depending upon such factors as rise-fall times and signal duration. The long term spectrum of white noise bursts, however, remains unaltered by interruptions and is commonly used for flutter fusion listening tasks. (See Pollack, 1969, for details on potential artifacts that may arise when using interrupted white noise).

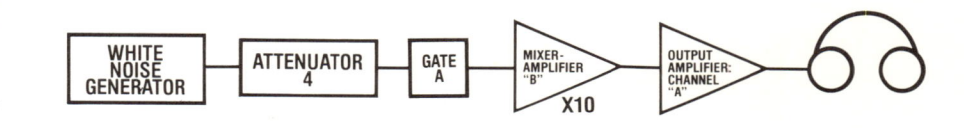

Procedure:
A white noise signal is passed through an Attenuator and Electronic Gate. The suggested programming instructions will produce interrupted noise bursts of either 25 *bursts per second (bps),* 50 bps, or 100 bps with sound duty cycles of 50%, 75%, and 90% as desired. Of course, virtually any other interruption rate or duty cycle may be chosen by slightly varying the memory commands and clock settings. The gated noise is then sent to a Mixer-Amplifier, set to provide 20 dB gain, and one Output Amplifier channel and headphone. (Note: It may prove convenient to program one Gate for one duty cycle value and the second Gate for a different setting. Alternating from one condition to the other would then be a matter of routing the Attenuator output from one Gate to the other.)

Exercises:
(1) After listening to gross changes in the bps rate (i.e., 25, 50, and 100 bps) and noting the flutter fusion effect for different on-off ratios, try to determine the exact bps values at which the sound appears continuous. This can be accomplished by gradually rotating the Period Per Step Control counterclockwise from, for example, 1 millisecond per memory address to 0.1 millisecond per address (i.e., from 10 bps to 100 bps).

(2) Repeat exercise #1 for various Electronic Gate rise/fall times and note how the sound percept changes. How do you explain what you hear?

(3) Repeat exercise #1 for several different sensation levels and note if signal intensity noticeably affects flutter fusion.

INTERRUPTION RATE IN BURSTS PER SECOND	CLOCK SETTINGS IN MILLISECONDS		DUTY CYCLE (SOUND ON/OFF TIME RATIO)		
	RANGE SWITCH	PER/STEP CONTROL	50%	75%	90%
			[GATE ON FOR FOLLOWING MEMORY ADDRESSES]		
25 bps	X 0.1	4	00-49	00-74	00-89
50 bps	X 0.1	2	00-49	00-74	00-89
100 bps	X 0.1	1	00-49	00-74	00-89

PROGRAMMING INSTRUCTIONS

NOTES:

Selected References:

Abel, S.M. (1972). Discrimination of temporal gaps. *J. Acoust. Soc. Am.*, **52**, 519-524.

Dannenbring, G.L. and Bregman, A.S. (1976). Effect of silence between tones on auditory stream segregation. *J. Acoust. Soc. Am.*, **59**, 987-989.

Gerber, S.E. (1967). Flutter perception in normal listeners. *J. Speech Hear. Res.*, **10**, 319-322.

Gilliom, J.D. and Mills, W.M. (1976). Gap detection: two-channel detection of the missing event. *J. Acoust. Soc. Am.*, **60**, 395-404.

Goldstein, M., Jr. (1957). Pitch judgments for repeated bursts of tone and noise. *J. Acoust. Soc. Am.*, **29**, 184(A).

Green, D.M. (1974). Temporal auditory acuity. *Psychol. Rev.*, **78**, 540-551.

Harris, G.G. (1963). Periodicity perception by using gated noise. *J. Acoust. Soc. Am.*, **35**, 1229-1233.

Leshowitz, B. (1971). Measurement of the two-click threshold. *J. Acoust. Soc. Am.*, **49**, 462-466.

Miller, G.A. and Heise, G.A. (1950). The trill threshold. *J. Acoust. Soc. Am.*, **22**, 637-638.

Miller, G.A. and Taylor, W.G. (1948). The perception of repeated bursts of noise. *J. Acoust. Soc. Am.*, **20**, 171-182.

Nábelek, I.V., Nábelek, A.K., and Hirsh, I.J. (1970). Pitch of tone bursts of changing frequency. *J. Acoust. Soc. Am.*, **48**, 536-553.

Penner, M.J. (1975). Persistence and integration: two consequences of a sliding integrator. *Percept. Psychophys.*, **18**, 114.

Plomp, R. (1964). Rate of decay of auditory sensation. *J. Acoust. Soc. Am.*, **36**, 277-282.

Pollack, I. (1969). Periodicity pitch for interrupted white noise — fact or artifact? *J. Acoust. Soc. Am.*, **45**, 237-238.

Pollack, I. (1971a). Spectral basis of auditory "jitter" detection. *J. Acoust. Soc. Am.*, **50**, 555-558.

Pollack, I. (1971b). Amplitude and time jitter thresholds for rectangular-wave trains. *J. Acoust. Soc. Am.*, **50**, 1133-1142.

Pollack, I. (1971c). Discrimination of the interval between two brief pulses. *J. Acoust. Soc. Am.*, **50**, 1203-1204.

Shonle, J.I. and Horan, K.E. (1976). Trill threshold revisited. *J. Acoust. Soc. Am.*, **59**, 469-471.

Symmes, D., Chapman, L., and Halstead, W. (1955). The fusion of intermittent white noise. *J. Acoust. Soc. Am.*, **27**, 741-748.

Williams, K.N. and Perrott, D.R. (1972). Temporal resolution of tonal pulses. *J. Acoust. Soc. Am.*, **51**, 644-647.

EXPERIMENT V-5: ACOUSTIC TEMPORAL ORDER

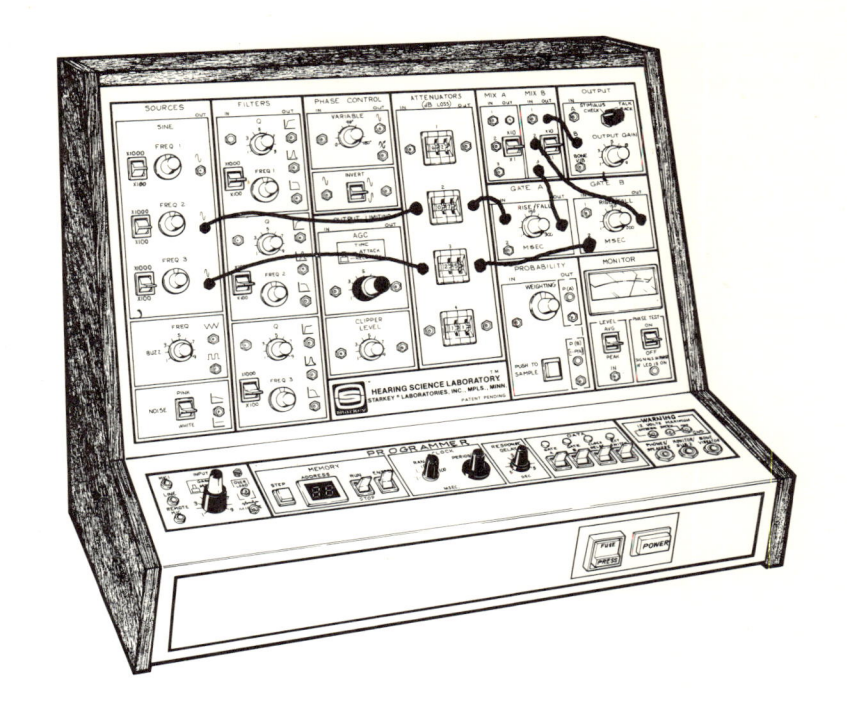

Purpose:
To examine the ability of a listener to identify the order of occurrence of stimuli in a sequence of acoustic events.

Background Principle:
Under certain test conditions, a rapid sequence of sound stimuli may appear as a continuous or single acoustic event, rather than as a series of discrete signals. Laboratory Experiments IV-2 and IV-3, for example, deal with the consonant or dissonant perceptions associated with "high-speed" objective beats. See Also Laboratory Experiments V-4, VII-2, and VII-5 on the fusion of multiple clicks into a single sound image.

The question arises as to what minimum temporal separation must exist between two sounds for a listener to recognize not only their individuality but their order as well. In the present experiment, the listener will be required to identify the order of occurrence for two different frequency tones, one of which leads the other in onset.

Procedure
Two pure tone signals, having different frequencies, are sent from Sine Wave Generators 2 and 3 through separate Attenuators and Electronic Gates, after which they are combined within Mixer-Amplifier "B" and delivered to one Output Amplifier channel and headphone. The suggested programming instructions in this acoustic temporal order listening task permit the experimenter to vary the temporal separation between the signal **onsets** by simply choosing the appropriate Programmer Clock settings as described in the exercises below.

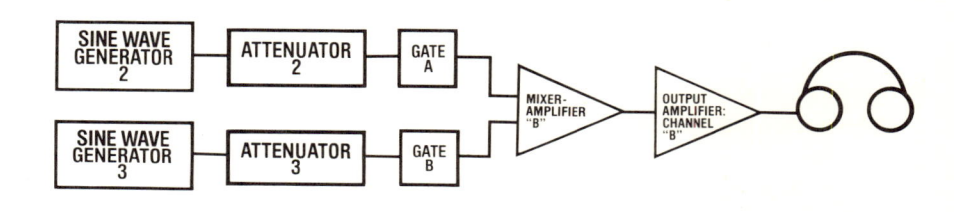

Exercises
(1) The test tone frequencies used originally by Hirsh (1959) for this listening task shared a frequency ratio of 6/5 (i.e., a minor third) or this musical interval raised two or four octaves.

Sample frequencies included:

F_1	F_2
250 Hz	300 Hz
250 Hz	1200 Hz
1000 Hz	1200 Hz
1000 Hz	4800 Hz

The relative onset time of the two tones was varied between −60 and +60 milliseconds in steps of 20 milliseconds (i.e., either the low or high frequency component would at various times lead or follow the other). Note in the suggested programming instructions that these variations in onset time can be created by assigning an individual memory address with a Clock duration value of 60, 40, and 20 milliseconds, respectively. The two signals will next remain on for 0.5 second and switch off simultaneously. The rise/fall time for each Electronic Gate should be set to roughly 40 milliseconds to avoid audible clicks. The order of the stimuli occurrence is reversed during the second programming sequence. A two second pause separates the different tone sequences.

The subject is required to report whether he or she heard the lower or the higher pitch tone first. Present each test condition ten times to the listener and record the number of correct judgments made of the actual pitch sequence delivered. Consider each of the following questions in your analysis of the test results:

(A) Is the perception of temporal order affected by the frequency separation of the stimuli?

(B) Do the sensation levels of the stimuli affect the results or the ease of the listening task?

(2) Repeat exercise #1 with a white noise signal instead of one of the tones. Record any similarities or differences in the subject's performance because of this new test condition.

(3) Repeat exercise #1 after re-programming a silent interval between the offset of the first tone and the onset of the second tone in the sequence. The number of memory addresses that are used for this interstimulus interval will govern the duration of the silent period. Contrast the accuracy of the subject's responses for this experimental task with that of exercise #1.

NOTES:

Selected References:

Babkoff, H. and Sutton, S. (1971). Monaural temporal interactions. *J. Acoust. Soc. Am.*, **50**, 459-465.

Bregman, A.S. and Campbell, J.L. (1971). Primary auditory stream segregation and perception of order in rapid sequences of tones. *J. Exp. Psychol.*, **89**, 244-249.

Broadbent, D.E. and Ladefoged, P.N. (1959). Auditory perception of temporal order. *J. Acoust. Soc. Am.*, **31**, 1539(L).

Divenyi, P.L. and Hirsh, I.J. (1974a). Identification of temporal order in three-tone sequences preceding a fourth tone. *J. Acoust. Soc. Am.*, **55**, 390(A).

Divenyi, P.L. and Hirsh, I.J. (1974b). Identification of temporal order in three-tone sequences. *J. Acoust. Soc. Am.*, **56**, 144-151.

Gescheider, G.A. (1967). Auditory and cutaneous apparent successiveness. *J. Exp. Psychol.*, **73**, 179-186.

Green, D.M. (1971). Temporal auditory acuity. *Psychol. Rev.*, **78**, 540-551.

Green, D.M. (1973). Temporal acuity as a function of frequency. *J. Acoust. Soc. Am.*, **54**, 373-379.

Hirsh, I.J. (1959). Auditory perception of temporal order. *J. Acoust. Soc. Am.*, **31**, 759-767.

Hirsh, I.J. and Sherrick, C.E., Jr. (1961). Perceived order in different sense modalities. *J. Exp. Psychol.*, **62**, 423-432.

Leshowitz, B. and Hanzi, R. (1972). Auditory pattern discrimination in the absence of spectral cues. *J. Acoust. Soc. Am.*, **52**, 166(A).

Patterson, J.H. and Green, D.M. (1970). Discrimination of transient signals having identical energy spectra. *J. Acoust. Soc. Am.*, **48**, 894-905.

Patterson, J.H. and Green, D.M. (1971). Masking of transient signals having identical energy spectra. *Audiology*, **10**, 85-96.

Peters, R. (1964). Perceived order of tone pulses. *J. Acoust. Soc. Am.*, **36**, 1042(A).

Peters, R. (1967). Perceived order of tone pulses. *J. Acoust. Soc. Am.*, **42**, 1216(A).

Peters, R. and Wood, T.J. (1973a). Perception of temporal order for tones. *J. Acoust. Soc. Am.*, **53**, 311-312(A).

Peters, R. and Wood, T.J. (1973b). Perceived order of tone pulses. *J. Acoust. Soc. Am.*, **54**, 315(A).

Ptacek, P.H. and Pinheiro, M.L. (1971). Pattern reversal in auditory perception. *J. Acoust. Soc. Am.*, **49**, 493-498.

Ronken, D.A. (1970). Monaural detection of a phase difference between clicks. *J. Acoust. Soc. Am.*, **47**, 1091-1099.

Swisher, L. and Hirsh, I.J. (1972). Brain damage and the ordering of two temporally successive stimuli. *Neuropsychologia*, **10**, 137-152.

Thomas, I.B. and Fitzgibbons, P.J. (1971). Temporal order and perceptual classes. *J. Acoust. Soc. Am.*, **50**, 86-87.

Thomas, I.B., Hill, P.B., Carroll, F.S., and Garcia, B. (1970). Temporal order in the perception of vowels. *J. Acoust. Soc. Am.*, **48**, 1010-1013.

Warren, R.M. (1972). Perception of temporal order: special rules for the initial and terminal sounds of sequences. *J. Acoust. Soc. Am.*, **52**, 167(A).

Warren, R.M., Obusek, C.J., Farmer, R.M., and Warren, R.P. (1969). Auditory sequence: confusion of patterns other than speech and music. *Science*, **164**, 586-587.

Watson, C.S., Wroton, H.W., Kelly, W.J., and Benbassat, C.A. (1975). Factors in the discrimination of tonal patterns. I. Component frequency, temporal position, and silent intervals. *J. Acoust. Soc. Am.*, **57**, 1175-1185.

White, C.T. and Lichtenstein, M. (1963). Some aspects of temporal discrimination. In C.T. White and M. Lichtenstein (Eds.) *Perceptual and motor skills.* pp. 471-482. Southern University Press, Birmingham, Alabama.

Wier, C.C. and Green, D.M. (1975). Temporal acuity as a function of frequency difference. *J. Acoust. Soc. Am.*, **57**, 1512-1515.

EXPERIMENT V-6: AUDITORY NUMEROSITY

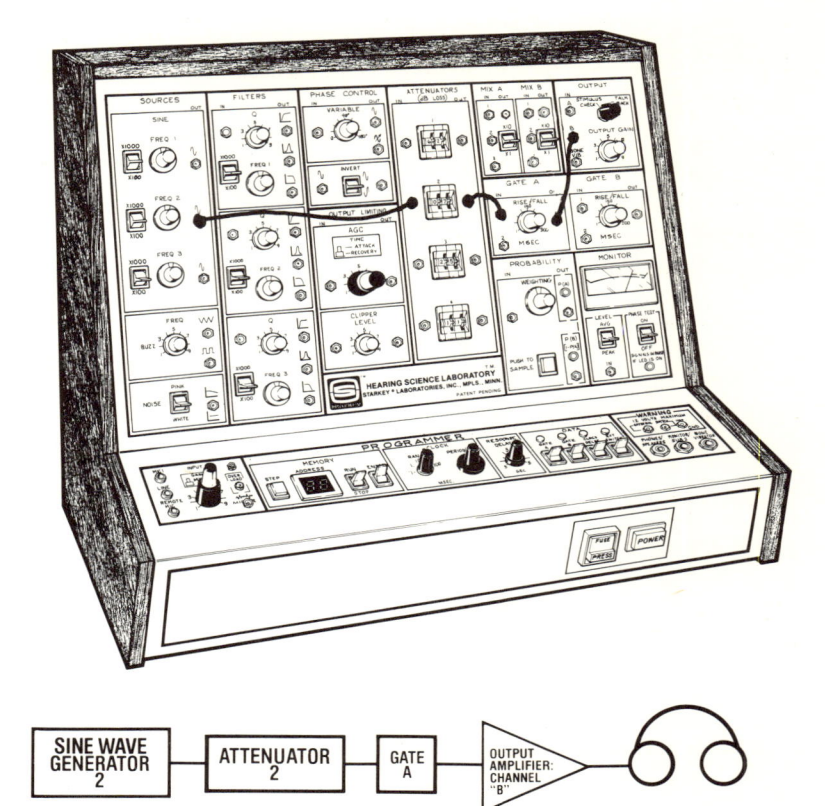

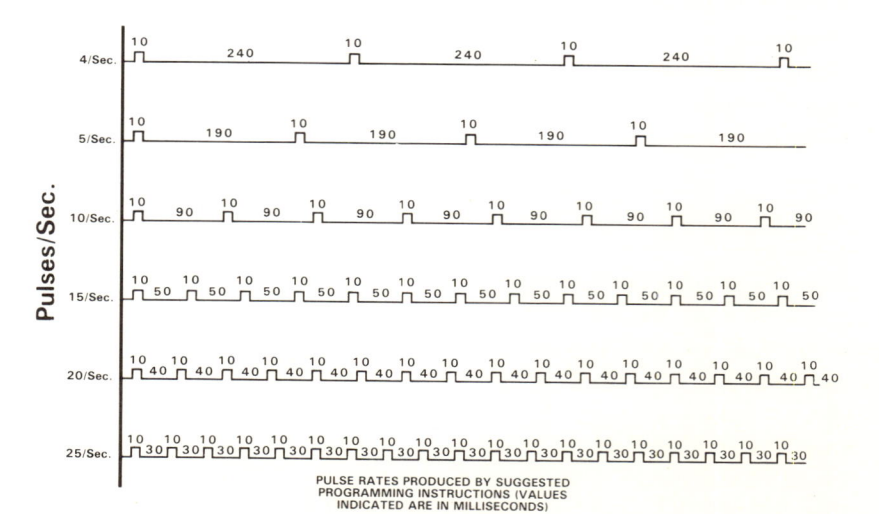

Purpose:
To examine the ability of a listener to estimate the number of events in an acoustic sequence.

Background Principle:
In Laboratory Experiment V-5, we noted that the auditory system is limited in its ability to identify the order of acoustic events. In the present demonstration we shall find that limits also exist for the number of discrete sounds that can be accurately counted within a given time period. The limited research which has explored this so-called *numerosity* phenomenon indicates that subjects in general tend to underestimate the number of stimuli in an acoustic sequence. A listener's ability to count tone bursts

tends to be fairly accurate below five pulses per second, but repetition rates between five and ten per second lead to numerous errors. Higher pulse rates (e.g., up to 30 per second) are typically estimated to be well below the actual number of events in the tone series, and subjects rarely report hearing more than ten pulses per second.

Procedure:

Sine Wave Generator #2 provides the test tone stimulus which is passed through Attenuator #2 and Electronic Gate "A". The suggested programming instructions will create pulsed tones having a duration of 10 milliseconds each and repetition rates ranging from four pulses per second to twenty-five per second, as desired. The tone bursts are then routed through one Output Amplifier channel and headphone.

Each test trial is preceded by a 1.5 second silent interval and a half-second warning light (provided by a series-connected bulb and battery that is controlled by the Programmer External Switch memory channel).

Exercises:

(1) Select an initial tone frequency near 1000 Hz and a test stimulus level that is roughly 40 dB above the listener's threshold. For each test condition, the subject must estimate the number of tone bursts that are presented.

(2) Repeat exercise #1 for several test tone frequencies and Sensation Levels and note any change in the subject's "accuracy of report."

(3) Repeat the basic listening task for a variety of durations for the tone pulse silent intervals and note if increasing or decreasing these values affects the subject's performance.

NOTES:

Selected References:

Cheatham, P.G. and White, C.T. (1954). Temporal numerosity: III. Auditory perception of number. *J. Exp. Psychol.*, **47**, 425-428.

Garner, W.R. (1951). The accuracy of counting repeated short tones. *J. Exp. Psychol.*, **41**, 310-316.

Gerber, S.E. (1974). Auditory temporality. In S.E. Gerber (Ed.) *Introductory Hearing Science.* pp. 172-186. Saunders Co., Philadelphia.

Perrott, D.R. and Williams, K.N. (1971). Auditory temporal resolution: gap detection as a function of interpulse frequency disparity. *Psychonomic Science*, **25**, 73-74.

Taubman, R.E. (1950). Studies in judged number: III. The judgment of auditory number. *J. Gen. Psychol.*, **43**, 167-194.

White, C.T. (1963). Temporal numerosity and the psychological unit of duration. *Psychol. Monogr.*, **77**, No. 12, 575.

EXPERIMENT V-7: DIFFERENTIAL SENSITIVITY FOR DURATION

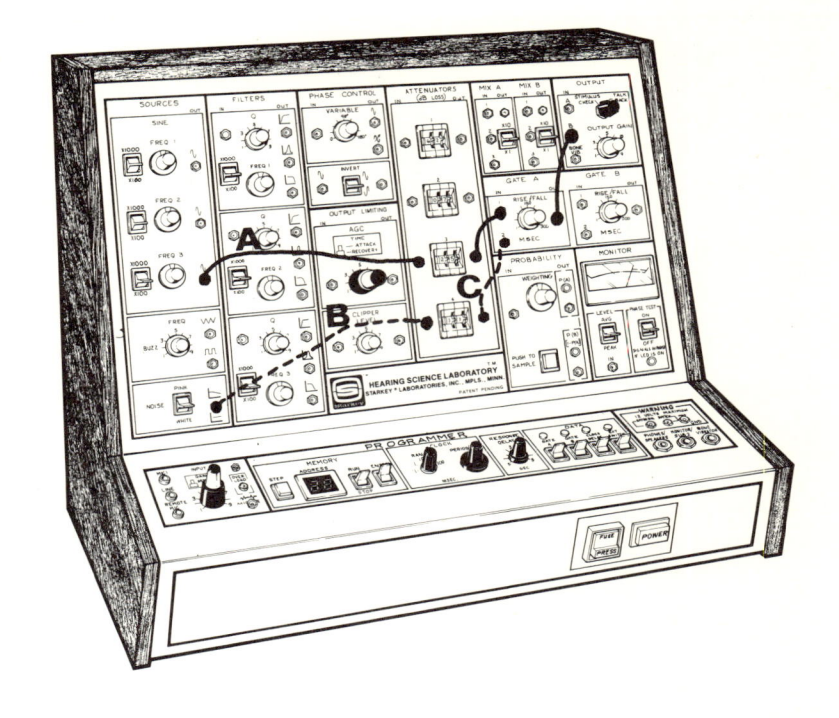

Purpose:
To demonstrate the ability of a listener to detect differences in the duration of brief sounds.

Background Principle:
Relatively tiny differences in the duration of speech sounds can alter stress and inflection patterns and thereby influence linguistic interpretation. Questions remain, however, as to the precise value of the smallest noticeable difference in duration. Different test procedures, interstimulus silent intervals, and standard and comparison tone levels are variables which can affect experimental results in this area. In the present demonstration, we shall explore this phenomenon by comparing a "standard" duration signal with a series of increasing duration comparison tones.

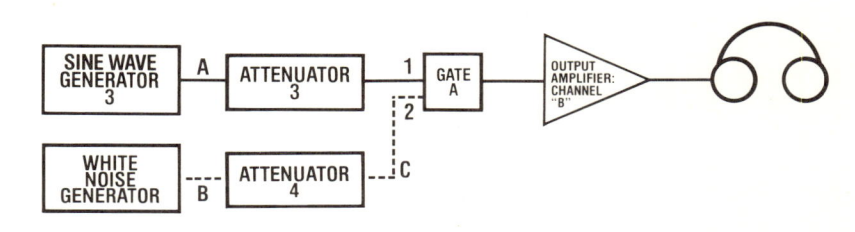

Procedure:
A pure tone signal is passed through an Attenuator and Electronic Gate before being sent to one Output Amplifier channel and headphone. A white noise may also be used as the stimulus for this listening task. This is achieved by disconnecting the pure tone connection (i.e., wire "A") and attaching wires "B" and "C" which route the noise to the second Input Jack of the Electronic Gate. The suggested programming instructions permit the "standard" test signal to switch on for 40 milliseconds, after which a one-half second interstimulus silent interval occurs followed by a variable duration "comparison" tone. By entering or erasing additional "switch-on" commands for Electronic Gate "A", the duration of the comparison signal may be changed in one millisecond increments as desired (see the programming suggestions table). Note that a two second pause is programmed to precede each test trial.

Exercises:
(1) Select an initial test tone frequency near 1000 Hz and an Attenuator #3 setting that produces a roughly 50 dB Sensation Level stimulus. Begin the comparison task with both signals equal in duration (i.e., 40 milliseconds each). The subject should always report whether the signals are the same or different. After some initial practice trials, enter additional switch-on commands to the Gate "A" Programmer Channel for memory addresses 81-95 (i.e., add up to 15 milliseconds to the duration of the comparison tone). The subject should be able to report that the two stimuli are different. For subsequent test trials, erase switch-on commands from the memory, two addresses at a time, until the subject cannot detect a difference in duration.

(2) Exercise #1 should be repeated for a variety of stimulus frequencies, and sensation levels and differences in test results should be noted.

(3) Repeat exercise #1, using white noise instead of a pure tone signal and contrast the subject's performance with the two types of stimuli.

(4) Repeat the basic comparison task with different standard signal durations (e.g., 100 msec, 150 msec, 250 msec, et al.) and comparison signal increments (e.g., steps of 5 or 10 milliseconds). Can you observe the presence of a possible trading relationship between the value of the JND for duration and the duration of the standard signal itself?

NOTES:

Selected References:

Abel, S.M. (1972a). Duration discrimination of noise and tone bursts. *J. Acoust. Soc. Am.,* **51,** 1219-1223.

Abel, S.M. (1972b). Discrimination of temporal gaps. *J. Acoust. Soc. Am.,* **52,** 519-524.

Chistovitch, L.A. (1959). Discrimination of the time interval between two short acoustic pulses. *Soviet Physics: Acoustics,* **6,** 480-484.

Creelman, C.D. (1962). Human discrimination of auditory duration. *J. Acoust. Soc. Am.,* **34,** 582-593.

Creelman, C.D. (1964). Human discrimination of auditory duration. In J.A. Swets (Ed.) *Signal detection and recognition by human observers.* Chapter 12, pp. 265-290. Wiley, New York.

Green, D.M. (1971). Temporal auditory acuity. *Psychol. Rev.,* **78,** 540-551.

Henry, F. (1948). Discrimination of the duration of a sound. *J. Exp. Psychol.,* **38,** 734-743.

Massaro, D.W. (1972). Perceptual images, processing time, and perceptual units in auditory perception. *Psychol. Rev.,* **79,** 124-145.

Rochester, S. (1971). Detection and duration discrimination of noise increments. *J. Acoust. Soc. Am.,* **49,** 1783-1789.

Ruhm, H.B., Mencke, E.O., Braxton, M., Cooper, W.A., Jr., and Rose, D.E. (1966). Differential sensitivity to duration of acoustic signals. *J. Speech Hear. Res.,* **9,** 371-384.

Masking Phenomena VI

EXPERIMENT VI-1: TONE-ON-TONE MASKING

Purpose:
To determine the threshold shift produced by the presence of one tone upon another.

Background Principle:
In Laboratory Experiment IV-1, we observed that the ear has a limited ability to analyze a complex sound into its component frequencies. We will now explore the fact that when the level of one stimulus is greater than another's, the weaker sound may not be perceived at all. The listening difficulties produced by this *masking* phenomenon are commonly encountered within such noisy environments as cocktail parties and city traffic. In a number of studies on masking, one pure tone has been used to mask another. Consider, for example, the masking effect that a 500 Hz, 80 dB *Sensation Level (SL)* tone has upon the perceptibility of several barely audible tones of differing frequency. (Note: the reference for dB SL is the subject's own threshold level at a given frequency.) One finds that the presence of the 500 Hz masker renders many of the other tones inaudible; their magnitudes must be increased by various amounts in order for them to be perceived again. The difference between a tone's threshold level in quiet and in the presence of a masking stimulus is called the *threshold shift*. The curves shown in Figure "A" display the threshold shift produced by a 500 Hz masking tone at several different magnitudes. Notice that when the 500 Hz masker is quite intense (e.g., at 80 dB SL), a substantial amount of threshold shift occurs for those tones having frequencies **above** the masker frequency, but little or no threshold shift is produced for those tones below 500 Hz; this is termed the *upward spread of masking*. When, however, the masking tone is quite weak (e.g., 20 dB SL), its masking influence extends symmetrically slightly above and below the masker frequency.

Procedure:
The *masking tone* from Sine Wave Generator #1 is passed through Attenuator #1 and into Mixer-Amplifier "A". The various *signal* tones that will be masked are obtained from Sine Wave Generator #2 and pass through Attenuator #2 as well as Electronic Gate "A", which is programmed to pulse the masked signal on and off, repeatedly. This pulsed signal should be easy to identify against the background of a masking stimulus that is on continuously. Both signals are combined within Mixer-Amplifier "A" and sent to Output Amplifier channel "A", which powers one headphone.

Exercises:
(1) Adjust the masking tone generator to a frequency near 500 Hz. Set the signal tone to an initial frequency that is substantially higher than that of the masker (e.g., 2000 or 4000 Hz). Find the threshold of audibility for each

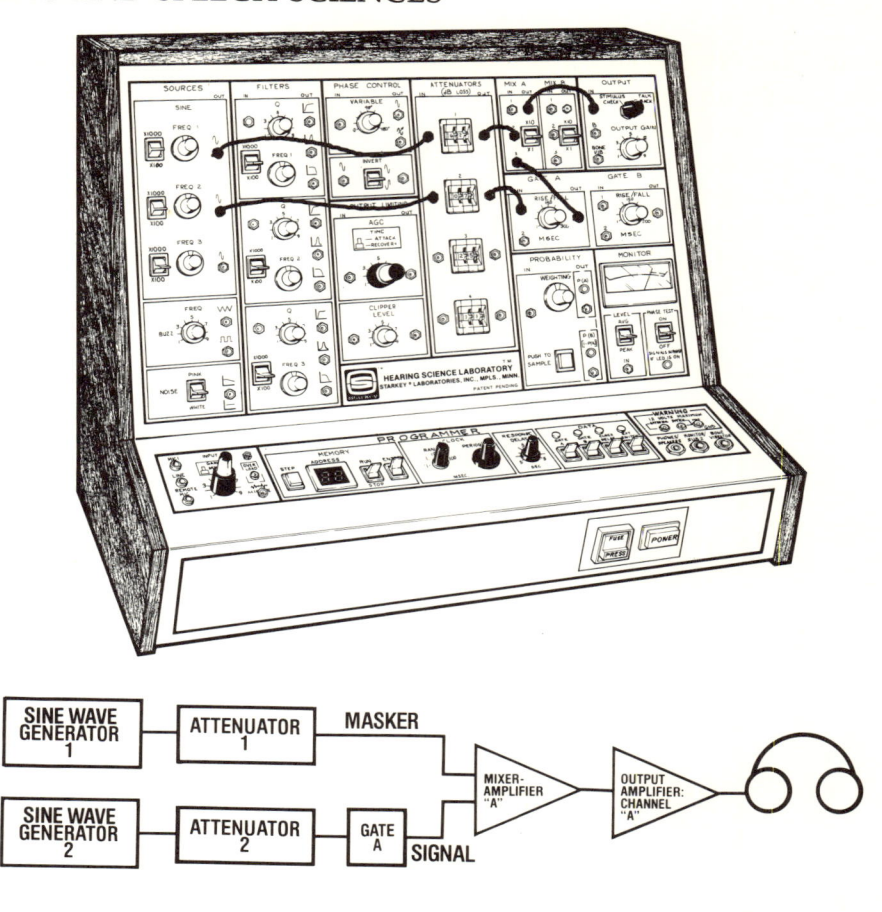

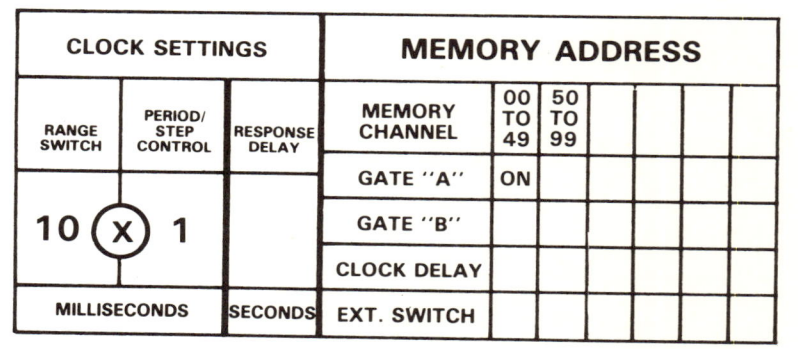

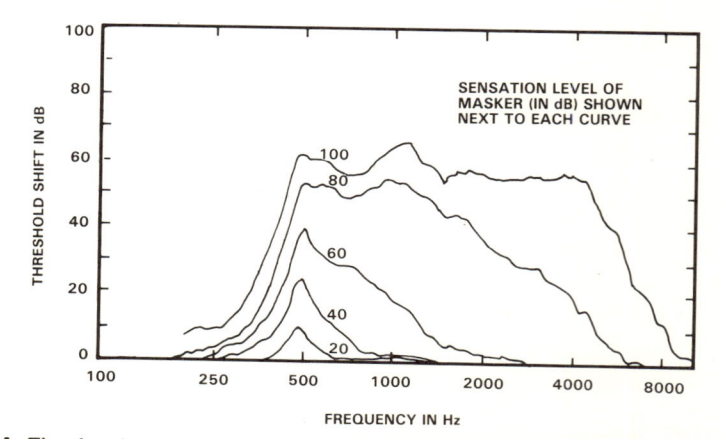

FIGURE A: The threshold shift produced by a 500 Hz masker tone will depend upon the frequency of the masked signal and the level of the masker stimulus. Note the "upward spread of masking" for higher level maskers and the relatively symmetrical masking effect for the less intense masking stimulus. (After Ehmer, 1959a).

tone alone. Next, set the masking tone to a level that is 60 dB more intense than its threshold value (i.e., 60 dB less attenuation for 60 dB SL). During the test, the experimenter gradually increases the intensity level of the pulsing signal tone until the subject reports its reappearance. The difference between the Attenuator settings, with and without the presence of the masking tone, is the subject's threshold shift (in dB) for the particular test conditions.

(2) Repeat exercise #1 for several different signal frequencies. Plot the threshold shift values you obtain upon the graph shown in Figure "B."

(3) Repeat exercise #2 with a 500 Hz masking stimulus only 20 dB more intense than its threshold level. Is the second masking curve you obtain more symmetrical than the first?

NOTES:

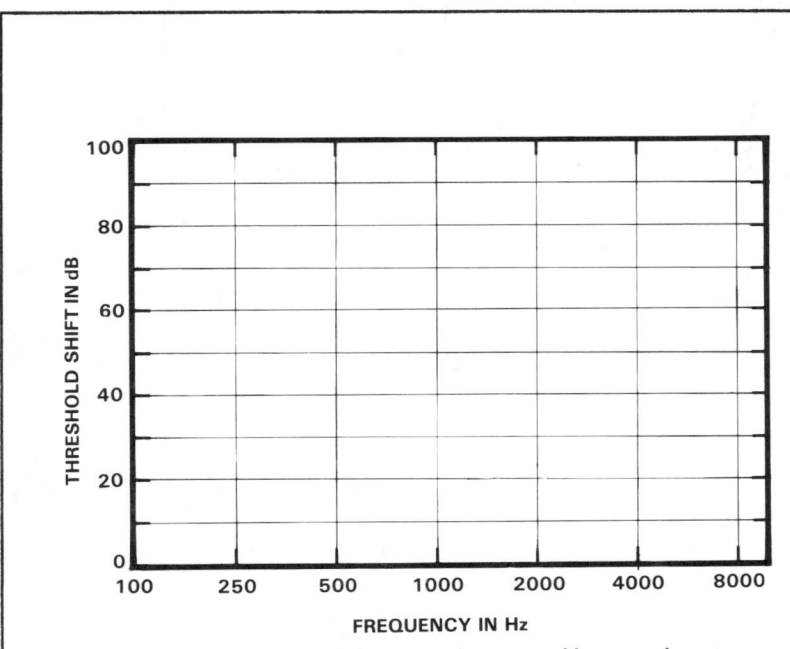

FIGURE B: Data graph for tone-on-tone masking experiment.

Selected References:

Carter, N.L. and Kryter, K.D. (1962). Masking of pure tones and speech. *J. Aud. Res.*, **2**, 66-98.

Clack, T.D. (1968). Aural harmonics: preliminary time-intensity relationships using the tone-on-tone masking technique. *J. Acoust. Soc. Am.*, **43**, 283-288.

Clack, T.D. (1975). Some influences of subjective tones in monaural tone-on-tone masking. *J. Acoust. Soc. Am.*, **57**, 172-180.

Ehmer, R.H. (1959a). Masking patterns of tones. *J. Acoust. Soc. Am.*, **31**, 1115-1120.

Ehmer, R.H. (1959b). Masking by tones vs. noise bands. *J. Acoust. Soc. Am.*, **31**, 1253-1256.

Garner, W.R. and Miller, G.A. (1947). The masked threshold of pure tones as a function of duration. *J. Exp. Psychol.*, **37**, 293-303.

Green, D.M. (1965). Masking with two tones. *J. Acoust. Soc. Am.*, **37**, 802-813.

Green, D.M. (1969). Masking with continuous and pulsed sinusoids. *J. Acoust. Soc. Am.*, **46**, 939-946.

Jeffress, L.A. (1975). Masking of tone by tone as a function of duration. *J. Acoust. Soc. Am.*, **58**, 399-403.

Leshowitz, B. and Cudahy, E. (1972). Masking with continuous and gated sinusoids. *J. Acoust. Soc. Am.*, **51**, 1921-1929.

Leshowitz, B. and Wightman, F.L. (1971). On-frequency masking with continuous sinusoids. *J. Acoust. Soc. Am.*, **49**, 1180-1190.

Small, A. (1959). Pure tone masking. *J. Acoust. Soc. Am.*, **31**, 1619-1625.

Vogten, L.L.M. (1978). Simultaneous pure-tone masking: The dependence of masking asymmetries on intensity. *J. Acoust. Soc. Am.*, **63**, 1509-1519.

Wegel, R.L. and Lane, C.E. (1924). The auditory masking of one pure tone by another and its probable relation to the dynamics of the inner ear. *Physics Review*, **23**, 266-285. Also in J.D. Harris (Ed.) *Forty germinal papers in human hearing*. J. Aud. Res., Groton, Connecticut. (1969).

Wightman, F.L. (1969). Binaural masking with sine-wave maskers. *J. Acoust. Soc. Am.*, **45**, 72-78.

EXPERIMENT VI-2: THE CRITICAL BAND

Purpose:
To examine the selectivity of the hearing mechanism.

Background Principle:
Experiments that employ pure tones for both masker and masked stimuli are plagued by the presence of such two-tone interactions as beats and difference tones. In an attempt to avoid these experimental artifacts, researchers have used various types of complex, "noisy" stimuli as maskers. The *critical bandwidth* is a term used to describe certain properties of the ear, especially seen in particular masking experiments. Theorists have often characterized our hearing mechanism to be similar in nature and performance to a network of filters. The critical bandwidth is a description of the selectivity of these hypothetical filters toward various forms of auditory stimulation. In one demonstration of this concept, a tone is presented to a listener within a background of narrow band noise. As the bandwidth of the masking noise is gradually increased, with its overall energy level kept constant, the tone undergoes an ever greater threshold shift — until a certain bandwidth is reached. Beyond this "critical bandwidth" limit, no further threshold shift occurs at moderate intensity levels. In this type of experiment, the critical bandwidth of the ear, at specific test tone frequencies, may be defined by the number of hertz within the widest, maximally effective masking noise band. Actual critical bandwidths range between 100 to 200 Hz for stimuli below 1000 Hz and between 200 to 3500 Hz for stimuli above 1000 Hz. A relatively simple technique for obtaining indirect estimates of the critical bandwidth is to compare the masked threshold level for a tone to the energy per cycle, or *spectrum level,* in a given wide band masking noise. The difference in decibels between these two quantities (actually the ratio formed by their respective energies) is known as the *critical ratio.* The spectrum level of a masker may be determined from the overall sound pressure level of the noise by employing the following relationship:

Spectrum Level = Overall Sound Pressure Level − 10 log (Noise Bandwidth)

An 80 dB SPL noise for example, having a bandwidth of 10,000 Hz, would have a spectrum level of:

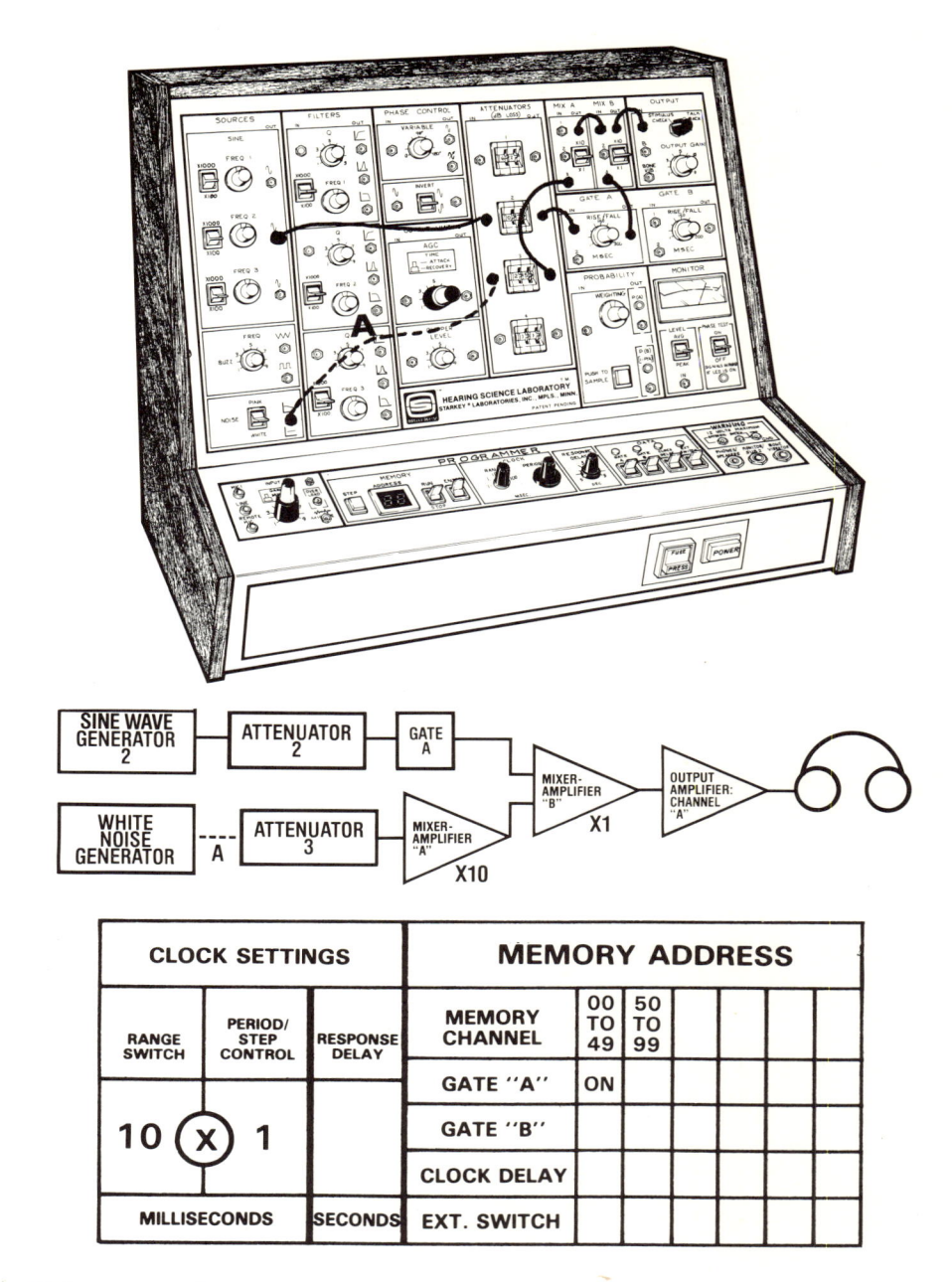

$$\text{dB SL} = 80 - 10\,(\log 10{,}000)$$
$$= 80 - 10\,(4)$$
$$= 40 \text{ dB Spectrum Level}$$

If, for a tone of 1000 Hz, the masked threshold level for a listener were 58 dB SPL with this particular noise, then the critical ratio would be:

Critical Ratio (in dB) = Masked Threshold − Noise Spectrum Level
18 dB = 58 dB SPL − 40 dB Spectrum Level

The corresponding critical bandwidth estimate for this critical ratio may be computed from the following relationship:

$$\log (\text{Critical Bandwidth}) = \frac{\text{Critical Ratio}}{10}$$

Thus, for our example:

$$\log (\text{Critical Bandwidth}) = \frac{18}{10} = 1.8$$

With the aid of a log table or calculator, we find that the number whose log is 1.8 (i.e., the *antilog* of 1.8) is 63. The estimated critical bandwidth is, therefore, 63 Hz. Direct measurements of the critical bandwidth, however, have revealed that the critical ratio is roughly 2.5 times smaller than the actual critical bandwidth for frequencies above 200 Hz (the actual critical bandwidth at 1 KHz would therefore be approximately 160 Hz). Accounts of how this disparity arose from the mistaken research assumptions and data of early investigations may be found within the selected reference section below.

Procedure:

The white noise masker is sent through Attenuator #3, Mixer-Amplifier "A", Mixer-Amplifier "B", and one Output Amplifier and headphone. The pure tone signal is passed through its own Attenuator, an Electronic Gate, and Mixer-Amplifier "B" where it is combined with the noise. The suggested programming instructions will permit the tone to repeatedly pulse for 0.5 sec. and off for the same duration.

Exercises:

Select a pure tone frequency near 1000 Hz. Set the Mixer-Amplifier "A" Gain Switch to the *X* 10 (i.e., 20 dB Gain) position. With dashed circuit wire "A" temporarily disconnected and with the tone Attenuator set to 50 dB attenuation, adjust the Output Gain Control Knob until the subject's threshold, in quiet, is obtained for the pulsed tone. If available, a sound level meter and artificial ear may be used to accurately measure the various tone and noise sound pressure levels in this exercise. Otherwise, use the approximate values shown in Table I below. Set the noise Attenuator to 00 dB and reconnect wire "A". Raise the level of the tone by decreasing the Tone Attenuator settings until the subject detects the signal in the background of loud noise. The masked threshold (in dB SPL) is equal to the sound pressure level of the tone-in-quiet plus the additional number of dB required to hear the tone-in-noise. Assume that the bandwidth of the noise reaching the listener is 6000 Hz (i.e., the approximate bandwidth which the headphone will pass). Measure the overall SPL of the noise or use the third column of Table I for an approximate value.

Table I

Output Amplifier Gain Control Position	Approximate Tone Output (in dB SPL) (For 50 dB Atten.)	Approximate Noise Output (in dB SPL) (For 0 dB Atten. and 20 dB Gain)
3	28	85
4	31	88
5	34	91
6	37	94
7	40	97
8	43	100
9	46	103

As described in the Background Principle Section above, calculate the spectrum level of the noise from its dB SPL and bandwidth values (Note: the log of 6000 is 3.78). Subtract the spectrum level from the subject's masked threshold level to compute the critical ratio. Finally, calculate the estimate of the critical bandwidth from the critical ratio. If your results are far from roughly 160 Hz, list the several variables which may have contributed to the discrepancy.

NOTES:

Selected References:

van den Brink, G. (1964). Detection of tone pulses of various durations in noise of various bandwidths. *J. Acoust. Soc. Am.*, **36**, 1206-1211.

Greenwood, D.D. (1961). Auditory masking and the critical band. *J. Acoust. Soc. Am.*, **33**, 484-502.

Haggard, M.P. (1974). Feasibility of rapid critical bandwidth estimates. *J. Acoust. Soc. Am.*, **55**, 304-308.

Kaplan, H.L. (1975). The five distractors experiment: exploring the critical band with contaminated white noise. *J. Acoust. Soc. Am.*, **58**, 404-411.

Moore, B.C.J. (1975). Mechanisms of masking. *J. Acoust. Soc. Am.*, **57**, 391-399.

Patterson, R.D. (1976). Auditory filter shapes derived with noise stimuli. *J. Acoust. Soc. Am.*, **59**, 640-654.

Plomp, R. (1964). The ear as a frequency analyzer. *J. Acoust. Soc. Am.*, **36**, 1628-1636.

Reed, C.M. and Bilger, R.C. (1973). A comparative study of S/N$_0$ and E/N$_0$. *J. Acoust. Soc. Am.*, **53**, 1039-1044.

Sharf, B. (1970). Critical bands. In J.V. Tobias (Ed.) *Foundations of modern auditory theory*. Vol. I. Academic Press Inc., New York

Soderquist, D.R. (1970). Frequency analysis and the critical band. *Psychon. Sci.*, **21**, 117-119.

Srinivasan, R. (1971). Auditory critical bandwidth for short-duration signals. *J. Acoust. Soc. Am.*, **50**, 616-622.

Swets, J.A., Green, D.M., and Tanner, W.P., Jr. (1962). On the width of critical bands. *J. Acoust. Soc. Am.*, **34**, 108-113.

Zwicker, E., Flottorp, G., and Stevens, S.S. (1957). Critical bandwidth in loudness summation. *J. Acoust. Soc. Am.*, **29**, 548-557.

Zwicker, E. and Fastl, H. (1972). On the development of the critical band. *J. Acoust. Soc. Am.*, **52**, 699-702.

EXPERIMENT VI-3: THE RELATIONSHIP BETWEEN MASKING LEVEL AND THRESHOLD SHIFT

Purpose:
To demonstrate the relationship between the level of a white noise masking stimulus and the threshold shift it produces.

Background Principle:
As discussed in the preceding experiment, only a relatively narrow range of noise frequencies within some "critical band" is necessary to mask a pure tone. What masking effect, then, would a white noise (having equal energy per cycle) exert upon the detection of tonal or speech stimuli. A simple and classic experiment reveals that for simultaneous presentations of a signal and moderate level white noise, a *linear*, or one to one, correspondence exists between a change in masker level and the threshold shift it produces (see Figure "A").

Procedure:
The white noise masking stimulus is passed through an Attenuator and into a Mixer-Amplifier. The pure tone signal that is to be masked is sent to its own Attenuator and then to Electronic Gate "A" which will switch the tone on and off, once a second, in accordance with the suggested programming instructions. Both the noise and tone are combined within the Mixer-Amplifier and delivered to one Output Amplifier channel and headphone.

Exercises:
(1) Use an initial tone frequency near 1000 Hz. Set the signal and noise Attenuators to supra-threshold levels that permit the tone to remain just barely audible. Now increase the level of the noise by a fixed amount (e.g., 10 dB less attenuation). The tone should no longer be detected. Compensate for the additional masking level by increasing the magnitude of the tone in one decibel steps. Does the tone reappear when its level is increased by about 10 dB? Repeat these noise and tone increments for additional tone frequencies to satisfy yourself that each additional decibel of masking energy shifts the threshold of the tone by an equivalent amount.

(2) Repeat exercise #1 for live or recorded speech signals. Do you find, as did Hawkins and Stevens (1950), that the one to one relationship between masking level and threshold shift is also evident for connected discourse?

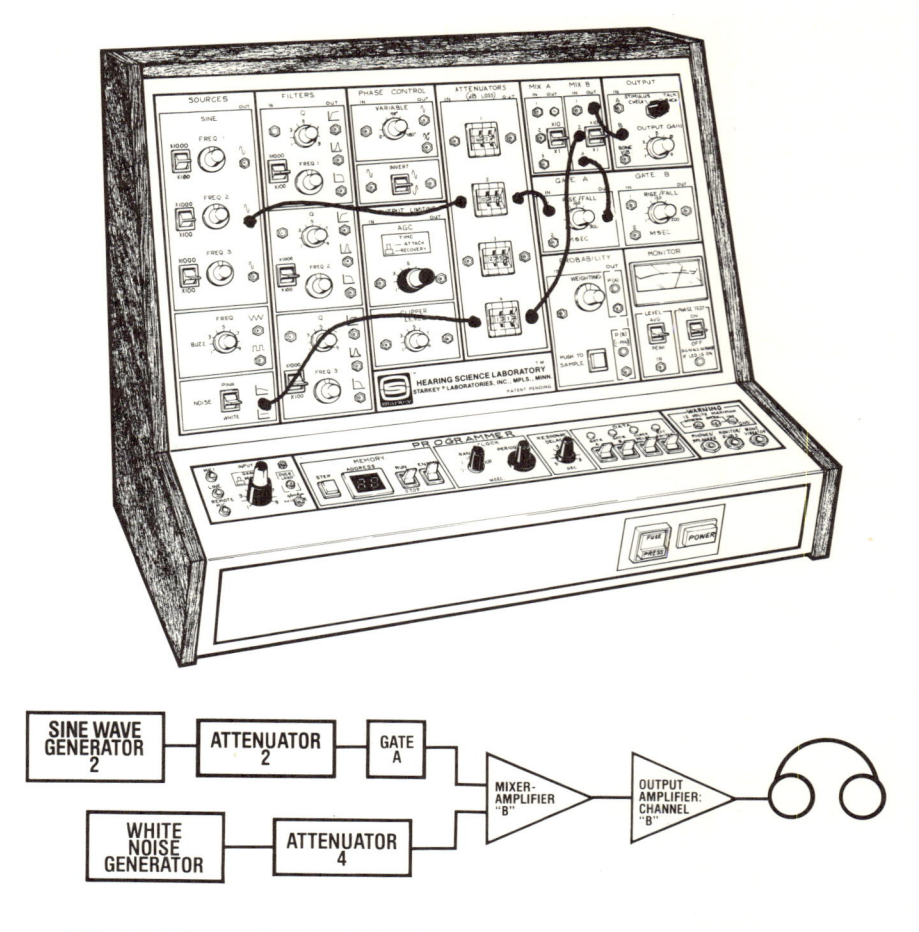

FIGURE A: A linear relationship exists between the level of a white noise masker and the pure tone threshold shift it produces. (After Hawkins and Stevens, 1950).

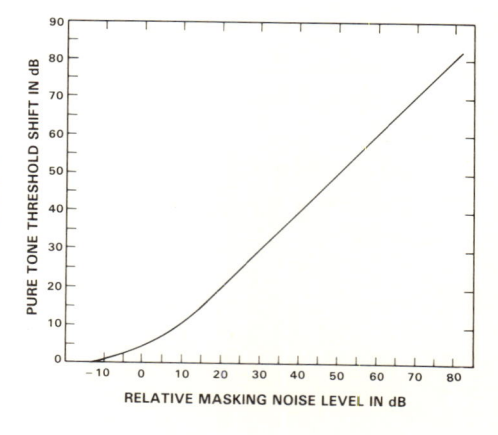

NOTES:

Selected References:

Bilger, R.C. and Hirsh, I.J. (1956). Masking of tones by bands of noise. *J. Acoust. Soc. Am.*, **28**, 623-630.

Bourbon, W.T., Evans, T.R., and Deatherage, B.H. (1968). Effects of intensity on "critical bands" for tonal stimuli as determined by band-limiting. *J. Acoust. Soc. Am.*, **43**, 56-59.

Campbell, R.A. (1964). Masker level and noise signal detection. *J. Acoust. Soc. Am.*, **36**, 570-575.

Greenwood, D.D. (1961). Auditory masking and the critical band. *J. Acoust. Soc. Am.*, **33**, 484-502.

Hawkins, J.E., Jr. and Stevens, S.S. (1950). The masking of pure tones and of speech by white noise. *J. Acoust. Soc. Am.*, **22**, 6-13.

Miller, G.A. (1947). Sensitivity to changes in the intensity of white noise and its relation to masking and loudness. *J. Acoust. Soc. Am.*, **19**, 609-619.

Moore, B.C.J. (1975). Mechanisms of masking. *J. Acoust. Soc. Am.*, **57**, 391-399.

EXPERIMENT VI-4: CENTRAL MASKING

Purpose:
To note the threshold shift of a tone in one ear when a masker is introduced to the contralateral ear.

Background Principle:
It is possible to raise the threshold of a tone in one ear slightly by delivering another stimulus (tone or noise) to the contralateral ear. This phenomenon has been called *central masking,* for the effect is believed to arise from some process within the central nervous system. Central masking threshold shifts can occur even though the masking stimulus level is less than the magnitude at which the sound crosses through the skull to the opposite side of the head (see Laboratory Experiment VII-9). The degree of threshold shift that occurs with central masking is typically no greater than 10 decibels, and the effect is most pronounced when pulsed, rather than when continuous maskers are employed.

Procedure:
The pure tone test signal is passed through an Attenuator, Electronic Gate "A", and Output Amplifier channel "A" which powers one of the headphones. The white noise masking stimulus is routed through its own Attenuator, Electronic Gate "B", Output Amplifier channel "B", and the second headphone. The Electronic Gates are programmed to provide a simultaneous onset for the tone and noise. The tone remains on for 10 milliseconds, while the noise remains on for 250 milliseconds. A two second pause separates the test stimuli presentations. Note that a bulb and battery may be connected in series with the External Switch memory channel Output Jacks so that a warning light will define the listening interval for the subject (see Laboratory Experiment II-2).

CLOCK SETTINGS				MEMORY ADDRESS			
RANGE SWITCH	PERIOD/ STEP CONTROL	RESPONSE DELAY	MEMORY CHANNEL	00	1 TO 24	25	26 TO 99
10	×1	2	GATE "A"	ON			
			GATE "B"	ON	ON		
			CLOCK DELAY			ON	
MILLISECONDS		SECONDS	EXT. SWITCH	ON	ON		

Exercises:
(1) Adjust the frequency control to an initial value near 1000 Hz. The listener's responsibility is to report when the tone is just barely audible (i.e., at 0 dB Sensation Level). For each of the test conditions listed below, the experimenter will record that tone Attenuator setting at which the subject's 0 dB Sensation Level is obtained.

A. Steady Tone in Quiet
The Programmer should be stopped at memory address 00 which permits both the tone and noise to remain on continuously. Set both Attenuators to 60 dB. Temporarily disconnect one end of dashed circuit wire "A", thereby eliminating the noise, and obtain the listener's threshold in quiet for the tone by varying the Output Amplifier Gain Control Knob. (Note: If more signal level is needed, pass each stimulus through a separate 20 dB Gain Mixer-Amplifier). Next, obtain the subject's threshold for the noise alone by reconnecting dashed wire "A" and disconnecting wire "B." These 0 dB SL values will serve as reference points for the signal and masker.

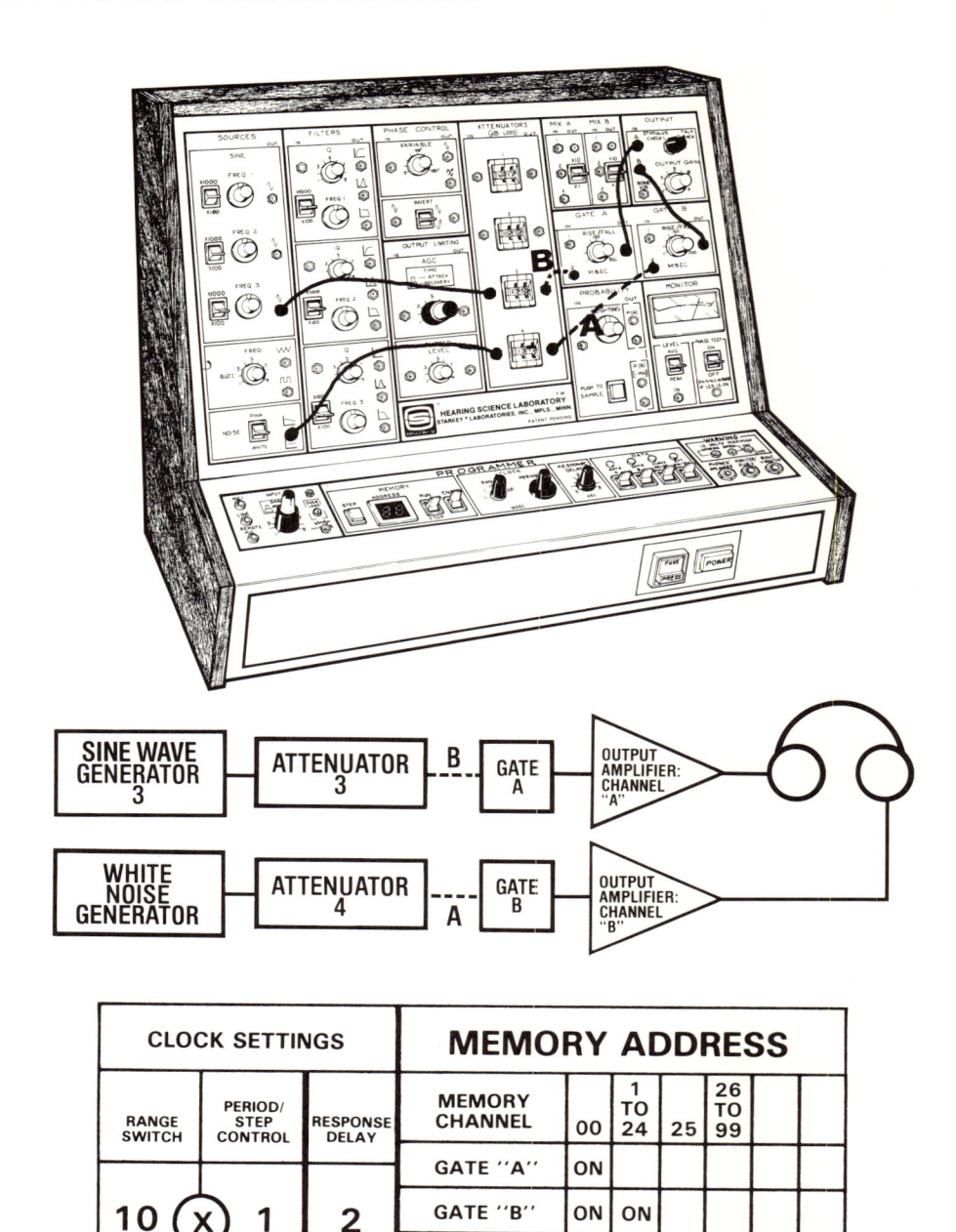

B. Steady Tone in Background of Steady Contralateral Noise
With the Programmer Clock stopped at memory address 00, reconnect both dashed circuit wires and gradually increase the noise level to an Attenuator setting which masks out the 0 dB Sensation Level tone obtained for exercise #1A. Once the tone has been masked, increase its level until it becomes audible again. The difference in dB between this new Attenuator setting and the original level is the amount of threshold shift produced by central masking.

C. **Pulsed Tone in Quiet**
With the Programmer Clock running, disconnect dashed circuit wire "A" and determine the pulsed tone threshold.

D. **Pulsed Tone within Steady Contralateral Noise**
With the Programmer Clock running, disconnect dashed circuit wire "A" at Electronic Gate "B" and route it directly to Output Amplifier channel "B." This permits the noise to remain on continuously. Recheck the pulsed tone threshold and note any threshold shift that occurs.

E. **Pulsed Tone with Pulsed Noise**
With the Programmer Clock running, reconnect dashed circuit wire "A" to Electronic Gate "B." Set the noise Attenuator to a value that is 60 dB above the threshold for the noise obtained in exercise #1A.

Contrast the efficacy of the masking stimulus for the various test conditions.

(2) Repeat exercise #1E for several noise levels (e.g., 50, 40, 30, and 20 dB SL).

(3) Repeat exercise 1E with the tone burst delayed in onset by 20, 40, and 60 milliseconds behind the onset of the noise masker. This is easily accomplished by reprogramming Gate "B" to switch on at memory addresses: 02, 04, and 06, respectively, rather than at address 00.

(4) Repeat exercise #1 for a very low frequency tone, such as 250 Hz. Do the differences between the masking test conditions still occur?

NOTES:

Selected References:

Dirks, D.D. and Malmquist, C. (1964). Changes in bone conduction thresholds produced by masking in the nontest ear. *J. Speech Hear. Res.*, **7**, 271-278.

Dirks, D.D. and Malmquist, C. (1965). Shifts in air conduction thresholds produced by pulsed and continuous contralateral masking. *J. Acoust. Soc. Am.*, **37**, 631-637.

Ingham, J.G. (1957). The effect upon monaural sensitivity of continuous stimulation of the opposite ear. *Q.J. Exp. Psychol.*, **9**, 52-60.

Ingham, J.G. (1959). Variations in cross masking with frequency. *J. Exp. Psychol.*, **58**, 199-205.

Sherrick, C.E. and Mangabeira-Albernaz, P.L. (1961). Auditory threshold shifts produced by simultaneously pulsed contralateral stimuli. *J. Acoust. Soc. Am.*, **33**, 1381-1385.

Zwislocki, J.J. (1953). Acoustic attenuation between the ears. *J. Acoust. Soc. Am.*, **25**, 752-759.

Zwislocki, J.J. (1971). Central masking and neural activity in the cochlear nucleus. *Audiology*, **10**, 48-59.

Zwislocki, J.J. (1972). A theory of central auditory masking and its partial validation. *J. Acoust. Soc. Am.*, **52**, 644-659.

Zwislocki, J.J., Buining, E., and Glantz, J. (1968). Frequency distribution of central masking. *J. Acoust. Soc. Am.*, **43**, 1267-1271.

Zwislocki, J.J., Damianopoulos, E.N., Buining, E., and Glantz, J. (1967). Central masking: some steady-state and transient effects, *Percept. Psychophys.*, **2**, 59-64.

EXPERIMENT VI-5: FORWARD AND BACKWARD MASKING

Purpose:
To examine the threshold shift for a signal that precedes or follows a masking stimulus.

Background Principle:
In previous experiments, both the masking and masked stimuli were presented simultaneously to the listener. It is also possible to create a threshold shift when the masker precedes or follows the signal. These two phenomena are known respectively as *forward masking* and *backward masking* (see Figure "A"). The most influential variable in forward and backward masking appears to be the duration of the silent interval between the masker and signal, often termed Δt. If this value exceeds roughly 100 milliseconds (depending upon the specific test situation), little or no forward or backward masking will occur. The precise nature of these phenomena is still open to speculation.

Procedure:
The pure tone signal to be masked is sent through an Attenuator and then passed through Electronic Gate "A". The white noise used as the masking stimulus for this experiment is also sent through its own Attenuator and then to Electronic Gate "B". The suggested programming instructions permit the two Gates to switch on and off in two different sequences. The noise precedes the signal tone for the forward masking task but will follow the tone in the backward masking condition. A two second pause for the listener's response is provided after each test configuration by the Programmer Delay Channel. The output from each Gate is combined within a Mixer-Amplifier and then delivered to one Output Amplifier channel and headphone.

Exercises:
(1) Select 1000 Hz as your initial signal tone frequency. Set the noise Attenuator to read 65 dB. With the Programmer Clock stopped at any Memory Address for which the noise is continuously on, adjust the Output Amplifier Gain Control Knob until the noise is just barely audible to the listener. We shall consider this point his threshold (i.e., 0 dB Sensation Level) for the noise. If the noise Attenuator is then set to read 00, a fixed noise level of roughly 65 dB Sensation Level will be provided to the observer. While the Programmer is running through either the forward or backward masking test sequences, disconnect the noise output wire ("A") and adjust the tone Attenuator until the subject's threshold for the signal-in-quiet is determined. Then, reconnect the noise and readjust the tone Attenuator until the subject's signal-in-noise threshold is obtained. Note the difference in level settings. For the particular programming instruc-

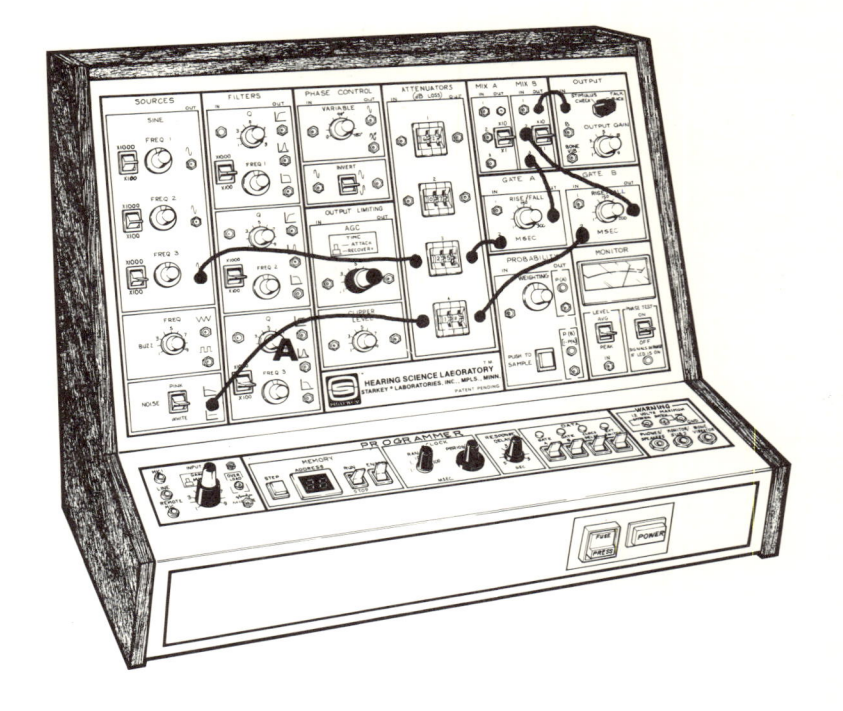

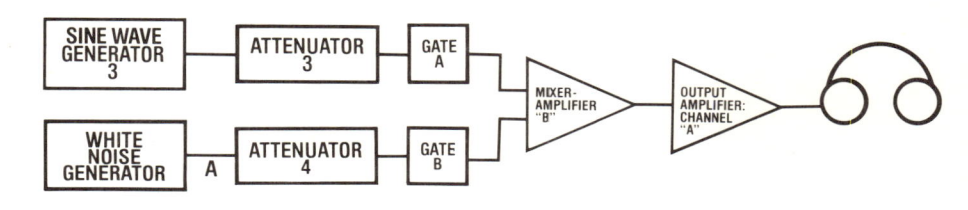

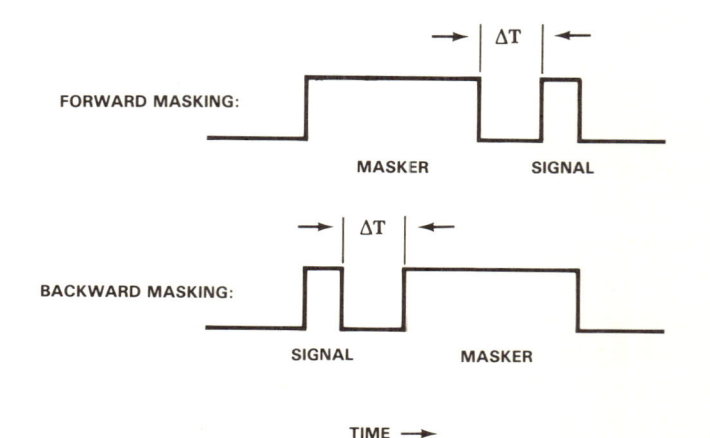

FIGURE A: The sequence of events in forward and backward masking listening tasks.

tions shown above, the duration of the tone, silent interval, and masking noise will be 40, 2, and 150 milliseconds, respectively. For these temporal conditions, you may find that there will be up to 20 dB more of a threshold shift produced by backward masking than by forward masking.

(2) Repeat the forward and backward masking tasks for the various parameter values shown below. Note which variable seems to exert the greatest and least effect upon the threshold shift of the tone.

Tone Duration	Masker Intensity	Silent Interval Duration (Δt)	Tone Freq.
10 & 80 msec.	20 & 40 dB SL	10, 20, 40, & 100 msec.	200 Hz & 4 kHz

(3) Use another pure tone as the masking stimulus instead of the white noise masker. Do you find that the forward and backward masking effects for two tones are similar to the earlier, simultaneous "tone on tone" masking experiment?

NOTES:

Selected References:

Deatherage, B.H. and Evans, T.R. (1969). Binaural masking: backward, forward, and simultaneous effects. *J. Acoust. Soc. Am.*, **46**, 362-371.

Dirks, D.D. and Bower, D. (1970). Effect of forward and backward masking on speech intelligibility. *J. Acoust. Soc. Am.*, **47**, 1003-1008.

Elliott, L.L. (1962a). Backward masking: monotic and dichotic conditions. *J. Acoust. Soc. Am.*, **34**, 1108-1115.

Elliott, L.L. (1962b). Backward and forward masking of probe tones of different frequencies. *J. Acoust. Soc. Am.*, **34**, 1116-1117.

Elliott, L.L. (1969). Masking of tones before, during, and after brief silent periods in noise. *J. Acoust. Soc. Am.*, **45**, 1277-1279.

Elliott, L.L. (1971). Backward and forward masking. *Audiology*, **10**, 65-76.

Leshowitz, B. and Cudahy, E. (1972). Masking with continuous and gated sinusoids. *J. Acoust. Soc. Am.*, **51**, 1921-1929.

Massaro, D.W. (1975). Backward recognition masking. *J. Acoust. Soc. Am.*, **58**, 1059-1065.

Patterson, J.H. (1971). Additivity of forward and backward masking as a function of signal frequency. *J. Acoust. Soc. Am.*, **50**, 1123-1125.

Penner, M.J. (1974). Effect of masker duration and masker level on forward and backward masking. *J. Acoust. Soc. Am.*, **56**, 179-182.

Penner, M.J., Robinson, C.E., and Green, D.M. (1972). The critical masking interval. *J. Acoust. Soc. Am.*, **52**, 1661-1668.

Pickett, J. (1959). Backward masking. *J. Acoust. Soc. Am.*, **31**, 1613-1615.

Plomp, R. (1964). Rate of decay of auditory sensation. *J. Acoust. Soc. Am.*, **36**, 277-282.

Pollack, I. (1973). Forward, backward and combined masking: implications for an auditory integration period. *Qtly J. Exp. Psychol.*, **25**, 424-432.

Robinson, C.E. and Pollack, I. (1971). Forward and backward masking: testing a discrete perceptual-moment hypothesis in audition. *J. Acoust. Soc. Am.*, **50**, 1512-1519.

Robinson, C.E. and Pollack, I. (1973). Interaction between forward and backward masking: a measure of the integrating period of the auditory system. *J. Acoust. Soc. Am.*, **53**, 1313-1316.

Scharf, B. (1971). Fundamentals of auditory masking. *Audiology*, **10**, 30-40.

Smiarowski, R.A. and Carhart, R. (1975). Relations among temporal resolution, forward masking, and simultaneous masking. *J. Acoust. Soc. Am.*, **57**, 1169-1174.

Wilson, R.H. and Carhart, R. (1971). Forward and backward masking: interactions and additivity. *J. Acoust. Soc. Am.*, **49**, 1254-1263.

EXPERIMENT VI-6: PULSATION THRESHOLD (THE "CONTINUITY EFFECT")

Purpose:
To demonstrate that the temporal character of a pulsating signal may be altered by the presence of a non-simultaneous masking stimulus.

Background Principle:
In most masking experiments, the "masker," such as a noise, is presented at the same time as the "signal" that is to be detected (e.g., a pure tone or speech). The "masked threshold" refers to a shift in the detectability of the signal (see, for example, Laboratory Experiments VI-1 thru VI-4). In the present demonstration, however, we are concerned with a non-simultaneous sequence of stimuli in which a pulsed masker influences the perception of the temporal characteristics of a pulsating signal. When, for example, a pulsating 1000 Hz tone signal is alternated with fixed level white-noise bursts, the tone indeed appears to pulsate for high sensation levels (e.g., > 40 dB Sensation Level) but loses degrees of its interrupted character at lower signal levels (e.g., between 10 and 40 dB Sensation Level). The masking effects of the noise burst in this procedure are not measured by a change in the detection threshold of the signal, as noted above for simultaneous masking procedures. Rather, the perception of the test signal can be altered, sounding as if it is on **continuously.** The name given to this phenomenon is, therefore, *pulsation threshold,* or the *continuity effect.* Pulsation threshold is taken to be the highest level at which the test signal is perceived to be continuous (although it is always really alternating with the masker).

Procedure:
The pure tone signal from Sine Wave Generator #2 is sent through an Attenuator and Electronic Gate "A." The output from the White Noise Generator is routed through Attenuator #4 and Gate "B." The outputs from both Gates are combined within Mixer-Amplifier "B" and then delivered to one Output Amplifier channel and headphone (or loudspeaker). The suggested programming instructions will alternate the two Gates (and their respective signals) on and off for periods of 125 milliseconds each. Adjust the Rise/Fall Time Control Knob of each Gate to the first counterclockwise dial scale marking (i.e., ≃ 40 msec.) so as to reduce audible transients during the demonstration.

Exercises:
(Note: Pulsation threshold is a subtle effect that requires practice listening within a quiet environment. An observer's level of "selective concentration" for the effect will also be found to influence test results.)

(1) Set Attenuator #4 to a value of 5 dB and the Output Amplifier Gain Control Knob to dial scale position "5". Select an initial test tone frequency near 1000 Hz. Vary the level of the tone signal between Attenuator #2 settings of 5 and 40 dB while the Programmer Clock is running. Note the level at which the signal pulsations cease and a continuous tone is perceived. Alternately remove and reconnect circuit wire "A" which carries the white noise masker. Note how the signal pulsations reappear when the noise is removed.

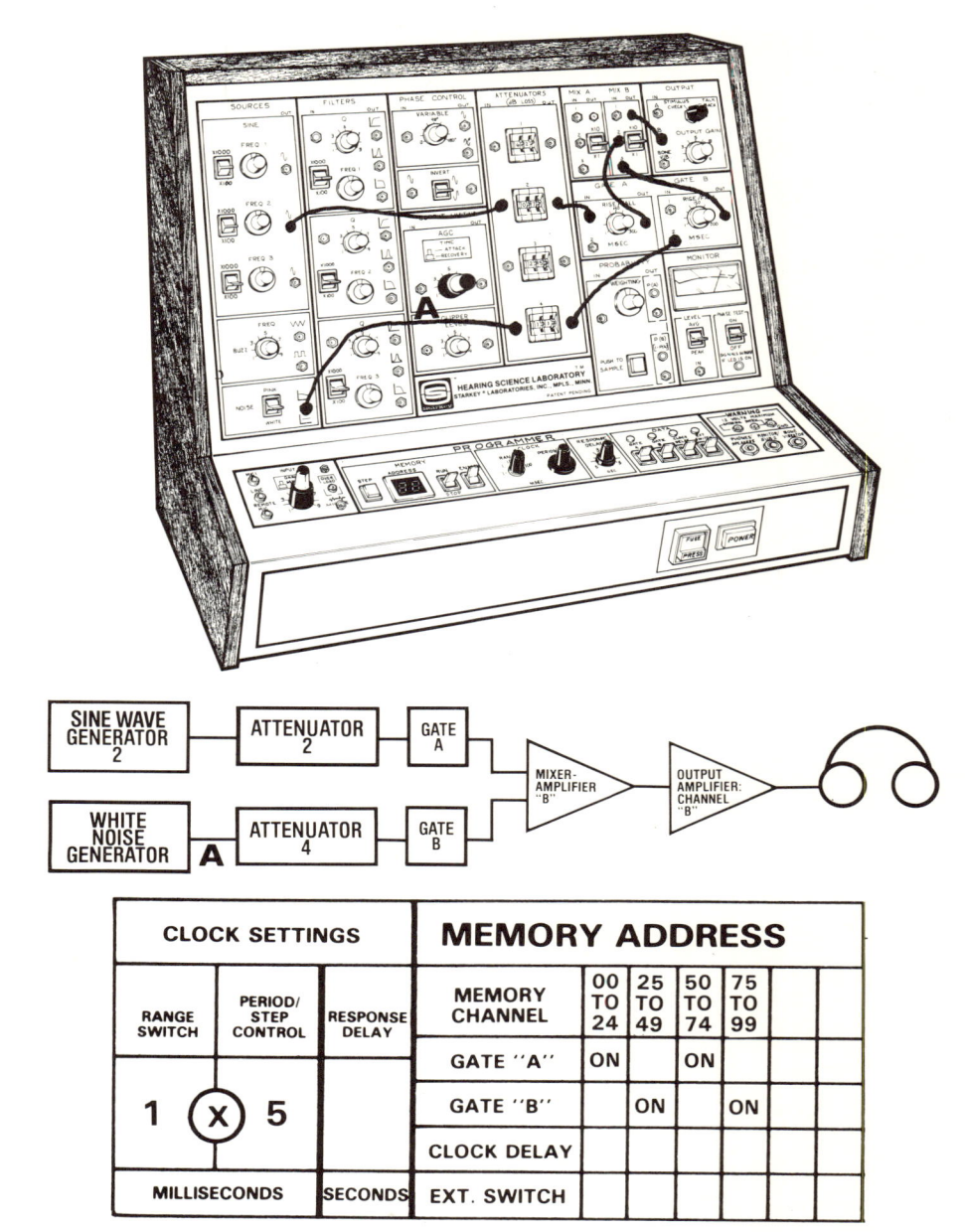

(2) Repeat exercise #1 with a variety of tone signal frequencies and record the different Attenuator settings which produce the "continuity effect." Plot the pulsation threshold levels for a listener as a function of signal frequency on the axes provided in Figure "A".

(3) Repeat exercise #1 with a pulsating tonal masker instead of white noise bursts. Perform this task with a variety of signal tone frequencies and levels. In each instance determine pulsation thresholds with masking tones that are below, near, and above the test signal in frequency. Summarize and record the effects you observe.

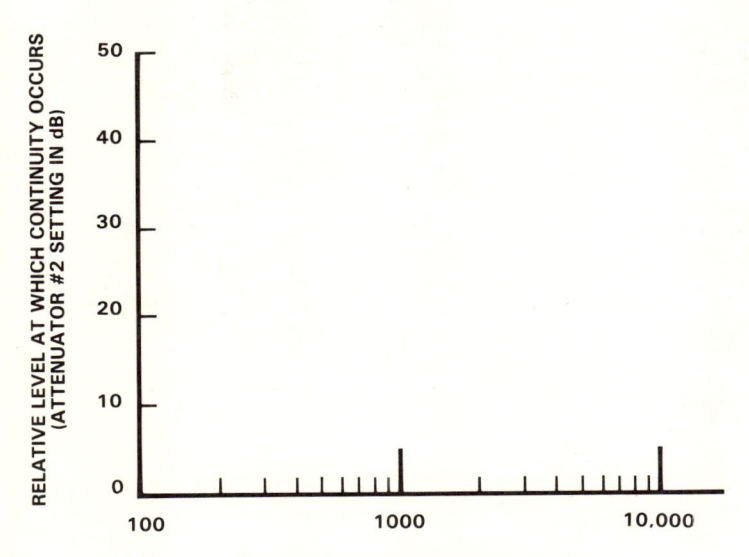

NOTES:

FIGURE A: Data graph for plotting a subject's pulsation threshold at different frequencies for the same white noise masker.

(Y-axis: RELATIVE LEVEL AT WHICH CONTINUITY OCCURS (ATTENUATOR #2 SETTING IN dB); X-axis: FREQUENCY OF TONE SIGNAL IN HERTZ)

Selected References:

Elfner, L.F. and Homick, J.L. (1967). Continuity effects with alternately sounding tones under dichotic presentation. *Percept. Psychophys,* **2**, 34-36.

Elfner, L.F. (1969). Continuity in alternately sounded tone and noise signals in a free field. *J. Acoust. Soc. Am.,* **46**, 914-917.

Elfner, L.F. (1971). Continuity in alternately sounded tonal signals in a free field. *J. Acoust. Soc. Am.,* **49**, 447-449.

Thurlow, W.R. (1957). An auditory figure-ground effect. *Am. J. Psychol.* **70**, 653-654.

Thurlow, W.R. and Elfner, L.F. (1959). Continuity effects with alternately sounding tones. *J. Acoust. Soc. Am.,* **31**, 1337-1339.

Thurlow, W.R. and Marten, A.E. (1962). Perception of steady and intermittent sounds with alternating noise-burst stimuli. *J. Acoust. Soc. Am.,* **34**, 1853-1858.

Verschuure, J., Rodenburg, M., Maas, A. J. J. (1976). Presentation conditions of the pulsation threshold method. *Acustica*, **35**, 47-54.

EXPERIMENT VI-7: TWO-TONE SUPPRESSION

Purpose:
To demonstrate the phenomenon of monaural "unmasking" which can occur during non-simultaneous masking conditions.

Background Principle:
In Laboratory Experiment VI-3, we observed that increasing the level of a masking stimulus caused a corresponding *threshold shift*, or increase in the detection threshold level, for a masked tone signal. An unusual exception to this classical finding can take place, under certain conditions, if the masker and signal stimuli are presented in non-simultaneous listening tasks (e.g., those in Laboratory Experiments VI-5 and VI-6). Specifically, the introduction of an additional, different frequency tone component to the masker can actually decrease its masking efficacy upon the test signal. This results in a decrease in the signal threshold in forward masking, or lowered level of subjective signal continuity in pulsation threshold. The underlying causes for this "unmasking" phenomenon are as yet unknown, but it has been suggested that the internal activity produced by the original masker tone may actually be reduced, or *suppressed*, through the addition of the second masker tone component.

One means of demonstrating *two-tone suppression* is to compare a subject's pulsation threshold under two different listening conditions (see Houtgast, 1972). Initially, a 1000 Hz, 40 dB Sensation Level (SL) **masker** will be permitted to continuously alternate with a 1000 Hz tone **signal**. The tone signal level is varied until a continuous sound percept is noted. For this elementary reference listening condition, the subject's pulsation threshold is actually his threshold for detecting the presence of amplitude modulation. Continuity occurs when the signal level is set about 2 dB higher than the masker level. A second masker component, fixed at 60 dB SL but variable in frequency, is then added to the original 1000 Hz, 40 dB SL masker. Remarkably, adding this second tone "suppresses" the efficacy of the original masker component and pulsations, rather than continuity, are perceived by the listener. The tone signal level is then decreased in order to restore subjective continuity. The amount of this decrease quantifies, in dB, the suppression effect and will depend upon the particular frequency relationship between the masker tone components. As noted in Laboratory Experiment VI-6, a quiet background and listener concentration are important to the observance of this subtle effect.

Procedure:
The output from Sine Wave Generator #1 is split into two portions to provide the 1000 Hz signal and the 1000 Hz component of the two-tone masking stimulus. The level and switching control for the 1000 Hz signal is achieved by the action of Attenuator #2 and Electronic Gate "B", respec-

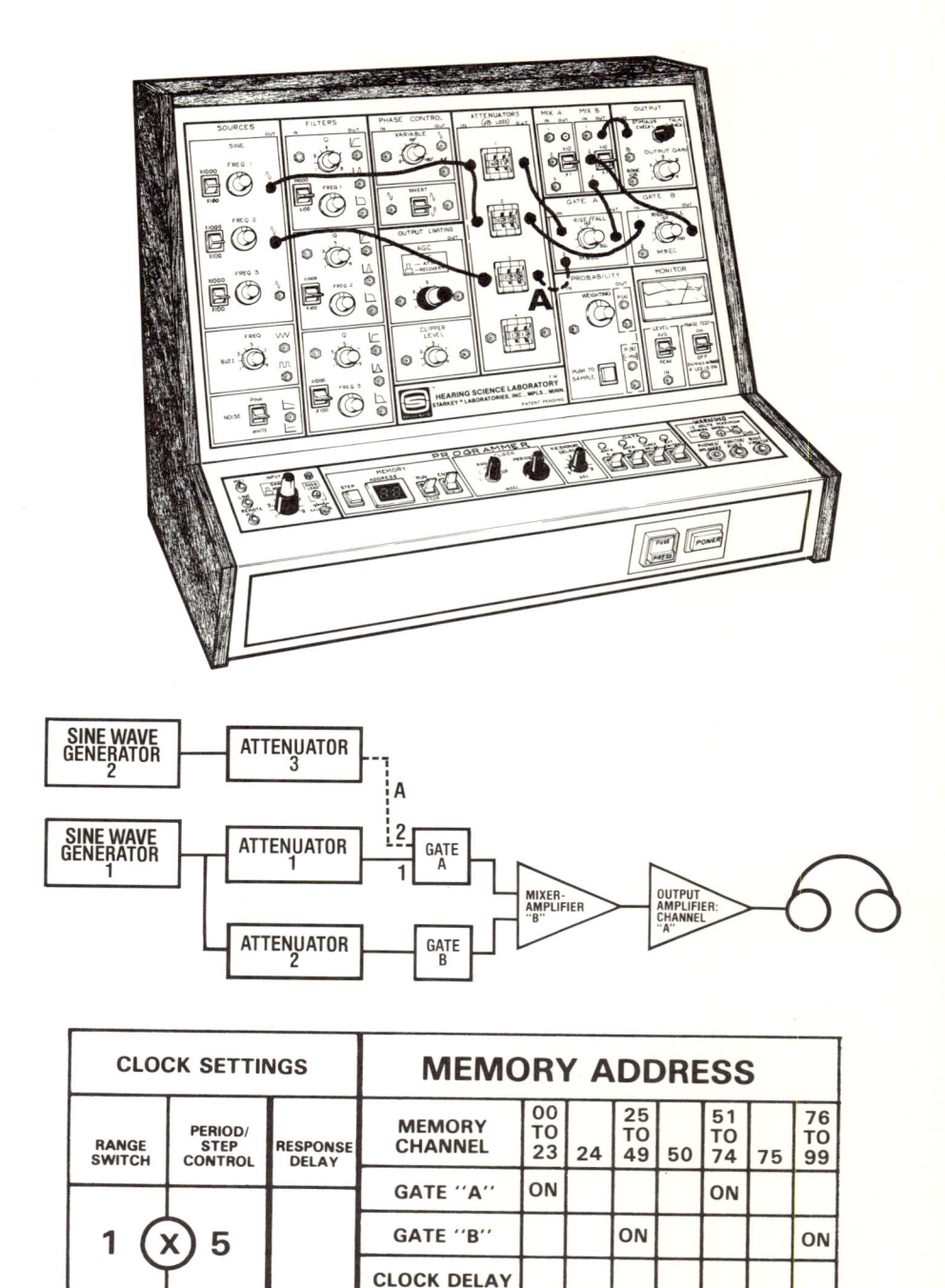

CLOCK SETTINGS			MEMORY ADDRESS					
RANGE SWITCH	PERIOD/ STEP CONTROL	RESPONSE DELAY	MEMORY CHANNEL	00 TO 23	24	25 TO 49	50	51 TO 74	75	76 TO 99
1	X 5		GATE "A"	ON				ON		
			GATE "B"			ON				ON
			CLOCK DELAY							
MILLISECONDS		SECONDS	EXT. SWITCH							

tively. Attenuator #1 and Gate "A" control the 1000 Hz component of the two-tone masker. The output from Sine Wave Generator #2 provides the second frequency component of the masker and is routed through Attenuator #3 and combined with the 1000 Hz masker within Gate "A." The outputs from both Gates are combined within Mixer-Amplifier "B" and delivered to one Output Amplifier channel and headphone. The suggested programming instructions will permit both Gates and their respective stimuli to switch on and off for durations of roughly 120 milliseconds each. The rise/fall time for both Gates should be adjusted so as to minimize any audible transients or overlapping of masker and signal waveforms.

Exercises:

(1) In accordance with the discussion above, set Sine Wave Generator #1 near 1000 Hz. The Output Amplifier Gain Control Knob and Attenuator #1 should be set to provide the 1000 Hz, 40 dB SL masker component. With the Programmer Clock running and dashed circuit wire "A" disconnected, adjust the tone signal level with Attenuator #2 until the subject reports hearing a pulsed tone against a continuous background. This is the listener's pulsation threshold. For signal levels above or below this landmark value, the two tones will seem to alternate. Set Sine Wave Generator #2 near 1200 Hz and adjust Attenuator #3 to be 20 dB lower than Attenuator #1 (i.e., the 2nd masker component should be fixed near 60 dB SL). Now connect dashed circuit wire "A" and note if the pulsating character of the 1000 Hz signal re-emerges. Some experimentation with the various levels may be necessary until the effect becomes apparent. Finally, decrease the signal level with Attenuator #2 until continuity reappears and record the difference in decibels between the two pulsation thresholds.

(2) Repeat exercise #1 for several 2nd masker tone component frequencies and note if the "monaural release from masking" is more pronounced when masker component #2 is higher or lower in frequency than masker component #1.

NOTES:

Selected References:

Abbas, P.J. and Sachs, M.B. (1976). Two-tone suppression in auditory-nerve fibers: extension of a stimulus-response relationship. *J. Acoust. Soc. Am.*, **59**, 112-122.

Carterette, E.C., Friedman, M.P., and Lowell, J.D. (1969). Mach bands in hearing. *J. Acoust. Soc. Am.*, **45**, 986-998.

Houtgast, T. (1972). Psychophysical evidence for lateral inhibition in hearing. *J. Acoust. Soc. Am.*, **51**, 1885-1894.

Houtgast, T. (1973). Psychophysical experiments on "tuning curves" and "two-tone inhibition." *Acustica*, **29**, 168-179.

Houtgast, T. (1974). Lateral suppression and loudness reduction of a tone in noise. *Acustica*, **30**, 214-221.

Legouix, J., Remond, M., and Greenbaum, H. (1973). Interference and two-tone inhibition. *J. Acoust. Soc. Am.*, **53**, 409-419.

Rainbolt, H. and Small, A.M. (1972). Mach bands in auditory masking: an attempted replication. *J. Acoust. Soc. Am.*, **51**, 567-574.

Sachs, M.B. and Kiang, N.Y.S. (1968). Two-tone inhibition in auditory nerve fibers. *J. Acoust. Soc. Am.*, **43**, 1120-1128.

Sachs, M.B. and Abbas, P.J. (1976). Phenomenological model for two-tone suppression. *J. Acoust. Soc. Am.*, **60**, 1157-1163.

Shannon, R.V. (1976). Two-tone unmasking and suppression in a forward-masking situation. *J. Acoust. Soc. Am.*, **59**, 1460-1470.

Small, A.M. (1975). Mach bands in auditory masking revisited. *J. Acoust. Soc. Am.*, **57**, 251-252.

Tyler, R.S. and Small, A.M. (1977). Two-tone suppression in backward masking. *J. Acoust. Soc. Am.*, **62**, 215-218.

Binaural Hearing
VII

EXPERIMENT VII-1: BINAURAL SUMMATION

Purpose:
To compare and contrast the loudness of a tone when listening with one and both ears.

Background Principle:
Numerous studies have confirmed that the auditory abilities of a listener are quite different (and almost always enhanced) when two ears, rather than one, are utilized. A tone, for example, that is just barely audible when delivered monaurally will increase in perceived loudness when routed to both ears simultaneously. This binaural enhancement corresponds to an intensity level increment of roughly three to six decibels. The effect, known as *binaural summation,* becomes even more noticeable when stimuli levels substantially above the subject's threshold are employed. Note that although loudness has increased, the binaural effect is less than double the monaural percept (10 dB would roughly correspond to a doubling in loudness).

Procedure:
The output from one Sine Wave Generator is sent through Attenuator #4 and into both Electronic Gates. The signal that emerges from Gate "A" is routed to two separate Attenuators and Output Amplifier channels, one for each headphone. The output from Gate "B" is delivered to only one Attenuator, Output Amplifier channel, and headphone. The suggested programming instructions permit the listener to contrast the loudness of the stimulus first in one ear, followed by the binaural test condition. The Programmer Delay Channel provides a 0.5 second pause after each test condition in the sequence.

Exercises:
(1) With the Programmer Clock stopped at Memory Address 00 (i.e., Gate "B" on) and the tone present in one ear, adjust Attenuator #3 until the signal is barely audible. Next, start the Clock and adjust Attenuators 1 and 2 by equal amounts (always maintaining identical level settings) until the binaural and monaural listening conditions sound the same in loudness. Try this with an initial tone frequency of 1000 Hz and note the difference in decibels, if any, between the summated and single tone situations.

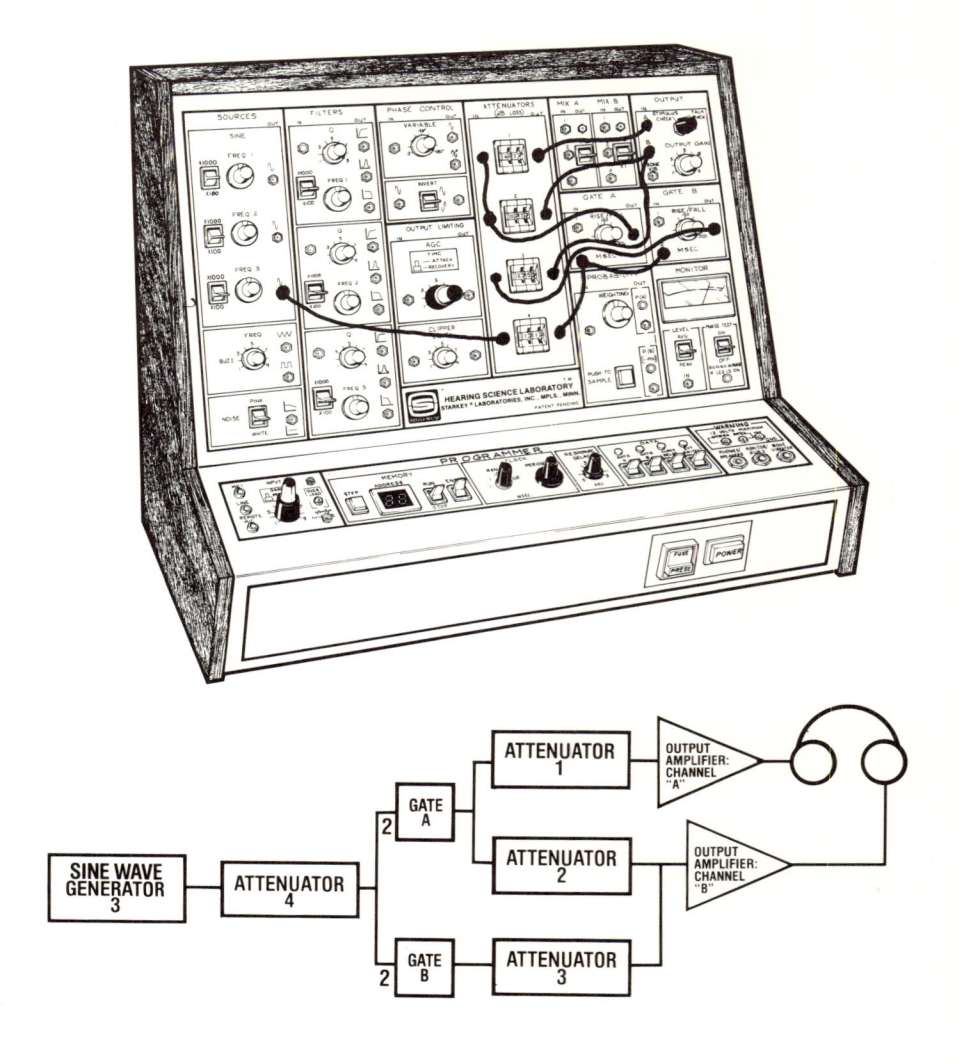

(2) Repeat exercise #1 for tones of various frequencies and sensation levels (Note: you may use Attenuator #4 as a "master" level control for the signals). Is binaural summation more pronounced at certain frequencies or signal levels?

(3) Repeat exercise #1 with such non-sinusoidal stimuli as white noise or speech and contrast these results with those obtained for exercise #1.

NOTES:

Selected References:

Caussé, R. and Chavasse, P. (1942). Différence entre l'ecoute binauriculaire et monauriculaire pour la perception des intensitiés supraliminaires. *Comptes Rendus de Société Biologie,* **86,** 405.

Elmasian, R. and Galambos, R. (1975). Loudness enhancement: monaural, binaural, and dichotic. *J. Acoust. Soc. Am.,* **58,** 229-234.

Galambos, R., Bauer, J., Picton, T., Squires, K., and Squires, N. (1972). Loudness enhancement following contralateral stimulation. *J. Acoust. Soc. Am.,* **52,** 1127-1130.

Hirsh, I.J. (1948). Binaural summation — a century of investigation. *Psychol. Bull.,* **45,** 193-206.

Irwin, R.J. (1965). Binaural summation of thermal noises of equal and unequal power in each ear. *Am. J. Psychol.,* **78,** 57-65.

Levelt, W.J.M., Riemersma, J.B., and Bunt, A.A. (1972). Binaural additivity of loudness. *Brit. J. Math. Statist. Psychol.,* **25,** 51-68.

Reynolds, G.S. and Stevens, S.S. (1960). Binaural summation of loudness. *J. Acoust. Soc. Am.,* **32,** 1337-1344.

Scharf, B. (1969). Dichotic summation of loudness. *J. Acoust. Soc. Am.,* **45,** 1193-1205.

Scharf, B. (1974). Loudness summation between tones from two loudspeakers. *J. Acoust. Soc. Am.,* **56,** 589-593.

Scharf, B. and Fishken, D. (1970). Binaural summation of loudness, reconsidered. *J. Exp. Psychol.,* **86,** 374-379.

Scharf, B. and Weissmann, S.M. (1970). Dichotic summation of loudness over time. *J. Acoust. Soc. Am.,* **47,** 96-97(A).

Simmons, F.B. (1965). Binaural summation of the acoustic reflex. *J. Acoust. Soc. Am.,* **37,** 834-836.

Smith, M.H. and Licklider, J.C.R. (1949). Statistical bias in comparisons of monaural and binaural supplementation. *Psychol. Bull.,* **36,** 378-384.

Treisman, M. and Irwin, R.J. (1967). Auditory intensity discriminal scale I. evidence derived from binaural intensity summation. *J. Acoust. Soc. Am.,* **42,** 586-592.

EXPERIMENT VII-2: BINAURAL FUSION OF PULSED STIMULI

Purpose:
To examine the effects of interaural time delay upon the lateralization of a fused sound image.

Background Principle:
Because of the separation between our two ears, the sounds that reach them travel dissimilar paths and typically differ in time of arrival and interaural intensity (see Laboratory Experiment VII-4). These separate signal inputs are normally merged into a single sound image by the two ears through a process described as *binaural fusion*. The simplest demonstration of binaural fusion may be achieved by simultaneously presenting the identical stimulus to each ear. A listener with normal hearing usually reports the presence of a single sound image within or near the head and roughly in line with the nose. By varying the interaural time of arrival of the binaural stimuli, the fused sound image can be shifted laterally within the subject's head. If, however, the time delay between the two signals exceeds a critical value, the fused image will split and be heard as two separate percepts — one at each ear. The size of this critical time delay varies with the particular stimulus employed (roughly 2-3 milliseconds for clicks and up to 15 milliseconds for speech signals).

Procedure:
Pairs of low pass noise bursts will serve as the test stimuli for demonstrating the fusion effect. The output of the White Noise Generator is sent through three cascaded Low Pass Filters to produce a 36 dB/octave rolloff (see Figure I-30A). The low pass noise is then routed through an Attenuator and into both Electronic Gates. The signal from each Gate enters a separate Output Amplifier channel and headphone. Adjust each Filter cutoff frequency to roughly 600 Hz and set each "Q"-control to its fully counterclockwise position. The suggested programming instructions permit the observation and comparison of five different experimental conditions. The sequence begins with the binaural noise pulses being switched on and off simultaneously. A fused sound image should appear near the center of the subject's head. In each subsequent test presentation, the two noise bursts will be separated by ever greater interaural time delays that will cause the fused image to lateralize toward one ear. A breakdown in fusion should occur at the maximum interaural delay, with each noise pulse appearing at a separate ear. The Programmer Delay Channel provides a 0.5 second pause between each experimental condition.

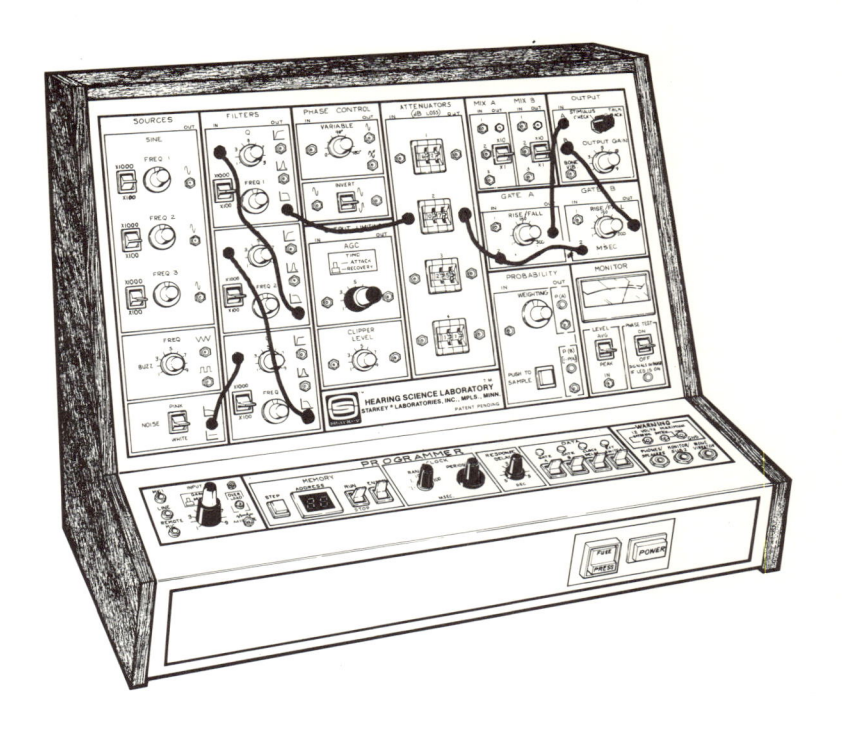

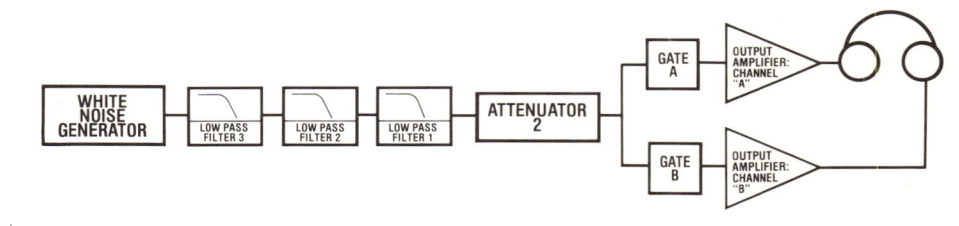

Exercises:
(1) Perform the demonstration described above for a variety of stimulus levels. Does the fused sound image more readily lateralize near threshold or supra-threshold levels?

(2) Use a 500 Hz tone instead of a noise as the pulsed stimulus. This can be achieved by connecting the Attenuator input wire directly to the output of one of the Sine Wave Generators. Can you account for the fact that the tonal fused image continually, and cyclically, returns to the center of your head?

NOTES:

Selected References:

Banks, M.S. and Green, D.M. (1973). Localization of high- and low-frequency transients. *J. Acoust. Soc. Am.*, **53**, 1432-1433.

van den Brink, G., Sintnicolaas, K., and van Stam, W.S. (1976). Dichotic pitch fusion. *J. Acoust. Soc. Am.*, **59**, 1471-1476.

Cherry, E.C. (1959). Two ears—but one world. In W.A. Rosenblith (Ed.) *Sensory Communications.* MIT Press, Cambridge, Massachusetts.

Cherry, E.C. and Sayers, B. Mc A. (1959). On the mechanism of binaural fusion. *J. Acoust. Am.*, **31**, 535.

David, E.E., Jr., Guttman, N., and van Bergeijk, W.A. (1958). On the mechanism of binaural fusion. *J. Acoust. Soc. Am.*, **30**, 801-802.

Dunn, B.E. (1971). Effect of unilateral masking on the lateralization of binaural pulses. *J. Acoust. Soc. Am.*, **50**, 483-489.

Leakey, D.M., Sayers, B. Mc A., and Cherry, C. (1958). Binaural fusion of low- and high-frequency sounds. *J. Acoust. Soc. Am.*, **30**, 222.

Perrott, D.R. and Barry, S.H. (1969). Binaural fusion. *J. Aud. Res.*, **3**, 263-269.

Perrott, D.R., Briggs, R., and Perrott, S. (1970). Binaural fusion: its limits as defined by signal duration and signal onset. *J. Acoust. Soc. Am.*, **47**, 565-568.

Perrott, D.R. and Williams, K.N. (1970). Effects of interaural frequency differences on the lateralization function. *J. Acoust. Soc. Am.*, **48**, 1022(L).

Teas, D.C. (1962). Lateralization of acoustic transients. *J. Acoust. Soc. Am.*, **34**, 1460-1465.

EXPERIMENT VII-3: TIME-INTENSITY TRADEOFF IN LATERALIZATION

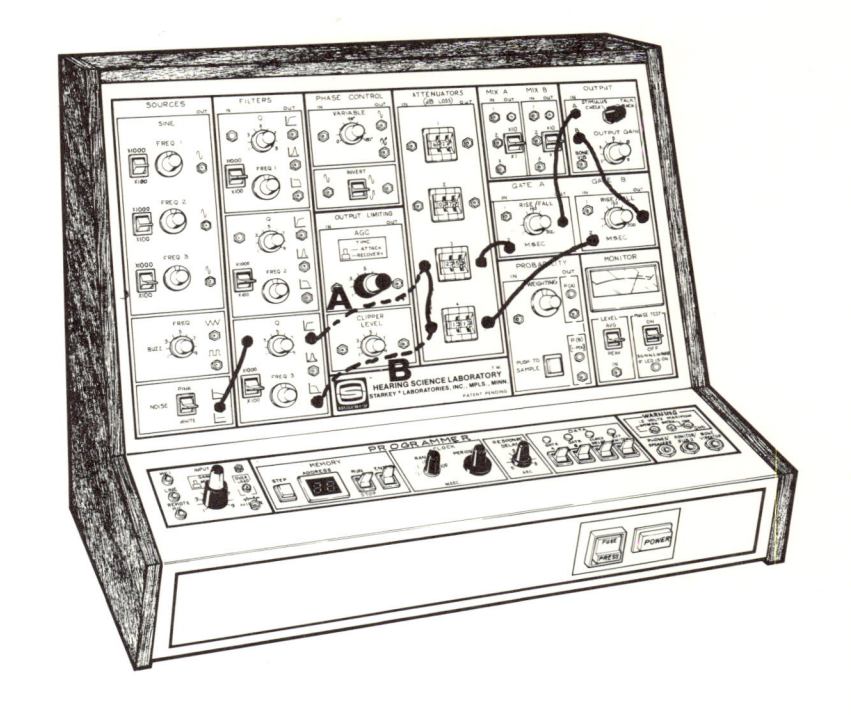

Purpose:
To observe the manner in which an intensity change can offset the temporal cues that produce the apparent lateral position of a dichotic pulse pair.

Background Principle:
In previous experiments, we have observed that the intensity, frequency, and temporal characteristics of a stimulus influence one another in a variety of ways. One binaural example of this interdependence is the manner in which an intensity change in a signal can compensate for the lateral shift caused by an interaural time delay between stimuli. The exact nature of this tradeoff between time and intensity is quite complex and appears to depend upon a multitude of stimuli factors. It has been determined in general that interaural intensity cues are most important for apparent lateral position when pure tone frequencies are higher than 1500 Hz. At much lower frequencies, it appears that temporal cues play the dominant role. Things are much more difficult to describe with non-pure tone stimuli.

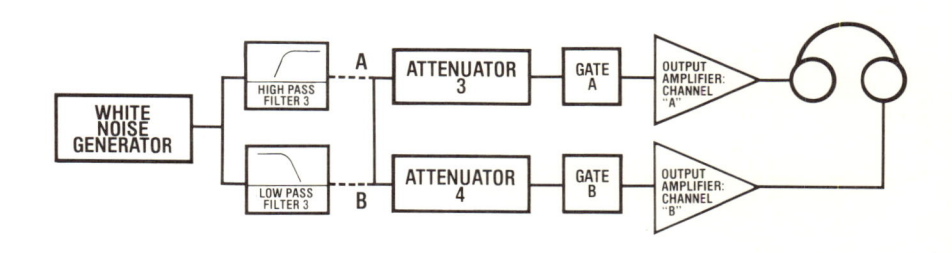

Procedure:
Pass a white noise signal through Filter #3. Set the Filter "Q" control fully counterclockwise. By connecting dashed circuit wire "A" or "B", respectively, either a high pass or low pass filtered noise signal can be produced. The selected noise is then sent to two different Attenuators. The outputs from these two Attenuators are delivered to separate Electronic Gates, Output Amplifier channels, and headphones. The suggested programming instructions will provide a dichotic noise pulse (i.e., different signals to each ear) to the listener which should fuse into a single click-like sound image within the head. The Programmer Delay Channel will permit a one second pause to occur after each test trial.

Exercises:
(1) Use a high pass filtered noise as the initial test stimulus. Adjust the Filter Frequency Control to a setting near 2000 Hz. After each experimental sequence, vary the level setting of one of the Attenuators in steps of 10 decibels each. Determine if the sound percept shifts about within the listener's head. Determine the intensity disparity, between the pulses reaching each ear, that is required to bring the sound image to the center of the subject's head.

(2) Repeat exercise #1 with low pass filtered noise pulses. Adjust the Filter Frequency Control to roughly 500 Hz. Can you determine which noise band frequencies are most readily influenced by the stimulus intensity changes?

(3) Repeat exercises #1 and #2 for a variety of stimuli and silent interval durations and compare and contrast the level settings required for centering of the fused sound image.

NOTES:

Selected References:

Babkoff, H., Sutton, S., and Barris, M. (1973). Binaural interaction of transients: interaural time and intensity asymmetry. *J. Acoust. Soc. Am.*, **53**, 1028-1036.

Bilsen, F.A. and Raatgever, J. (1973). Spectral dominance in binaural lateralization. *Acustica*, **28**, 131-132.

Blauert, J. (1972). On the lag of lateralization caused by interaural time and intensity differences. *Audiology*, **11**, 265-270.

Deatherage, B.H. and Hirsh, I.J. (1959). Auditory localization of clicks. *J. Acoust. Soc. Am.*, **31**, 486-492.

Domnitz, R. (1973). The interaural time JND as a simultaneous function of interaural time and interaural amplitude. *J. Acoust. Soc. Am.*, **53**, 1549-1552.

Gilliom, J.D. and Sorkin, R.D. (1972). Discrimination of interaural time and intensity. *J. Acoust. Soc. Am.*, **52**, 1635-1644.

Hafter, E.R. and Carrier, S.C. (1972). Binaural interaction in low-frequency stimuli: the inability to trade time and intensity completely. *J. Acoust. Soc. Am.*, **51**, 1852-1862.

Harris, G.G. (1960). Binaural interactions of impulsive stimuli and pure tones. *J. Acoust. Soc. Am.*, **32**, 685-692.

Henning, G. (1974). Detectability of interaural delay in high-frequency complex waveforms. *J. Acoust. Soc. Am.*, **55**, 84-90.

McFadden, D. and Pasanen, E.G. (1976). Lateralization of high frequencies based on interaural time differences. *J. Acoust. Soc. Am.*, **59**, 634-639.

Moushegian, G. and Jeffress, L.A. (1959). Role of interaural time and intensity differences in the lateralization of low-frequency tones. *J. Acoust. Soc. Am.*, **31**, 1441-1445.

Nuetzel, J.M. and Hafter, E.R. (1976). Lateralization of complex waveforms: effects of fine structure, amplitude, and duration. *J. Acoust. Soc. Am.*, **60**, 1339-1346.

Thurlow, W.R. and Jack, C.E. (1973). Some determinants of localization-adaptation effects for successive auditory stimuli. *J. Acoust. Soc. Am.*, **53**, 1573-1577.

Toole, F. (1970). In-head-localization of acoustic images. *J. Acoust. Soc. Am.*, **48**, 943-949.

Whitworth, R. and Jeffress, L.A. (1961). Time vs. intensity in the localization of tones. *J. Acoust. Soc. Am.*, **33**, 925-929.

Yost, W.A. (1976). Lateralization of repeated filtered transients. *J. Acoust. Soc. Am.*, **60**, 178-181.

Yost, W.A., Wightman, F.L., and Green, D.M. (1971). Lateralization of filtered clicks. *J. Acoust. Soc. Am.*, **50**, 1526-1531.

Young, L. and Carhart, R. (1974). Time-intensity trading functions for pure tones and a high-frequency AM signal. *J. Acoust. Soc. Am.*, **56**, 605-609.

EXPERIMENT VII-4: THE STEREOPHONIC EFFECT

Purpose:
To shift the perceived position of a fused sound image in three-dimensional space.

Background Principle:
The stimuli produced by a single loudspeaker in a *free sound field* (i.e., one without reflecting surfaces) reach our ears via two separate pathways. We may see from Figure "A" that sounds from the right channel speaker travel over paths A-B and A-D to arrive at the listener's right and left ears, respectively. It is important to note that because distance A-B is shorter than A-D, the signals will arrive first at the right ear. And due to the fact that sound intensity diminishes in accordance with the inverse-square of the distance traveled (i.e., twice the distance, ¼ the intensity; three times the distance, $1/9$ the intensity, etc.), we can expect the signal level at the left ear to be somewhat weaker than the right ear. Our binaural hearing mechanism utilizes these time-of-arrival and intensity differences as cues to form a single fused sound image that is perceived to be located at or near the actual source of the signal. In a similar fashion, the signals from the left channel speaker contain interaural intensity and time of arrival differences that create a fused sound image perceived to be located near the left speaker. When both speakers produce the same signals simultaneously, a *phantom sound image* is perceived to be located midway between the two speakers. The position of the sound image produced by this *stereophonic effect* can be shifted through the introduction of "interchannel" intensity or time of arrival differences which alter the original balanced signal condition. As with the case of the *lateralization* of fused sound images perceived within the head (see for example Laboratory Experiments VII-2 and 3), a trading relationship also exists between time and intensity cues for the *localization* of sound images perceived to be outside the head. Four or five times as much interchannel intensity or temporal disparity is needed, however, to produce a shift in localization equivalent to that for lateralization of sound images under headphone listening conditions.

Procedure:
Live voice signals from a microphone are sent through the Mic. 1 Input Preamplifier and separate Attenuators, Electronic Gates, and Output Amplifiers. These, in turn, power two loudspeakers. Space the speakers about six feet apart and station the listener midway between them and roughly six feet away. The suggested programming instructions will permit the speech to emerge first from one speaker at a time and then from both speakers simultaneously.

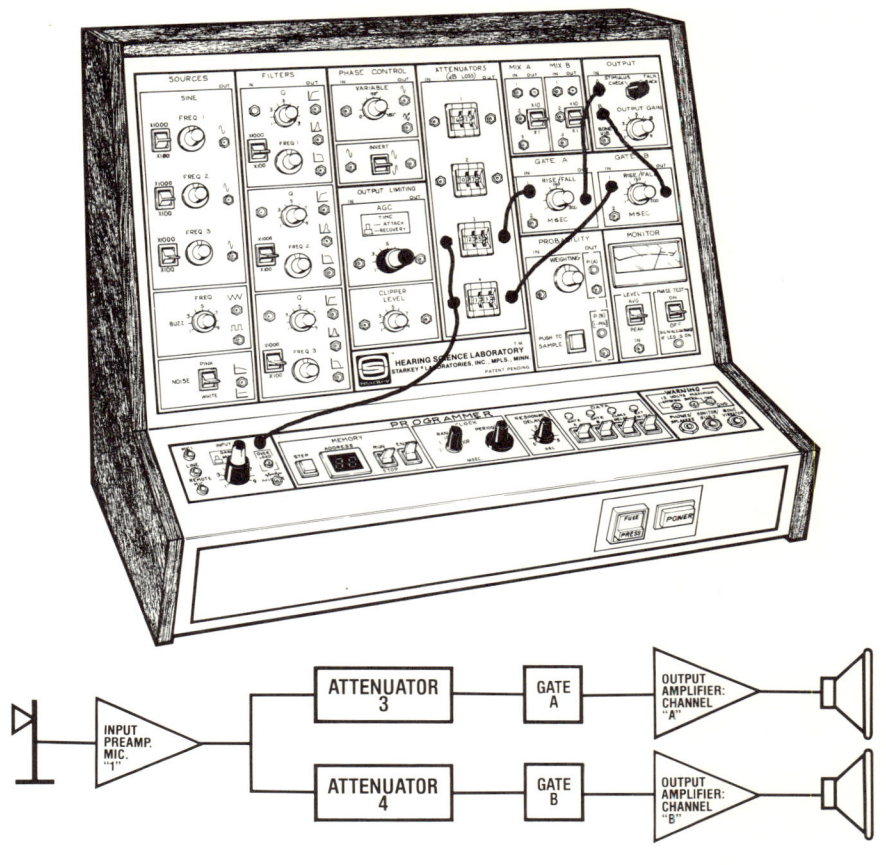

CLOCK SETTINGS			MEMORY ADDRESS				
RANGE SWITCH	PERIOD/ STEP CONTROL	RESPONSE DELAY	MEMORY CHANNEL	00	1	2	3 TO 99
			GATE "A"	ON		ON	
1	X 1	1	GATE "B"		ON	ON	
			CLOCK DELAY	ON	ON	ON	
MILLISECONDS		SECONDS	EXT. SWITCH				

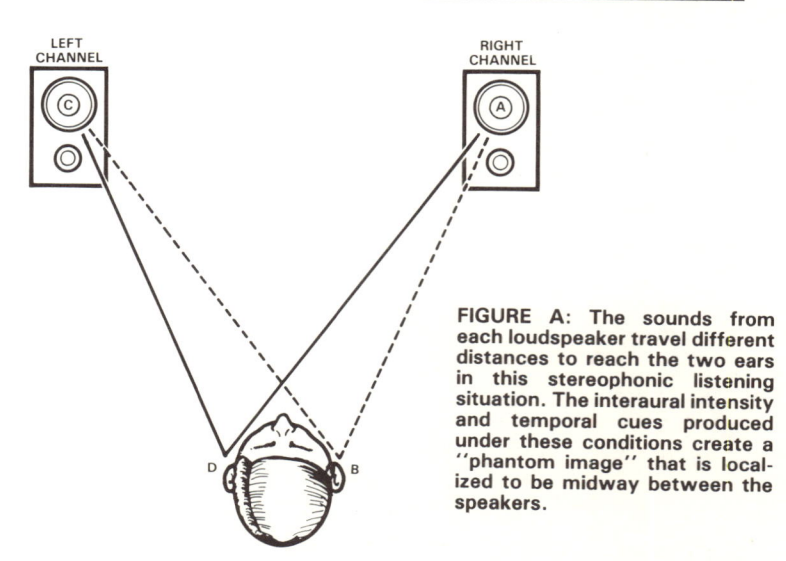

FIGURE A: The sounds from each loudspeaker travel different distances to reach the two ears in this stereophonic listening situation. The interaural intensity and temporal cues produced under these conditions create a "phantom image" that is localized to be midway between the speakers.

Exercises:

(1) Set both Attenuators to equal levels (e.g., 10 dB each) and note the changes in the position of the localized fused sound image during the various *monophonic* and stereophonic listening conditions. Next, set the Attenuators to a series of increasingly different levels (e.g., 10 dB and 20 dB, 10 dB and 30 dB, 10 dB and 40 dB) and note how these interchannel intensity differences affect the position of the stereophonic sound image.

(2) Repeat the exercises described in Laboratory Experiments VII-2 and VII-3, using loudspeakers instead of headphones, and note any differences between lateralization and localization effects.

NOTES:

Selected References:

Blauert, J. (1969). Sound localization in the median plane. *Acustica*, **22**, 205-213.

Damaske, P. (1971). Head-related two-channel stereophony with loudspeaker reproduction. *J. Acoust. Soc. Am.*, **50**, 1109-1115.

Elfner, L.F., Bothe, G.G., and Simrall, D.S. (1970). Monaural localization: effects of feedback, incentive, and interstimulus interval. *J. Aud. Res.*, **10**, 11-16.

Erulkar, S.D. (1972). Comparative aspects of spatial localization of sound. *Physiol. Rev.*, **52**, 237-360.

Feddersen, W.E. (1955). The localization of sound from two sources in phase opposition. *J. Acoust. Soc. Am.*, **27**, 208-209(A).

Gardner, M.B. (1969). Image fusion, broadening, and displacement in sound location. *J. Acoust. Soc. Am.*, **46**, 339-349.

Gardner, M.B. and Gardner, R.S. (1973). Problem of localization in the median plane: effect of pinnae cavity occlusion. *J. Acoust. Soc. Am.*, **53**, 400-408.

Hanson, R.L. and Kock, W.E. (1957). Interesting effect produced by two loudspeakers under free space conditions. *J. Acoust. Soc. Am.*, **29**, 145(L).

Harris, J.D. (1972). A florilegium of experiments on directional hearing. *Acta Otolar. Suppl.*, **298**, 26.

Hebrank, J. and Wright, D. (1974). Spectral cues used in the localization of sound sources on the median plane. *J. Acoust. Soc. Am.*, **56**, 1829-1834.

Jeffress, L.A. and Taylor, R.W. (1961). Lateralization versus localization. *J. Acoust. Soc. Am.*, **33**, 482-483.

Plenge, G. (1974). On the differences between localization and lateralization. *J. Acoust. Soc. Am.*, **56**, 944-951.

Sandel, T.T., Teas, D.C., Feddersen, W.E., and Jeffress, L.A. (1955). Localization of sound from single and paired sources. *J. Acoust. Soc. Am.*, **27**, 842-852.

Searle, C.L., Braida, L.D., Cuddy, D.R., and Davis, M.F. (1975). Binaural pinna disparity: another auditory localization cue. *J. Acoust. Soc. Am.*, **57**, 448-455.

Searle, C.L., Braida, L.D., Davis, M.F., and Colburn, H.S. (1976). Model for auditory localization. *J. Acoust. Soc. Am.*, **60**, 1164-1175.

Snow, W.B. (1953). Basic principles of stereophonic sound. *J. Soc. Motion Pictures Television Engrs*, **61**, 567-589.

Thurlow, W.R. and Mergener, J.R. (1970). Effect of stimulus duration on localization of direction of noise stimuli. *J. Speech Hear. Res.*, **13**, 826-838.

Toole, F.E. (1970). In-head-localization of acoustic images. *J. Acoust. Soc. Am.*, **48**, 943-949.

Wright, D., Hebrank, J.H., and Wilson, B. (1974). Pinna reflections as cues for localization. *J. Acoust. Soc. Am.*, **56**, 957-962.

EXPERIMENT VII-5: THE PRECEDENCE EFFECT

Purpose:
To examine the ability of the binaural hearing mechanism to tune out unwanted signals.

Background Principle:
In most listening situations, sounds reflect off hard surfaces to reach our ears from many directions. Despite this jumble of echoes, we can discern what is being said and where the sound is coming from. This *echo suppression* is due to the fact that the binaural hearing mechanism attends to the first signal to reach the ears and, in general, discounts subsequent arrivals. Four clicks may be used to demonstrate this so-called *precedence effect.* The first and second clicks are delivered, respectively, to the left and right ears. The third and fourth clicks are sent, in reverse order, to the right and left ears (see Figure "A"). If only the first pair of stimuli were presented, a listener would probably note the presence of a single fused click image near the left ear. The second pair alone would have produced a click image near the right ear. When both sets of clicks occur in sequence, the subject still reports the image to be near the left (i.e., where the first signal arrives). The precedence effect may not take place if the second pair of stimuli (1) lag behind the first pair by more than a few milliseconds or (2) are larger than the first pair by more than 15 dB in level. Were it not for this phenomenon of precedence, conversation, even in a quiet room, would be a confusing bedlam of overlapping echoes.

Procedure:
The clicks used in this experiment are actually produced by tonal signals that have very brief durations. The pure tone stimulus is first sent to separate Attenuators so that the magnitude of the clicks that reach the ears may be adjusted. The output from each Attenuator enters separate Electronic Gates, Output Amplifier channels, and headphones. Use a test tone frequency near 500 Hz and adjust both Attenuators to identical settings which provide clearly audible clicks for the listener. The suggested programming instructions will create three different experimental sequences of events. The first pair of binaural clicks will create a fused sound image near one headphone, whereas the second set of pulses will produce an image that lateralizes toward the opposite headphone. The third sequence includes all four clicks, as shown in Figure "A". The Programmer Delay Channel provides a one second pause between each of the three listening conditions to facilitate comparisons. Slowly vary the Programmer Clock settings from about 10 milliseconds per Memory Address to 0.1 milliseconds per Memory Address and note the changes in the perception of the clicks.

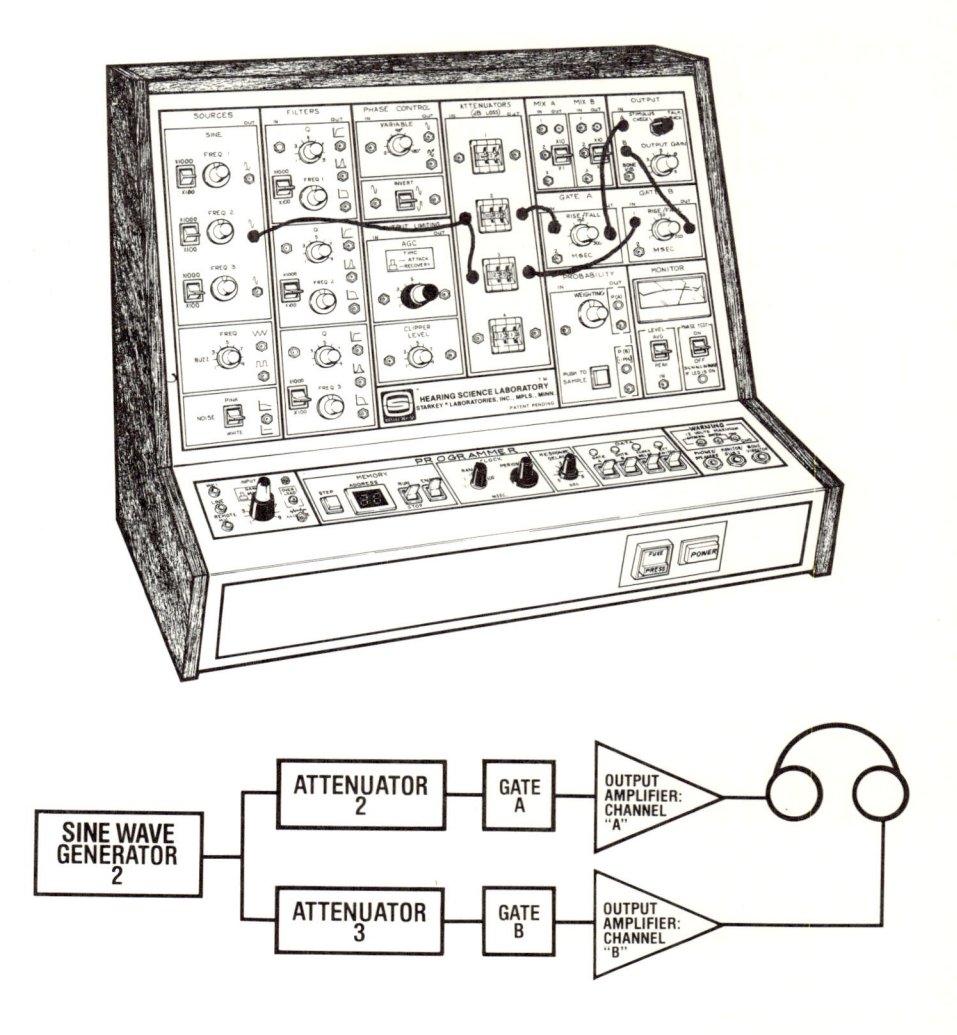

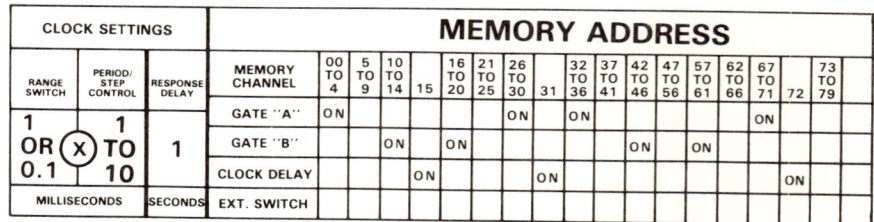

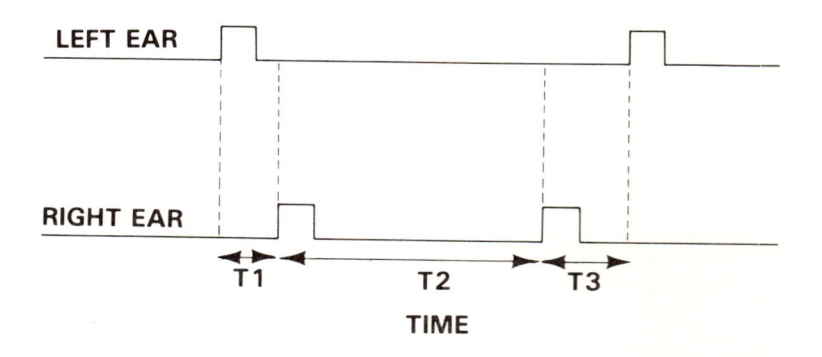

FIGURE A: A series of clicks may be used to demonstrate the precedence effect. The binaural hearing mechanism tends to disregard those pulses that arrive after the first stimulus, and the listener perceives a single fused sound image associated with the initial pair of clicks. (From Levitt, H. and Voroba, B. (1974). Binaural Hearing. In S.E. Gerber (Ed.) *Introductory Hearing Science,* Saunders, Philadelphia.)

Exercises:

(1) The crucial variable in this demonstration is the duration of the interclick silent intervals. After demonstrating the basic phenomenon, reprogram the Gates for increases in interclick delays of 10, 20, 30, 40, and 80 milliseconds. Try to determine the values at which precedence occurs and breaks down into separate click images at each ear.

(2) Route the output signals from the Hearing Science Laboratory to separate loudspeakers and repeat exercise #1. Is the precedence effect more noticeable under these listening conditions?

NOTES:

Selected References:

Blauert, J. (1971). Localization and the law of the first wavefront in the median plane. *J. Acoust. Soc. Am.,* **50,** 466-470.

Fay, R.D. and Hall, W.M. (1956). Historical note on the Haas effect. *J. Acoust. Soc. Am.,* **28,** 131-132.

Gardner, M.B. (1968). Historical background of the Haas and/or precedence effect. *J. Acoust. Soc. Am.,* **43,** 1243-1248.

Sandel, T.T., Teas, D.C., Feddersen, W.E., and Jeffress, L.A. (1955). Localization of sound from single and paired sources. *J. Acoust. Soc. Am.,* **27,** 842-852.

Snow, W.B. (1954). Effect of arrival time on stereophonic localization. *J. Acoust. Soc. Am.,* **26,** 1071-1074.

Wallach, H., Newman, E.B., and Rosenzweig, M.R. (1949). The precedence effect in sound localization. *Am. J. Psychol.,* **52,** 315-336.

EXPERIMENT VII-6: BINAURAL BEATS

Purpose:
To examine the binaural counterpart of the beat phenomenon.

Background Principle:
An unusual variation of the beat phenomenon (discussed in Laboratory Experiment IV-2) can be produced by delivering two pure tones of similar frequency to **separate** ears. Our binaural hearing mechanism somehow combines these tones in the neural pathways of the brain, and we perceive the presence of beats. This occurs despite the absence of any acoustic interaction between the tones. Oddly enough, this subjective beating effect can be noticed only for frequencies below roughly 1000 Hz.

Procedure:
Each pure tone signal is sent to a separate Attenuator. The output from Attenuator #1 is passed through Mixer-Amplifier "A" and Output Amplifier "A" which powers one headphone. The output from Attenuator #2 is divided into two branches, each of which is delivered to a separate Electronic Gate. The output from Gate "A" enters Mixer-Amplifier "A", whereas the signal from Gate "B" proceeds to Output Amplifier channel "B" and the second headphone. When Gate "A" is turned on by the Programmer, both tones will be combined within one ear. When Gate "B" is activated, the tones will appear in separate ears. The suggested programming instructions will permit the two Gates to switch on and off alternately. In this fashion, one may easily contrast the differences between the monaural, objective, and the binaural, subjective, beats conditions.

Exercises:
(1) Adjust the Frequency Controls of the two Sine Wave Generators to provide an initial tone pair separated by three or four Hz (e.g., 500 and 504 Hz). After noting the difference between the objective and subjective beats produced for these frequencies, try mid and high frequency tone pairs, such as 1000 & 1004 Hz and 6000 & 6004 Hz. Do you find that the binaural beating effect does not occur at high frequencies?

(2) Repeat exercise #1 for signal levels that are near the listener's thresholds for each frequency as well as for tone pairs substantially above threshold levels. Are binaural beats more readily detected at loud or soft sound levels?

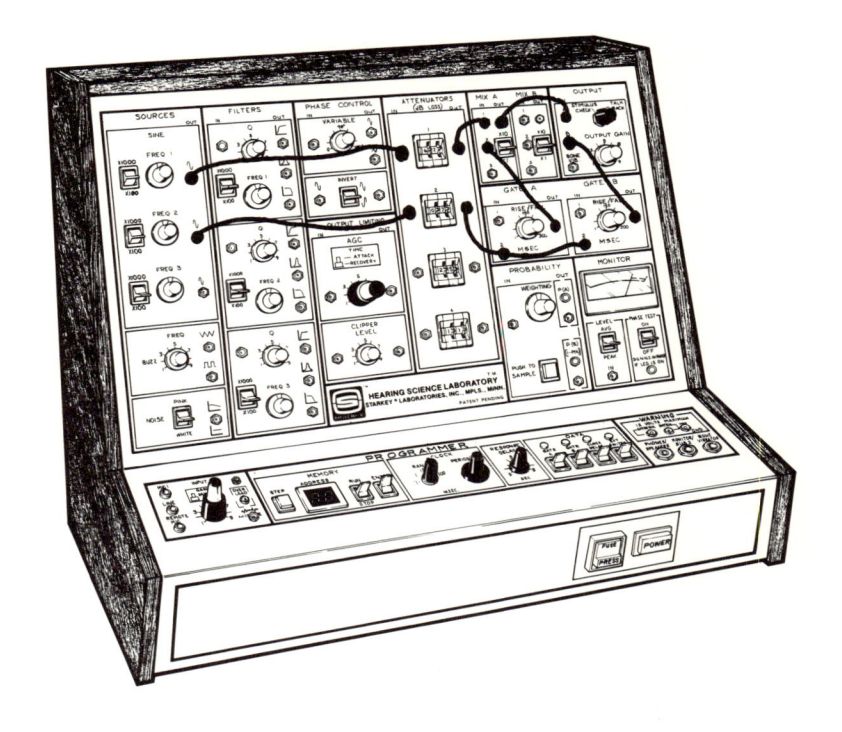

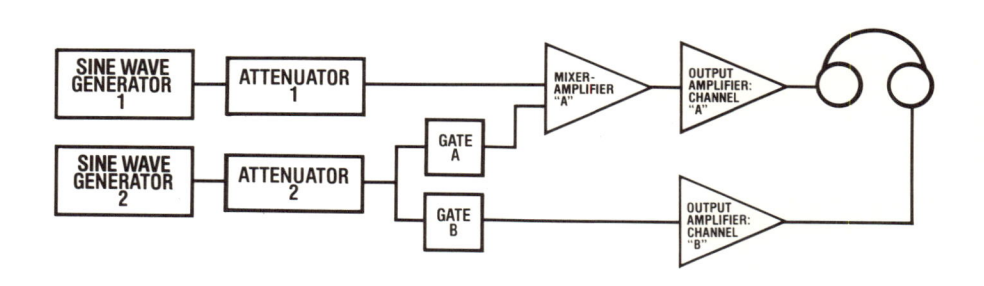

CLOCK SETTINGS			MEMORY ADDRESS			
RANGE SWITCH	PERIOD/STEP CONTROL	RESPONSE DELAY	MEMORY CHANNEL	00	1	2 TO 99
1	X 1	3	GATE "A"	ON		
			GATE "B"		ON	
			CLOCK DELAY	ON	ON	
MILLISECONDS		SECONDS	EXT. SWITCH			

NOTES:

Selected References:

von Békésy, G. (1960). *Experiments in hearing.* McGraw-Hill, New York.

Berger, K. (1966). Binaural pitch-matching with continuous tones. *J. Aud. Res.,* **6**, 87-90.

Fellows, S.A. (1967). The ability to perceive binaural beats by brain damaged and non-brain damaged adults. *J. Aud. Res.,* **7**, 387-390.

Lane, C.E. (1925). Binaural beats. *Phys. Rev.,* **26**, 401-412.

Licklider, J.C.R., Marill, T.M., and Neisser, U.R. (1954). Aural presentation of information. Final Report Contract No. AF-19 (604)-390, p. 31, (Also In J.D. Harris (Ed.). *Forty germinal papers in human hearing.* J. Audit. Res., Groton, Connecticut, 1969).

Licklider, J.C.R., Wesbster, J.C., and Hedlun, J.M. (1950). On the frequency limits of binaural beats. *J. Acoust. Soc. Am.,* **22**, 468-473.

Oster, G. (1973). Auditory beats in the brain. *Scientific Am.,* **229**, 76-84.

Perrott, D.R. and Nelson, M.A. (1969). Limits for the detection of binaural beats. *J. Acoust. Soc. Am.,* **46**, 1477-1481.

Perrott, D.R. (1970). A further note on "limits for the detection of binaural beats." *J. Acoust. Soc. Am.,* **47**, 663-664.

Tobias, J.V. (1972). Curious binaural phenomena. In J.V. Tobias (Ed.) *Foundations of modern auditory theory.* Vol. 2. Chapter 11, pp. 463-486, Academic Press, New York.

Wever, E.G. (1949). *Theory of hearing.* Chapter 17. Wiley, New York.

EXPERIMENT VII-7: MASKING LEVEL DIFFERENCES

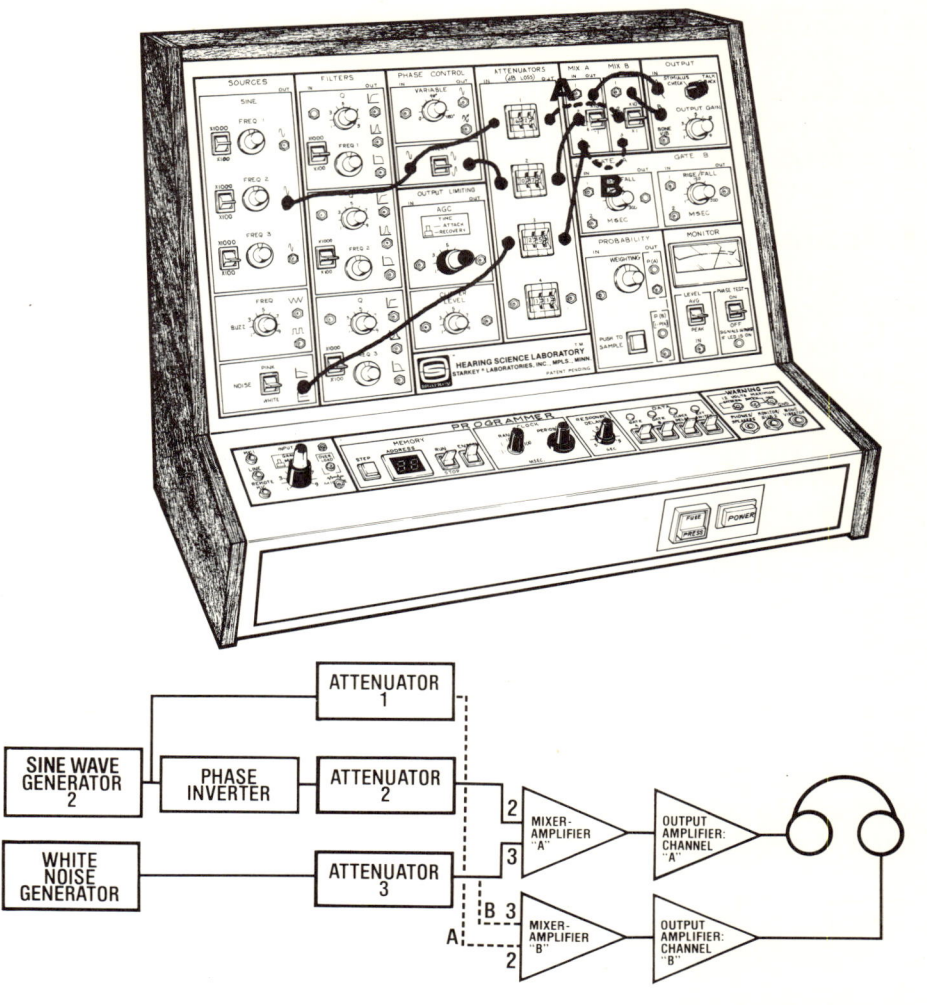

Purpose:
To demonstrate the binaural *release from masking* phenomenon.

Background Principle:
In addition to providing information as to the location of sounds within the environment, the binaural hearing mechanism suppresses interfering background noise. This process enhances the listener's ability to detect weak signals and can improve the intelligibility of speech stimuli. The several different listening situations that are described below illustrate some striking aspects of this phenomenon which has been variously called: binaural unmasking, release from masking, binaural analysis, and masking level differences (MLD's). We begin the demonstration by establishing a listener's masked threshold for a tone within a background of wide-band noise. Both the Signal (S) and the Noise (N) are delivered monaurally (m) to the subject. The signal and noise levels in this so-called *SmNm* listening condition are adjusted until the tone is just masked out by the noise. The same noise (in phase, or 0° phase difference) is then introduced to the opposite ear at the same time (i.e., the *SmNo* condition), and we find that the tone makes a startling reappearance. It is indeed striking that presenting more noise to the subject's ears should actually enhance detection. Masking has been "released" by the presence of the additional noise by as much as 5 to 15 dB. Perhaps even more surprising is the fact that the addition of the tone to the other ear (i.e., the *SoNo* condition) causes the signal to disappear again! This event would seem to conflict with the notion that two ears are always better than one. If the phase relationship between the two tones (or two noises) were to be inverted by 180°, the tone again emerges from the background of noise (i.e., the *SπNo* condition). The Masking Level Differences are usually specified in terms of the signal level (in decibels) required for detectability in one experimental condition relative to some reference test condition (typically the *SoNo* condition). At 500 Hz, an 8-10 dB MLD is not at all unusual. The advanced student is invited

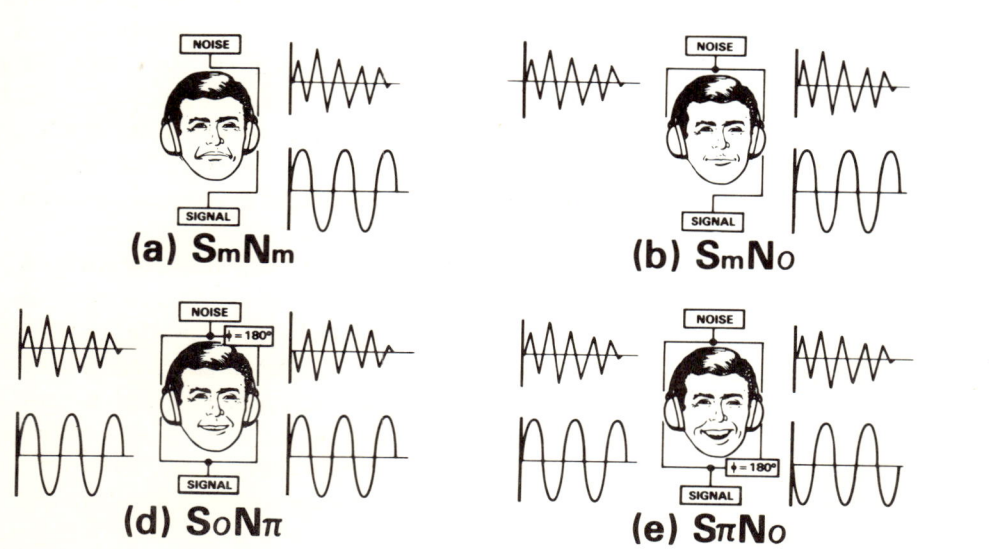

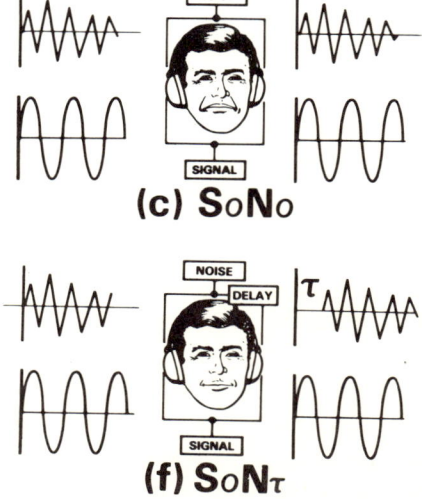

FIGURE A: A variety of masking level difference conditions are possible: (a) the *SmNm* listening condition (both signal and noise delivered monaurally). The tone is barely detectable. (b) The *SmNo* listening condition (signal monaural, noise in phase at both ears). The tone is clearly detectable. (c) The *SoNo* listening condition (signals binaurally in phase, noise binaurally in phase). The signal is again barely detectable. (d) The *SoNπ* listening condition (signals binaurally in phase, noise 180° or π radians binaurally out of phase). The signal is highly detectable. (e) The *SπNo* listening condition. This is the most detectable condition. (f) The *SoNτ* listening condition (signals binaurally in phase, noise delay to one ear). The signal detectability varies with the interaural delay. (After Levitt and Voroba, 1974).

to explore the several theories that have attempted to explain the underlying nature of the masking level differences between the various test conditions. Recent research (Quaranta and Cervellera, 1977) has tried to correlate the size of the MLD with certain central auditory pathologies. Release from masking of speech stimuli has also been accomplished.

Procedure:

The connections shown in the wiring guide and block diagram will permit the experimenter to demonstrate, in quick succession, the listening conditions described above. The pure tone signal is first passed through the Phase Inverter Switch before it enters Attenuator #2 (set the Phase Switch to the upper, non-inverting position until you are ready to try the final listening condition). The pure tone output from Sine Wave Generator #2 is also sent directly to Attenuator #1. Attenuators #1 and #2 must always be set to the identical level. The white noise signal is sent through Attenuator #3. The tone and noise waveforms that emerge from their corresponding Attenuators are combined within Mixer-Amplifier "A". Output Amplifier channel "A" receives the combined signals and routes them to one headphone. Note that the output wire from Mixer-Amplifier "B" is connected to Output Amplifier channel "B", which powers the second headphone. Connection of the dashed circuit wires permits either the tone (wire "A") or noise (wire "B") to enter the second channel and headphone. A fifth listening condition, in which the noise waveforms are phase-reversed, may be established by sending the wide-band noise, rather than the tone, into the phase reversal switch. When the Noise Generator output wire is disconnected, the Phase Tester module may be switched on to confirm and monitor the phase relationship of the pure tones delivered to the two headphones.

Exercises:

(1) Sequence of steps for Masking Level Difference demonstration:
    A. Connect all but the dashed wiring shown in the wiring guide and block diagram.
    B. Adjust the Sine Wave Generator to an initial setting near 500 Hz.
    C. Adjust the tone and noise Attenuators until the signal is just barely audible within the noise background.
    D. Add the noise to the second ear by connecting dashed circuit wire "B" between the third Input Jacks of both Mixer-Amplifiers. Note if the tone reappears.
    E. Add the tone to the second ear by connecting dashed circuit wire "A". Note if the tone gets fainter.
    F. Flip the Phase Reversal Switch to the invert position and note if the tone reappears.

(2) For each test condition, record the tone Attenuator settings at which the signal is just barely audible. The difference in decibels between the conditions is the measure of the masking level difference (e.g., MLD=threshold of tone for $SoNo$ condition minus threshold of tone for $S\pi No$ condition). Try the sequence of steps in exercise #1 for several different tone frequencies and background noise levels. Are masking level differences affected by frequency and magnitude factors?

Selected References:

Canahl, J.A., Jr. (1970). Binaural masking of a tone by a tone plus noise. *J. Acoust. Soc. Am.*, **47**, 476-479.

Durlach, N.I. (1972). Binaural signal detection: equalization and cancellation theory. In J.V. Tobias (Ed.) *Foundations of modern auditory theory.* Vol. 2. Academic Press Inc., New York.

Gerber, S.E., Jaffe, P.G., and Alford, B.L. (1971). Binaural threshold and interaural phase differences. *J. Aud. Res.*, **11**, 65-68.

Hirsh, I.J. (1948). The influence of interaural phase on interaural summation and inhibition. *J. Acoust. Soc. Am.*, **20**, 536-544.

Jeffress, L.A. (1972). Binaural signal detection: Vector theory. In J.V. Tobias (Ed.) *Foundations of modern auditory theory.* Vol. 2. Academic Press Inc., New York.

Jeffress, L.A. and McFadden, D. (1971). Differences of interaural phase and level in detection and lateralization. *J. Acoust. Soc. Am.*, **49**, 1169-1179.

Levitt, H. and Voroba, B. (1974). Binaural hearing. In S.E. Gerber (Ed.) *Introductory hearing science: physical and psychological concepts.* W.B. Saunders Co., Philadelphia.

McFadden, D., Jeffress, L.A., and Ermey, H.L. (1971). Differences of interaural phase and level in detection and lateralization: 250 Hz. *J. Acoust. Soc. Am.*, **50**, 1484-1493.

McFadden, D., Jeffress, L.A., and Lakey, J.R. (1972). Differences of interaural phase and level in detection and lateralization: 1000 and 2000 Hz. *J. Acoust. Soc. Am.*, **52**, 1197-1206.

McFadden, D. and Pasanen, E.G. (1974). High-frequency masking-level differences with narrow-band noise signals. *J. Acoust. Soc. Am.*, **56**, 1226-1230.

Quaranta, A. and Cervellera, G. (1977). Masking level differences in central nervous system diseases. *Archs Otolar.*, **103**, 482-484.

Punch, J. and Carhart, R. (1973). Influence of interaural phase on forward masking. *J. Acoust. Soc. Am.*, **54**, 897-904.

Robinson, D.E. and Dolan, T.R. (1972). Effect of signal frequency on the MLD for uncorrelated noise. *J. Acoust. Soc. Am.*, **51**, 1945-1946.

Robinson, D.E. and Trahiotis, C. (1972). Effects of signal duration and masker duration on detectability under diotic and dichotic listening conditions. *Percept. Psychophys.*, **12**, 333-334.

Schoeny, Z.G. and Carhart, R. (1971). Effects of unilateral Ménière's disease on masking-level differences. *J. Acoust. Soc. Am.*, **50**, 1143-1150.

Small, A.M. et al. (1972). MLDs in forward and backward masking. *J. Acoust. Soc. Am.*, **51**, 1365-1367.

Soderquist, D.R. and Lindsey, J.W. (1970). Masking-level differences as a function of noise spectrum level, frequency, and signal duration. *J. Aud. Res.*, **10**, 276-282.

Tillman, T.W., Carhart, R., and Nicholls, S. (1973). Release from multiple maskers in elderly persons. *J. Speech Hear. Res.*, **16**, 152-160.

Townsend, T.H. and Goldstein, D.P. (1972). Suprathreshold binaural unmasking. *J. Acoust. Soc. Am.*, **51**, 621-624.

Yost, W.A. (1972). Tone-on-tone masking for three binaural listening conditions. *J. Acoust. Soc. Am.*, **52**, 1234-1237.

EXPERIMENT VII-8: THE JND FOR DICHOTIC PHASE

Purpose:
To examine the sensitivity of the binaural hearing mechanism to changes in the interaural phase relationship between dichotic tone pulses.

Background Principle:
In Laboratory Experiment VII-3, we noted that interaural time of arrival differences between dichotically presented clicks can shift the apparent lateral position of a fused click image within the head. These temporal differences could also be defined in terms of the phase differences between two sound waveforms. Consider, for example, identical 1000 Hz tones which are switched on in succession one-half millisecond apart. It should be clear that since the period of a 1000Hz tone is one millisecond, the "starting phases" of the two signals will be one-half period or 180° out of phase with respect to each other

In the present experiment, a listener will be asked to compare a "diotic" pair of tone pulses (i.e., binaural signals which are identical in every respect) to a "dichotic" pair (i.e., disparate binaural signals) which share a non-zero interaural phase relationship.

Procedure:
Sine Wave Generator #3 provides a pure tone signal which is sent through an Attenuator and into both Electronic Gates. The output from Gate "A" is routed to the Adjustable Phase Shifter whose Reference and Variable Phase outputs are delivered to Mixer-Amplifier "A" and Attenuator #1, respectively.

Attenuator #1 may be used to equalize the Reference and Variable Phase output signal levels, if necessary. The signal leaving Attenuator #1 enters Mixer-Amplifier "B". The stimulus from Electronic Gate "B" is sent to both Mixer-Amplifiers which, in turn, present their outputs to separate Output Amplifiers and headphones. The suggested programming instructions will permit each tone pulse pair to switch on for roughly one second, separated by a one second silent interval. The entire sequence will then repeat itself every three seconds. Use the Monitor Level Meter to assure that the level of each test tone is identical (see Figure I-14 for proper connection to the Meter). Present a group of ten test trials for each randomly selected Phase Shifter setting. The subject should be required to report if the second dichotic pulse in sequence appeared to be shifted to the right or left of the first diotic pulse, which is typically perceived to be located in the listener's median plane (i.e., in line with the nose).

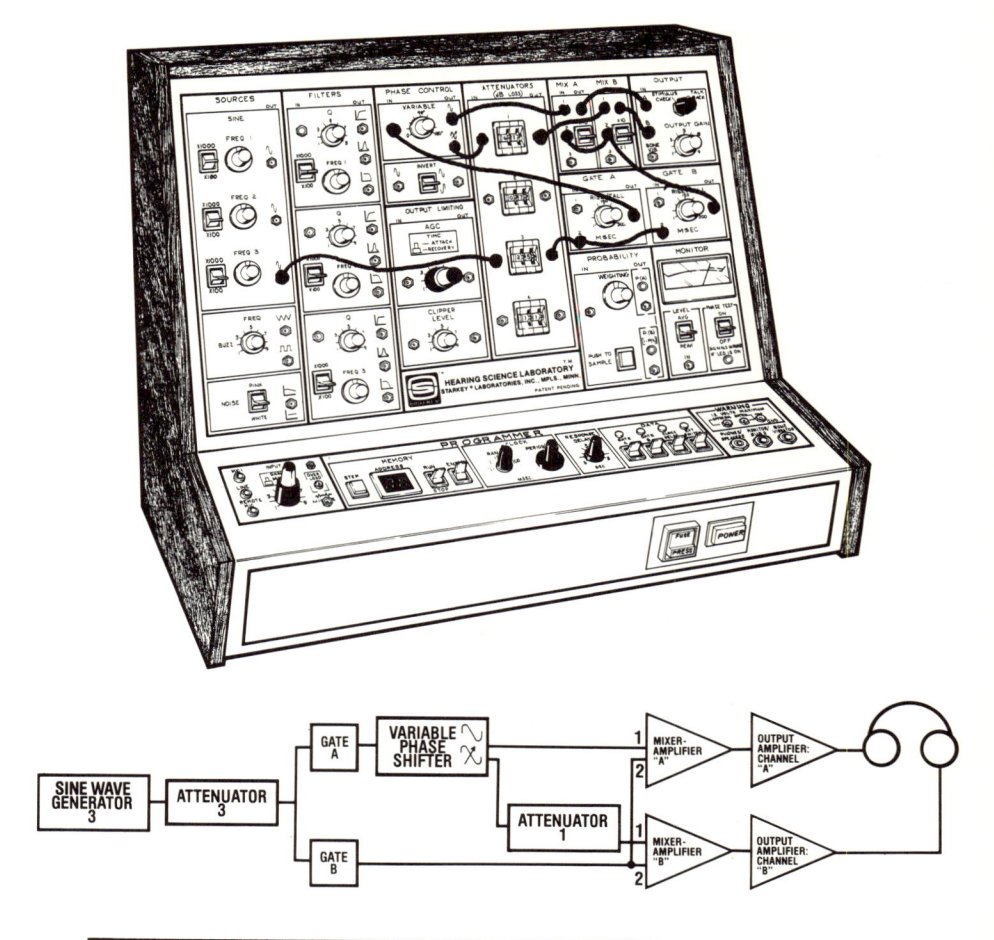

Exercises:
(1) Both the sensation level and frequency of the stimuli are variables which may affect the smallest dichotic phase difference which can be detected. Determine the minimum Phase Shifter Control Knob setting which produces a noticeable shift in the position of the binaural fused sound image for each of the following test stimuli conditions:

FREQUENCY OF TONE	SENSATION LEVELS OF TONE
250 Hz, 500 Hz, 1000 Hz	10, 30, 50 dB SL

(2) Repeat the listening tasks for 2000 and 4000 Hz. How do you explain the fact that no apparent shift in image position occurs?

NOTES:

Selected References:

Hafter, E.R. and De Maio, J. (1975). Difference thresholds for interaural delay. *J. Acoust. Soc. Am.*, **57**, 181-187.

Hershkowitz, R.N. and Durlach, N.I. (1969). Interaural time and amplitude JND's for a 500-Hz tone. *J. Acoust. Soc. Am.*, **46**, 1464-1467.

Jeffress, L.A., Blodgett, H.C., and Deatherage, B.H. (1952). The masking of tones by white noise as a function of the interaural phases of both components. *J. Acoust. Soc. Am.*, **24**, 523-527.

Jeffress, L.A. and McFadden, D. (1971). Differences of interaural phase and level in detection and lateralization. *J. Acoust. Soc. Am.*, **49**, 1169-1179.

Klumpp, R.G. and Eady, H.R. (1956). Some measurements of interaural time difference thresholds. *J. Acoust. Soc. Am.*, **28**, 859-860.

Licklider, J.C.R. and Webster, J.C. (1950). The discriminability of interaural phase relations in two-component tones. *J. Acoust. Soc. Am.*, **22**, 191-195.

McFadden, D. and Pasanen, E.G. (1976). Lateralization at high frequencies based on interaural time differences. *J. Acoust. Soc. Am.*, **59**, 634-639.

McFadden, D. and Sharpley, A.D. (1972). Detectability of interaural time differences and interaural level differences as a function of signal duration. *J. Acoust. Soc. Am.*, **52**, 574-576.

Mills, A.W. (1958). On the minimum audible angle. *J. Acoust. Soc. Am.*, **30**, 237-246.

Mills, A.W. (1972). Auditory localization. In J.V. Tobias (Ed.) *Foundations of modern auditory theory.* Vol. 2. Academic Press, New York.

Nordmark, J.O. (1976). Binaural time discrimination. *J. Acoust. Soc. Am.*, **60**, 870-880.

Tobias, J.V. and Schubert, E.D. (1959). Effective onset duration of auditory stimuli. *J. Acoust. Soc. Am.*, **31**, 1595-1605.

Tobias, J.V. and Zerlin, S. (1959). Lateralization threshold as a function of stimulus duration. *J. Acoust. Soc. Am.*, **31**, 1591-1594.

Wakeford, O.S. and Robinson, D.E. (1974). Detection of binaurally masked tones by the cat. *J. Acoust. Soc. Am.*, **56**, 952-956.

Yost, W.A. (1974). Discrimination of interaural phase differences. *J. Acoust. Soc. Am.*, **55**, 1299-1303.

Zurek, P.M. and Leshowitz, B.H. (1976). Interaural phase discrimination for combination tone stimuli. *J. Acoust. Soc. Am.*, **60**, 169-172.

Zwislocki, J. and Feldman, R.S. (1956). Just noticeable differences in dichotic phase. *J. Acoust. Soc. Am.*, **28**, 860-864.

EXPERIMENT VII-9: INTERAURAL ATTENUATION OF AIR CONDUCTION SIGNALS

Purpose:
To determine the acoustic isolation between the ears.

Background Principle:
High level acoustic stimuli delivered by a headphone to one ear will cross through the skull via bone conduction and may be detected by the opposite, non-test ear. Although it is possible to "remove" the non-test ear from a listening task by presenting it with an appropriate masking sound, the masker may also influence the ear under test through the physiological process of Central Masking (see Laboratory Experiment VI-4). Thus, *interaural attenuation (I.A.)*, or the degree to which sound energy is *absorbed* and changed to heat as it passes through the head, becomes an important consideration for clinical and laboratory studies in Hearing Science.

One way to determine the interaural attenuation of the skull for headphone listening is by the *method of compensation* (see Zwislocki, 1953). In this case, a high level, continuous tone is sent to one ear while a weaker signal having the same frequency is routed to the other ear. Ideally, the phase relationship between the weak signal and the attenuated *contralateralized* tone could be adjusted until both signals were 180° out-of-phase and completely canceled each other (see Laboratory Experiment I-1). Unfortunately, a listener would never notice the cancellation of the tone in one ear due to the ever present high level signal in the first. Zwislocki overcame this difficulty by making the weaker tone pulsate, thereby creating detectable loudness fluctuations. The underlying phenomena which relate to these particular experimental limitations and solutions were considered in Laboratory Experiments VII-1, on Binaural Summation, and Laboratory Experiment VII-2, on Binaural Fusion.

The subject was required to adjust the phase relationship between the tones until the overall loudness of the sound was softest when the signals were delivered to both ears and loudest when only the high level tone was presented. This occurs when the contralateralized and weak intermittent tones are 180° out-of-phase. Once this phase condition has been achieved, the subject then increases the level of the weak tone until no further pulsations in loudness can be discerned. The necessary signal levels for this steady loudness situation to occur are considered in Figure "A". It should be noted that the "compensating" intermittent tone must have twice the sound pressure (i.e., 6 dB more) than the contralateralized signal in order for the overall level (and loudness) to remain the same before and after superposition of the out-of-phase tones. In other words, the contralateralized tone is 6 dB less than the interrupted tone level. If, for example, the intermittent tone was 40 dB SPL for the steady loudness condition, the contralateralized signal must be 34 dB. And if the continuous high level

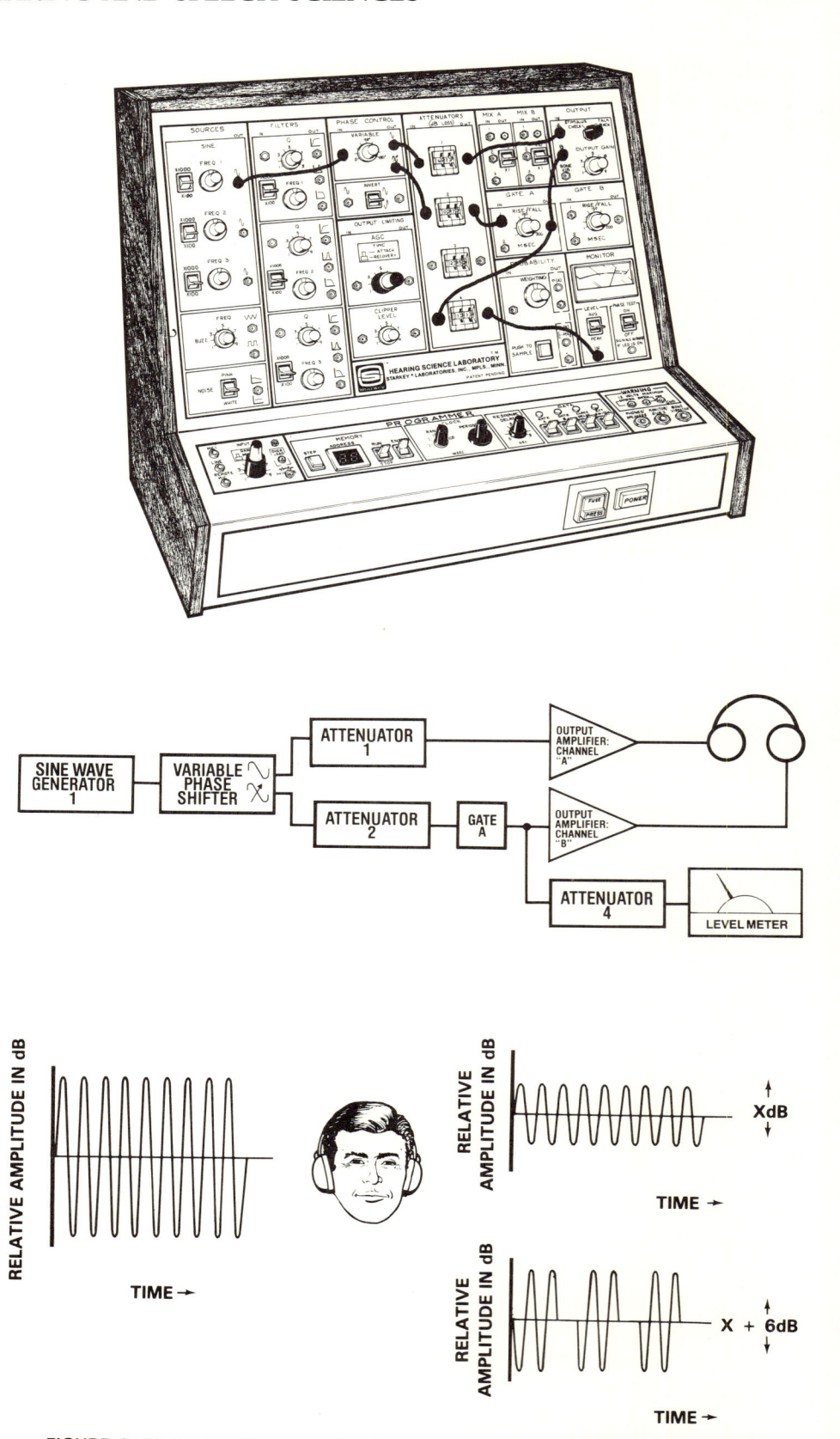

FIGURE A: Method of Compensation (Zwislocki, 1953). A high level continuous tone delivered to one ear crosses through the skull via bone conduction. A pulsed tone having the same frequency, but out-of-phase by 180° with respect to the attenuated contralateralized signal, is added to the other ear. As described in the text, the intermittent tone must be 6 dB greater in level than the contralateralized stimulus in order for the loudness percept to remain the same before and after superposition.

signal were originally 85 dB SPL, then the interaural attenuation of the skull for the frequency employed must be:

$$85 \text{ dB} - 34 \text{ dB} = 46 \text{ dB I.A.}$$

Experimenters have found that interaural attenuation varies between frequencies and subjects. In general, however, the skull provides a higher I.A. for higher frequency stimuli.

Procedure:

The output from Sine Wave Generator #1 is routed to the Variable Phase Shifter. The Reference Output signal is sent through Attenuator #1 and one Output Amplifier and headphone. The Variable Output signal is sent through Attenuator #2 and Electronic Gate "A" before being delivered to the second Output Amplifier channel and headphone. The gated signal is also passed through Attenuator #4 and the Level Meter so that the subject will be able to monitor when the intermittent signal has been presented. The suggested programming instructions will pulse the signal on and off every half-second. Set Attenuator #4 to a value which produces a mid-scale Meter reading whenever Gate "A" is switched on.

Exercises:

(1) Perform the listening task described in the Background Principle section above for tone frequencies near 200 Hz, 500 Hz, 1 kHz, 2 kHz, and 4 kHz. Record the I.A. values you obtain from a group of test subjects at each frequency and evaluate the degree of variability in your data. What factors do you think contribute most to differences in test data values?

(2) Based upon your reading of the Selected References, what transducers or techniques could you employ to increase the acoustic isolation between the ears?

NOTES:

Selected References:

von Békésy, G. (1948). Vibration of the head in a sound field and its role in hearing by bone conduction. *J. Acoust. Soc. Am.*, **20,** 749-760.

Liden, G. (1954). Speech audiometry. *Acta Oto-Lar.*, Suppl., **114,** 72-76. Stockholm.

Liden, G., Nilsson, G., and Anderson, H. (1959). Narrow-band masking with white noise. *Acta Oto-Lar.*, **50,** 116-124. Stockholm.

Littler, T.S., Knight, J.J., and Strange, P.H. (1952). Hearing by bone conduction and the use of bone conduction hearing aids. *Proc. Roy. Soc. Med.*, **45,** 783-790.

Studebaker, G.A. (1962). Placement of vibrator in bone-conduction testing. *J. Speech Hear. Res.*, **5,** 321-331.

Studebaker, G.A. (1964). Clinical masking of air- and bone-conducted stimuli. *J. Speech Hear. Dis.*, **29,** 23-35.

Studebaker, G.A. (1967). Clinical masking of the nontest ear. *J. Speech Hear. Dis.*, **32,** 360-371.

Teas, D.C. and Nielsen, D.W. (1975). Interaural attenuation versus frequency for guinea pig and chinchilla CM response. *J. Acoust. Soc. Am.*, **58,** 1066-1072.

Zwislocki, J. (1953). Acoustic attenuation between the ears. *J. Acoust. Soc. Am.*, **25,** 752-759.

Speech Perception VIII

EXPERIMENT VIII-1: SYNTHETIC VOWELS

Purpose:
To examine the electronic simulation of vowels.

Background Principle:
The larynx is the source of sound energy for the vowels of speech. A series of air puffs, generated by sub-laryngeal pressure, is rich with harmonics or multiples of the fundamental (i.e., lowest) frequency component of the sound. As this complex, buzz-like sound passes through the various chambers in our vocal tract (i.e., the oral, pharyngeal, and nasal cavities), changes occur in the relative amplitudes of its constituent frequencies. Certain frequencies are enhanced or resonated, while others are attenuated as a result of the specific size and shape of the vocal tract. Figures "A" and "B" display the relative amplitude of the pure tone components in the glottic buzz before and after passing through the vocal tract cavities for the vowel, /a/. The regions of maximum amplitude for the vowel are called *formants*. Researchers have shown that vowels may contain five or more of these frequency regions, but vowel recognition remains possible with only three or even two formants present. It is the particular frequency relationship between formant frequencies that determines the actual vowel that is produced, and the rapid process of speech production and recognition is extremely complex and difficult to analyze.

Procedure:
The output from the Square Wave Generator will provide the electronic analog of the laryngeal "buzz" source. Route the buzz signal through three Band Pass Filters. The resonant characteristics of the three filters modify the buzz waveform in a manner like that of the actual cavities within our vocal tracts. The Filter outputs are then sent to separate Attenuators so that their levels may be independently controlled. All three signals are then routed to Mixer-Amplifer "A", and the combined output is then sent to Mixer-Amplifier "B". Both Mixer-Amplifiers should be sent to the X 10 (20dB) Gain Switch position. The amplified signal is next sent to one Output Amplifier channel and headphone. Adjust the three Filter Frequency Controls in accordance with the formant frequencies needed for the particular English vowel you wish to synthesize (see Table I, below). Table I also shows the relative amplitudes for each of the three formants. Set the three Attenuators to the required values. For example, to simulate the vowel /a/ as in "hot", adjust the controls near the following settings:

	Filter Frequency	Attenuator Level (in dB)
Formant 1:	730 Hz	1
Formant 2:	1090 Hz	5
Formant 3:	2440 Hz	28

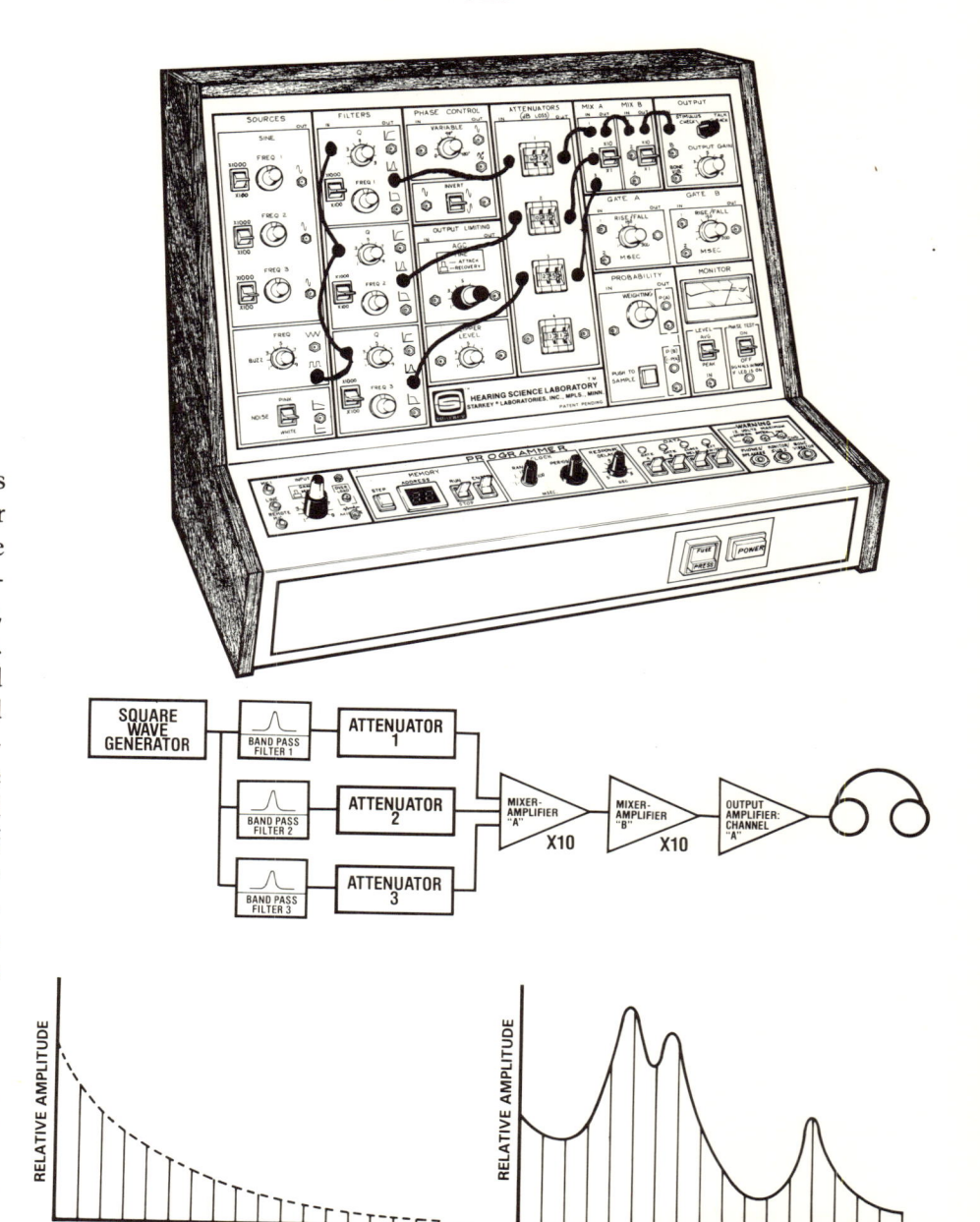

FIGURE A: Relative amplitude of the spectral components in the buzz-like sound of the larynx before its passage through the cavities in the vocal tract.

FIGURE B: The particular size and configuration of the vocal tract will selectively enhance certain frequencies in the laryngeal complex sound. The relative amplitudes and frequencies of the formants for the vowel, "ah," are indicated.

By slowly rocking the Frequency Knob of the Square Wave Generator around the required fundamental buzz frequency (i.e., 124 Hz for /a/), a slight pitch glide may be added to the vowel to make it sound more natural.

Exercises:
(1) Alternately unplug different Filter output wires and note the change in vowel quality. What effect does each of the formants have upon the recognition of the synthetic vowels?

(2) Use white noise as the source of energy for your vowels, instead of a square wave signal, and note if a recognizable vowel can be obtained. Can you account for your results?

TABLE 1: "Averages of fundamental and formant frequencies and formant amplitudes of vowels by 76 speakers." (Peterson and Barney, 1952). Note that the chart includes data for men's, women's, and childrens' vocalizations.

		i	I	ɛ	æ	ɑ	ɔ	ʊ	u	ʌ	ɜ
Fundamental frequencies (Hz)	M	136	135	130	127	124	129	137	141	130	133
	W	235	232	223	210	212	216	232	231	221	218
	Ch	272	269	260	251	256	263	276	274	261	261
Formant frequencies (Hz)											
F_1	M	270	390	530	660	730	570	440	300	640	490
	W	310	430	610	860	850	590	470	370	760	500
	Ch	370	530	690	1010	1030	680	560	430	850	560
F_2	M	2290	1990	1840	1720	1090	840	1020	870	1190	1350
	W	2790	2480	2330	2050	1220	920	1160	950	1400	1640
	Ch	3200	2730	2610	2320	1370	1060	1410	1170	1590	1820
F_3	M	3010	2550	2480	2410	2440	2410	2240	2240	2390	1690
	W	3310	3070	2990	2850	2810	2710	2680	2670	2780	1960
	Ch	3730	3600	3570	3320	3170	3180	3310	3260	3360	2160
Formant Amplitudes (dB)	L_1	−4	−3	−2	−1	−1	0	−1	−3	−1	−5
	L_2	−24	−23	−17	−12	−5	−7	−12	−19	−10	−15
	L_3	−28	−27	−24	−22	−28	−34	−34	−43	−27	−20

NOTES:

Selected References:

Bogert, B.P. (1953). On the bandwidth of vowel formants. *J. Acoust. Soc. Am.*, **25**, 791-792.

Dunn, H.K. (1950). The calculation of vocal resonances, and an electrical vocal tract. *J. Acoust. Soc. Am.*, **22**, 740-753.

Fant, C.G.M. (1956). On the predictability of formant levels and spectrum envelopes from formant frequencies. In M. Halle, H. Lund, and M. MacLean (Eds.) *For Roman Jakobson.* pp. 44-56. The Hague: Mouton.

Flanagan, J.L., Coker, C.H., Rabiner, L.R., Schafer, R.W., and Umeda, N. (1970). Synthetic voices for computers. *IEEE Spectrum*, **7**, 22-45.

Klein, W., Plomp, R., and Pols, L.C.W. (1970). Vowel spectra, vowel spaces and vowel identification. *J. Acoust. Soc. Am.*, **48**, 999-1009.

Liberman, A.M., Cooper, F.S., Shankweiler, D.P., and Studdert-Kennedy, M. (1967). Perception of the speech code. *Psychol. Rev.*, **74**, 431-461.

Peterson, G.E. and Barney, H.L. (1952). Control methods used in a study of the vowels. *J. Acoust. Soc. Am.*, **24**, 175-184.

Potter, R.K. and Peterson, G.E. (1948). The representation of vowels and their movement. *J. Acoust. Soc. Am.*, **20**, 528-535.

Scott, B.L. (1976). Temporal factors in vowel perception. *J. Acoust. Soc. Am.*, **60**, 1354-1365.

Stevens, K.N. and House, A.S. (1961). An acoustical theory of vowel production and some of its implications. *J. Speech Hear. Res.*, **4**, 303-320.

Stevens, K.N. and House, A.S. (1972). Speech Perception. In J.V. Tobias (Ed.), *Foundations of modern auditory theory.* Vol. 2. Academic Press, New York.

Stevens, K.N., Bastide, R.P., and Smith, C.P. (1955). Electrical synthesizer of continuous speech. *J. Acoust. Soc. Am.*, **27**, 207(A).

Stevens, K.N., Kasowski, S., and Fant, C.G.M. (1953). An electrical analog to the vocal tract. *J. Acoust. Soc. Am.*, **25**, 734-742.

Umeda, N. (1975). Vowel duration in American English. *J. Acoust. Soc. Am.*, **58**, 434-445.

Verbrugge, R.R., Strange, W., Shankweiler, D.P., and Edman, T.R. (1976). What information enables a listener to map a talker's vowel space? *J. Acoust. Soc. Am.*, **60**, 198-212.

Weibel, E.S. (1955). Vowel synthesis by means of resonant circuits. *J. Acoust. Soc. Am.*, **22**, 858-865.

EXPERIMENT VIII-2: THE ELECTROLARYNX

Purpose:
To produce speech sounds by mechanical (artificial) stimulation of the vocal tract.

Background Principle:
Some individuals who lose the normal vocalizing function of the larynx through disease or surgical removal may learn to communicate with *esophageal speech* (i.e., by forcing air into the esophagus and releasing it in a controlled manner). Unfortunately, this technique cannot be mastered by all laryngectomized persons. An *electrolarynx* is a device that electronically imitates the buzz-like sounds produced by the larynx. Pressing the electrolarynx against the neck and throat transmits the sound vibrations through the vocal tract. Movements of the *articulators*, such as the lips, tongue, and soft palate, will alter the resonant frequency characteristics of the vocal tract and transform the artificial buzz sound into recognizable speech sounds.

Procedure:
A harmonically rich square wave signal is routed to an Attenuator, a Mixer-Amplifier (set to 20 dB Gain), and the Bone Vibrator Output Amplifier. The Bone Vibrator itself is plugged into the appropriate Output Jack at the lower right hand portion of the front panel.

Exercises:
(1) Move the bone vibrator around on the neck to locate the area of contact which produces the loudest sound output from the subject's open mouth. The anterio-lateral surfaces of the thyroid cartilage are good places to try (see Figure "A"). The artificial larynx will sound less "mechanical" if the Square Wave Frequency Control Knob is rocked back and forth while the subject silently mouths words. The pitch glide produced by this rocking action will imitate the inflections of the natural voice.

(2) Repeat exercise #1 for both male and female speakers and note that the optimum frequencies for electrolarynx sound output are different for men and women. How can you account for this?

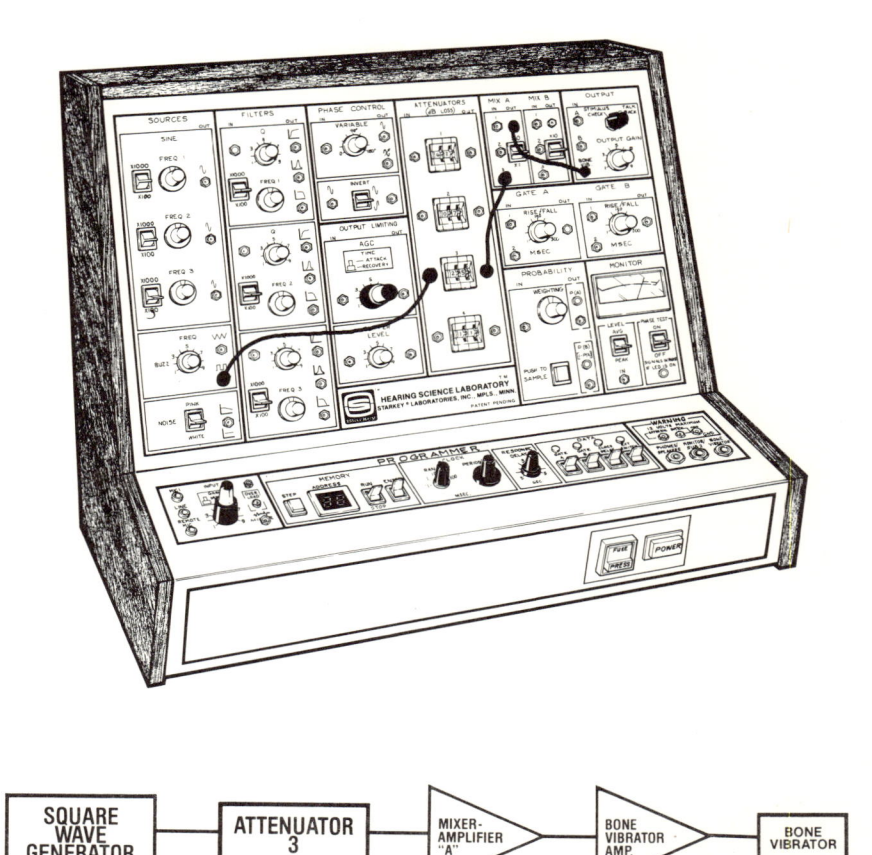

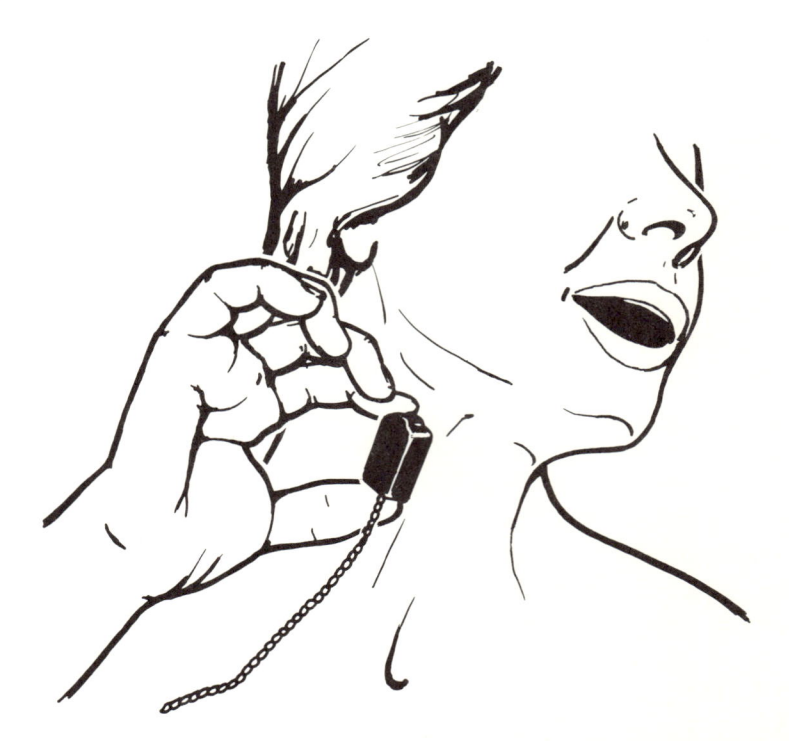

FIGURE A: Place the bone vibrator against the side of the neck and silently mouth words to create speech with the electrolarynx.

NOTES:

Selected References:

Flanagan, J.L. (1958). Some properties of the glottal sound source. *J. Speech Hear. Res.*, **1**, 99-116.

Gardner, W.H. and Harris, H.E. (1961). Aids and devices for laryngectomees. *Archs Otolar.*, **73**, 145.

Lauder, E. (1968). The laryngectomee and the artificial larynx. *J. Speech Hear. Dis.*, **33**, 147-157.

Lauder, E. (1970). The laryngectomee and the artificial larynx — a second look. *J. Speech Hear. Dis.*, **35**, 62-65.

Mathews, M.V., Miller, J.E., and David, E.E. (1961). An accurate estimate of the glottal waveshape. *J. Acoust. Soc. Am.*, **33**, 843 (A).

McCroskey, R.L. and Mulligan, M. (1963). The relative intelligibility of esophageal speech and artificial larynx. *J. Speech Dis.*, **28**, 37.

Miller, R.L. (1959). Nature of the vocal cord wave. *J. Acoust. Soc. Am.*, **31**, 667-677.

Sondhi, M.M. (1975) Measurement of the glottal waveform. *J. Acoust. Soc. Am.*, **57**, 228-232.

Yeni-Komshian, G.H., Weiss, M.S., and Heinz, J.M. (1975). Intelligibility of speech produced with an electronic artificial larynx. *J. Acoust. Soc. Am.*, **58**, S112.

EXPERIMENT VIII-3: THE PERFORMANCE-INTENSITY FUNCTION

Purpose:
To examine the intelligibility of speech stimuli at different signal magnitudes.

Background Principle:
A standard technique used to assess the intelligibility of speech requires the listener to write down or repeat aloud a list of words presented by the experimenter. The percentage of stimuli that are correctly identified at a particular stimulus intensity level is known as a *discrimination score*. The graph which portrays the relationship between these scores and stimulus levels is called a *performance intensity function,* formerly termed an *articulation gain function* (see Figure "A"). Note that the performance of a subject differs with the type of stimuli employed. The curve for monosyllables does not, for example, rise as abruptly as for *spondee* words, which contain two equally emphasized syllables. In 1947, researchers at the Harvard Psychoacoustics Laboratory compiled lists of spondee and so-called *phonetically balanced (PB)* words which remain in clinical and experimental use to this day. The *NU6 Lists,* developed at Northwestern University, are also in widespread use and are felt to have roughly the same frequency of occurrence in spoken English. A sampling of spondee and monosyllable words is provided in Table I. The level at which spondee words become intelligible 50% of the time is known as the *Threshold of Speech Intelligibility* or *Speech Reception Threshold (SRT).* For a listener with normal hearing, the maximum articulation score for monosyllable words (i.e., the so-called *PB max* point) lies roughly 30 to 40 dB SPL above the SRT. For some hearing impaired individuals, the PB max value may be less than 100%, with additional increases in signal level actually giving rise to a reduction in the subject's discrimination score or "rollover" (see curve "X" in Figure "A"). This is thought to be suggestive of retrocochlear lesions.

Procedure:
Live speech may be presented to a listener by passing a microphone signal through the Input Preamplifier channel, an Attenuator, Mixer-Amplifier, Output Amplifier, and headphone. The Mixer-Amplifier will be used for exercise #3 in which speech and noise waveforms are to be combined. Dashed circuit wire "A" provides the necessary connection for this task. The Level Meter may be used to monitor the speech or noise magnitudes by attaching dashed wire "B" to test points "X" or "Y", respectively. The subject's responses may be monitored by means of the talkback circuit discussed in Part I of this text and diagrammed in Figure I-43A. (Note: when presenting speech stimuli at high supra-threshold levels, there is a possibility that some speech sounds will lateralize across the head and be perceived

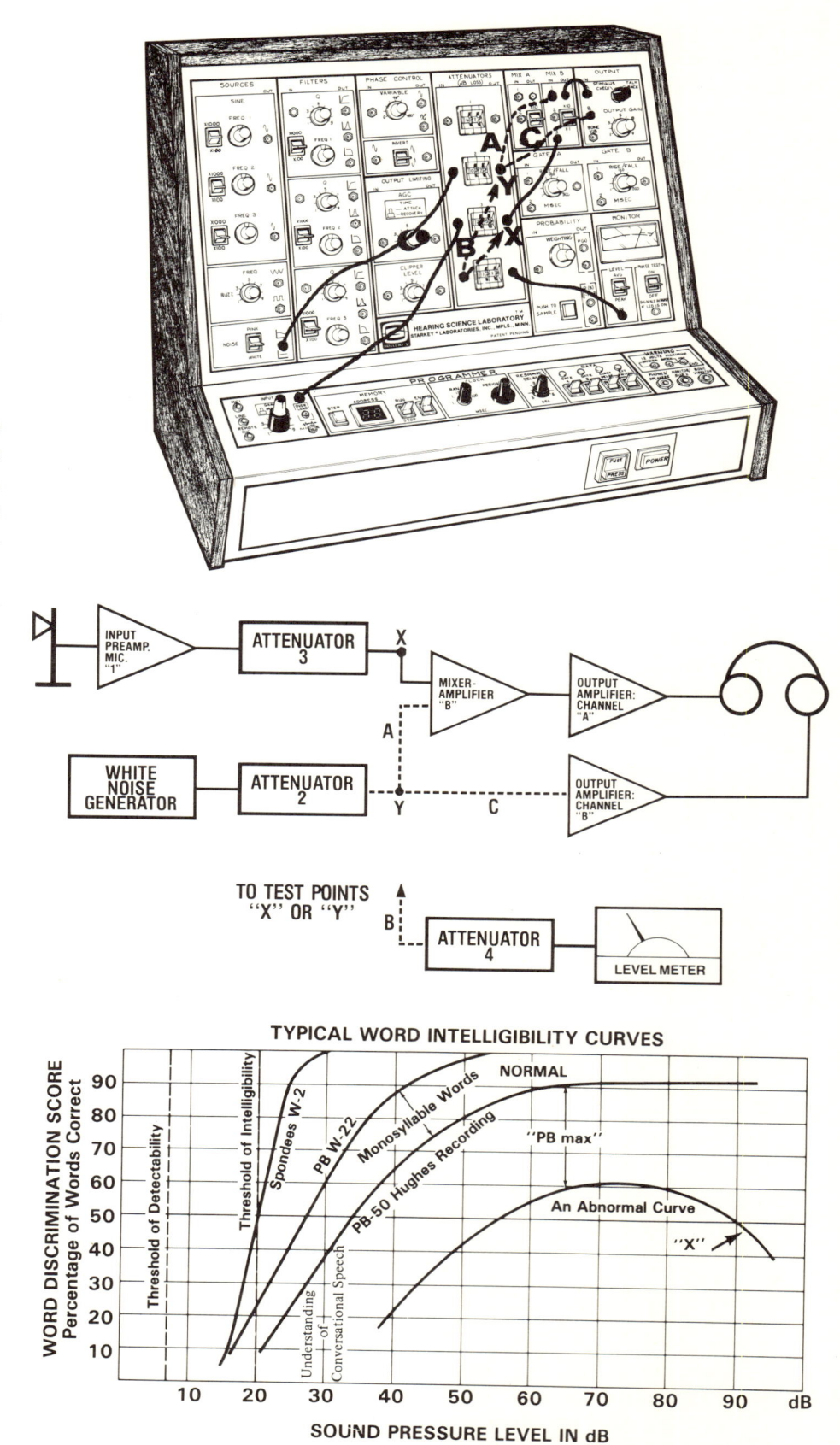

FIGURE A: A subject's word discrimination score depends upon the type of stimulus employed in addition to its sound pressure level. (From Davis, H. and Silverman, S.R. (Ed.). *Hearing and Deafness* (3rd ed.). Holt, Rinehart, Winston, New York, 1970).

by the non-test ear. To minimize this danger and remove the participation of the non-test ear from the listening task, it is necessary to introduce a wide-band masking noise into the non-test ear. This is accomplished by connecting dashed circuit wire "C," as shown in the wiring guide.

Exercises:

(1) Use the spondee and NU6 word lists shown below to determine the articulation scores of a listener for several different signal magnitudes. Plot your percentage correct scores on the graph shown in Figure "B."

(2) Obtain an estimate of a subject's SRT by means of a simple up-down procedure (see Laboratory Experiment II-4). Does this 50% response estimate agree with the 50% point on the graph obtained for exercise #1?

(3) Examine the change in a subject's discrimination score when various levels of white noise are combined with the speech stimuli in the same ear. Monitor the relative signal to noise levels with the Level Meter. At what *signal to noise ratio* does the speech become completely unintelligible?

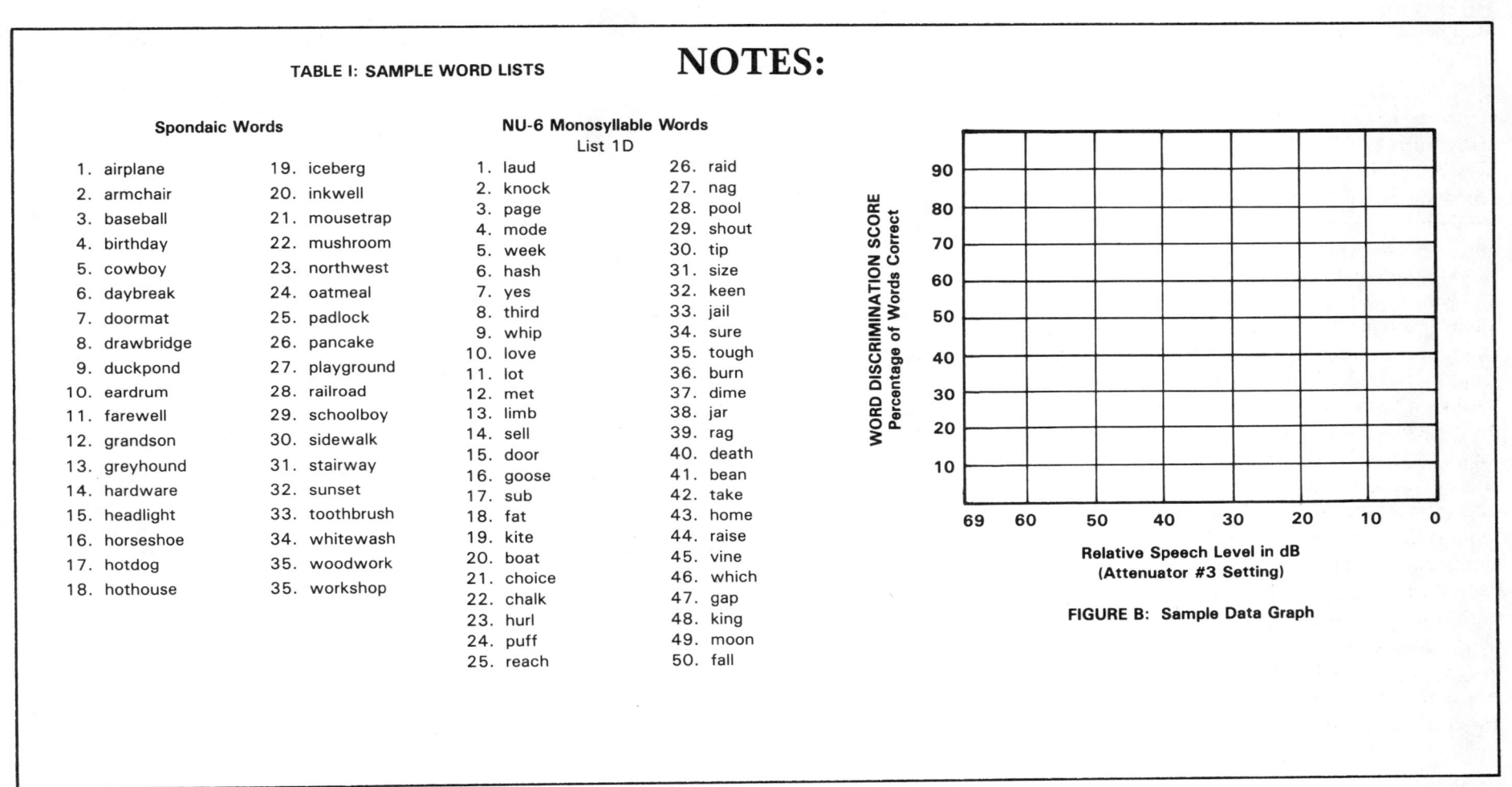

TABLE I: SAMPLE WORD LISTS

Spondaic Words

1. airplane	19. iceberg		
2. armchair	20. inkwell		
3. baseball	21. mousetrap		
4. birthday	22. mushroom		
5. cowboy	23. northwest		
6. daybreak	24. oatmeal		
7. doormat	25. padlock		
8. drawbridge	26. pancake		
9. duckpond	27. playground		
10. eardrum	28. railroad		
11. farewell	29. schoolboy		
12. grandson	30. sidewalk		
13. greyhound	31. stairway		
14. hardware	32. sunset		
15. headlight	33. toothbrush		
16. horseshoe	34. whitewash		
17. hotdog	35. woodwork		
18. hothouse	35. workshop		

NU-6 Monosyllable Words
List 1D

1. laud	26. raid
2. knock	27. nag
3. page	28. pool
4. mode	29. shout
5. week	30. tip
6. hash	31. size
7. yes	32. keen
8. third	33. jail
9. whip	34. sure
10. love	35. tough
11. lot	36. burn
12. met	37. dime
13. limb	38. jar
14. sell	39. rag
15. door	40. death
16. goose	41. bean
17. sub	42. take
18. fat	43. home
19. kite	44. raise
20. boat	45. vine
21. choice	46. which
22. chalk	47. gap
23. hurl	48. king
24. puff	49. moon
25. reach	50. fall

NOTES:

FIGURE B: Sample Data Graph

(Word Discrimination Score, Percentage of Words Correct, vs. Relative Speech Level in dB, Attenuator #3 Setting)

Selected References:

Bocca, E. and Calearo, C. (1963). Central hearing processes. In J. Jerger (Ed.) *Modern developments in audiology.* Academic Press Inc., New York.

Bode, D.L. and Carhart, R. (1974). Stability and accuracy of adaptive tests of speech discrimination. *J. Acoust. Soc. Am.,* **56,** 963-970.

Davis, H. and Silverman, S.R. (1970). *Hearing and deafness.* (3rd ed.) Holt, Reinhart and Winston, Inc., New York.

Egan, J.P. (1948). Articulation testing methods. *Laryngoscope,* **58,** 955-991.

French, N.R. and Steinberg, J.C. (1947). Factors governing the intelligibility of speech sounds. *J. Acoust. Soc. Am.,* **19,** 90-119.

Harris, J.D. (1965). Speech audiometry. In A. Glorig (Ed.) *Audiometry: principles and practices.* Williams and Wilkins Co., Baltimore, Maryland.

Jerger, J. and Jerger S. (1968). Progression of auditory symptoms in a patient with acoustic neurinoma. *Ann. Otol.,* **77,** 230-242.

Jerger, J. and Jerger, S. (1971). Diagnostic significance of PB word functions. *Archs Otolar.,* **93,** 573-580.

Jerger, J., Speaks, C., and Trammell, J.L. (1968). A new approach to speech audiometry. *J. Speech Hear. Dis.,* **33,** 318-328.

Lehiste, I. (Ed.) (1967). *Readings in acoustic phonetics.* MIT Press, Cambridge, Massachusetts.

Lehiste, I. and Peterson, G.E. (1959). Linguistic considerations in the study of speech intelligibility. *J. Acoust. Soc. Am.,* **31,** 280-286.

EXPERIMENT VIII-4: THE PERCEPTION OF LOW PASS AND HIGH PASS FILTERED SPEECH

Purpose:
To determine the intelligibility of filtered speech.

Background Principle:
Are some of the frequencies in speech more important than others for intelligibility? A number of experiments have shown that speech can be understood even though many of its component frequencies have been eliminated by passing the stimuli through an Electronic Filter. The curves shown in Figure "A" relate the percentage of monosyllabic words a listener correctly identifies to the cutoff frequencies of either high or low pass filters through which the speech is passed. It can be seen, from curve I, that when the cutoff frequency of a high pass filter is **low,** all the frequencies above this value will be passed by the device, and the speech will be quite intelligible. When the high pass filter cutoff is raised, however, speech becomes progressively less intelligible as fewer and fewer frequency components remain. The reverse description applies to the low pass filter curve (II) whose maximum intelligibility score occurs when the cutoff point is high, thereby permitting the many frequencies **below** this value to be passed. The curves intersect at a frequency of roughly 1800 Hz, indicating that the monosyllables are equally intelligible whether all components either above or below this frequency are passed. Note that for filter cutoffs below 1800 Hz, however, word intelligibility decreases for the low pass device. These data provide a partial answer to our opening question. The higher frequency components of speech, such as are contained within the consonants, would seem to be of greater importance to speech intelligibility.

Procedure:
The speech signals from a microphone are first sent to the Input Preamplifier and then through three series-cascaded Filters. Although a high pass filter configuration is shown on the wiring guide and block diagram, a low pass combination may also be created as shown in Figure I-30A in Part I of this text. Set all three Filter "Q"-controls fully counterclockwise and all Filter frequencies to the identical settings to achieve a 36 dB/octave rolloff. The filtered speech stimuli are then delivered to an Attenuator and one Output Amplifier channel and headphone.

Exercises:
(1) Perform a speech discrimination test using NU6 words for each of the following high and low pass filter cutoff frequencies:

Filter cutoff frequencies: 250, 500, 1000, 2000, and 4000 Hz.

Contrast the percentage of correct identifications for the high and low pass filter conditions at each cutoff frequency. Do your results agree with the basic relationship portrayed in Figure "A"? Set the Attenuator and Output Gain Control Knob to provide a most comfortable listening level for the subject.

(2) Repeat exercise #1 for several different speech levels and compare the test scores.

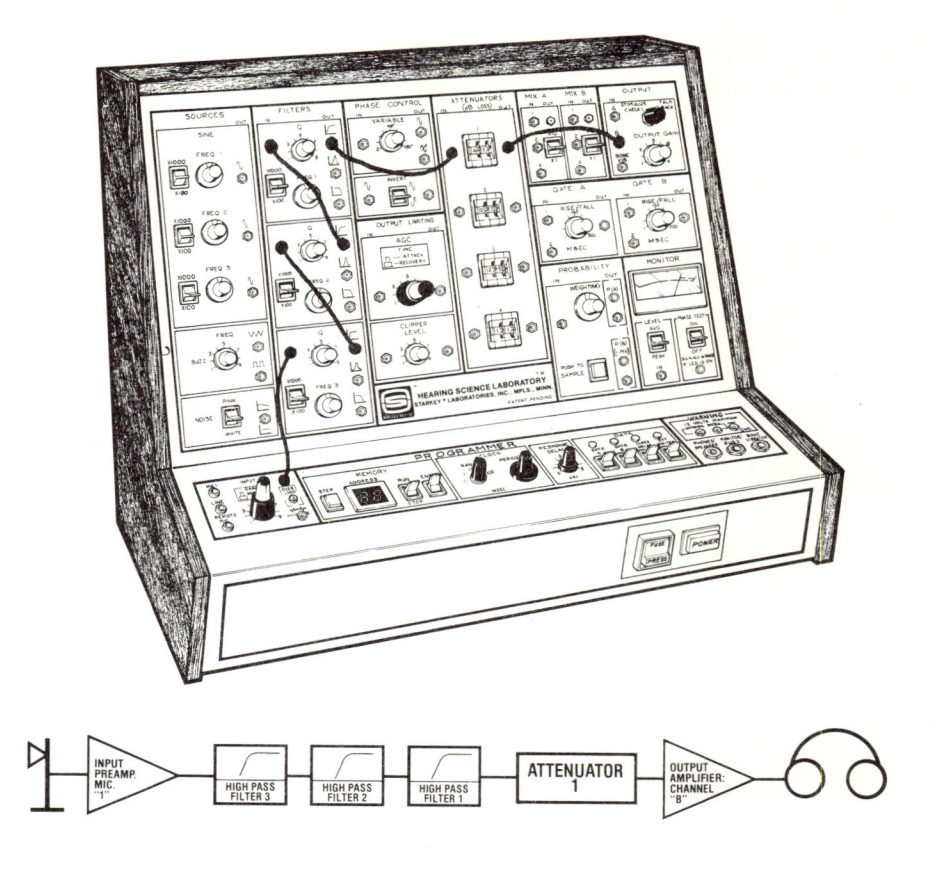

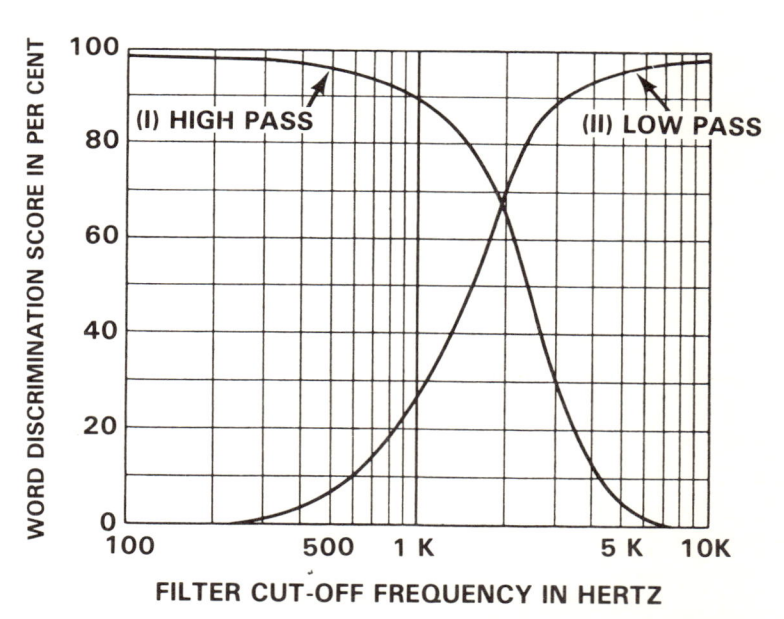

FIGURE A: When the higher frequencies of speech are filtered out of the signal, word discrimination scores decrease. (After French and Steinberg, 1947. From *The Speech Chain* by P.B. Denes and E.N. Pinson. © 1963 by Bell Telephone Laboratories, Inc. Reproduced by permission of Doubleday & Company, Inc.)

NOTES:

Selected References:

Ambrose, W.R. and Neal, W.R. (1973). The effects of frequency bandwidth on speech discrimination by hearing impaired subjects. *J. Aud. Res.,* **13,** 224-229.

Castle, W.E. (1963). Effects of selective narrow-band filtering on the perception by normal listeners of Harvard PB-50 word lists. *J. Speech Hear. Assoc., Virginia,* **5,** 12-21. Also in *J. Acoust. Soc. Am.,* **36,** 1047(A) (1964).

Chari, N.C.A., Herman, G., and Danhauer, J.L. (1977). Perception of one-third octave-band filtered speech. *J. Acoust. Soc. Am.,* **61,** 576-580.

Danaher, E.M. and Pickett, J.M. (1975). Some masking effects produced by low frequency vowel formants in persons with sensorineural hearing loss. *J. Speech Hear. Res.,* **18,** 261-271.

Fletcher, H. (1953). *Speech and hearing in communication.* chapter 10. Van Nostrand, New York.

French, N.R. and Steinberg, J.C. (1947). Factors governing the intelligibility of speech sounds. *J. Acoust. Soc. Am.,* **19,** 90-119.

Ling, D. (1964). Implications of hearing aid amplification below 300 cps. *Volta Rev.,* **66,** 723-729.

Lynn, G. and Gilroy, J. (1972). Neuro-audiological abnormalities in patients with temporal lobe tumors. *J. Neur. Sci.,* **17,** 167-184.

Miller, G.A. (1947). The masking of speech. *Psychol. Bull.,* **44,** 105-129.

Pollack, I. (1948). Effects of high-pass and low-pass filtering on the intelligibility of speech in noise. *J. Acoust. Soc. Am.,* **20,** 259-266.

Rosenthal, R.D., Lang, J.K., and Levitt, H. (1975) Speech reception with low frequency energy. *J. Acoust. Soc. Am.,* **57,** 949-955.

Ryals, B.M. and Asp, C.W. (1973). Intelligibility and tonality of 200 monosyllabic words (CID W-22) for 10 half-octave bandpass filtering conditions. *J. Acoust. Soc. Am.,* **54,** 300(A).

EXPERIMENT VIII-5: BINAURAL ALTERNATION OF SPEECH

Purpose:
To explore the effects of alternating speech stimuli between the ears.

Background Principle:
A speech signal that is switched from one ear to another will produce different perceptual effects when the rate of alternation is varied. At slow switching rates, the speech will appear to jump, or lateralize, from one ear to the other. As the switching rate increases to roughly four per second, a drop in speech intelligibility occurs, and the voice becomes garbled in quality. For switching periods shorter than about 100 milliseconds (a rate greater than 10 per second), this unusual distortion is replaced by increased intelligibility and the formation of a single fused sound image in the middle of one's head.

Procedure:
The live speech signals from a microphone are first sent to the Input Preamplifier and then to an Attenuator which controls the level of the stimuli. The output from the Attenuator branches into both Electronic Gates. Each gated signal enters a separate Output Amplifier channel and headphone. The simple Programmer instructions will permit the two Gates to switch on and off for equal durations governed by the Clock settings. Note: It is important that the speech signals either come from an individual other than the listening subject or that recorded stimuli be used. This is necessary to prevent the listener from hearing his own speech via bone conduction, which would confound the demonstration.

Exercises:
(1) Begin the listening task with a slow switching rate, such as two alternations per second, and gradually rotate the Programmer Period/Step Control to increase the speed of the Clock. Note the Clock settings at which both the decreased intelligibility and binaural fusion of the speech occur. Intelligibility may be assessed using the NU6 word lists.

(2) Alternately unplug and replace dashed circuit wire "A" shown in the wiring guide and block diagram. This will permit a comparison to be made between the effects of binaural switched speech and monaural interrupted speech.

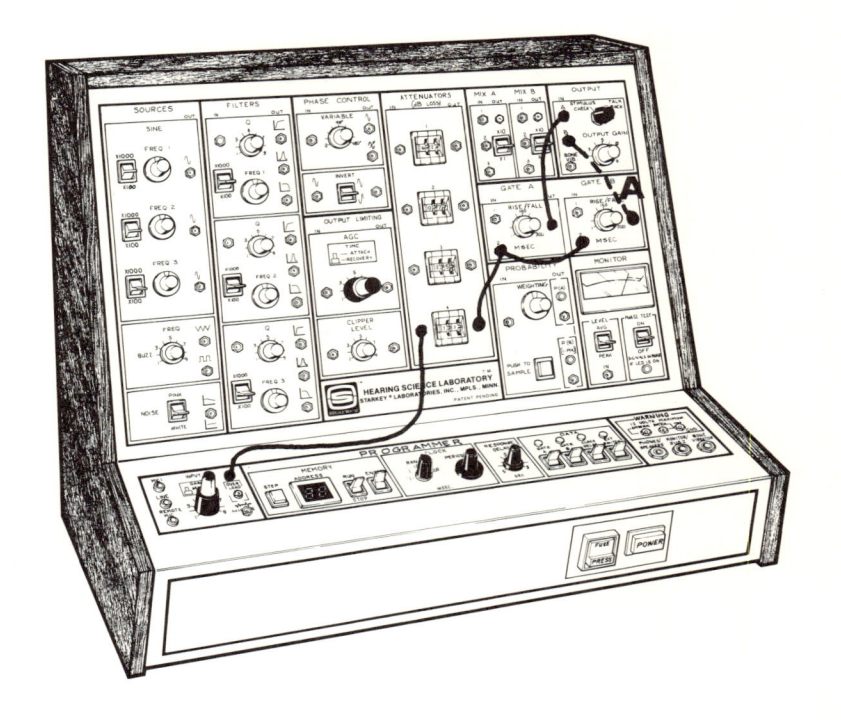

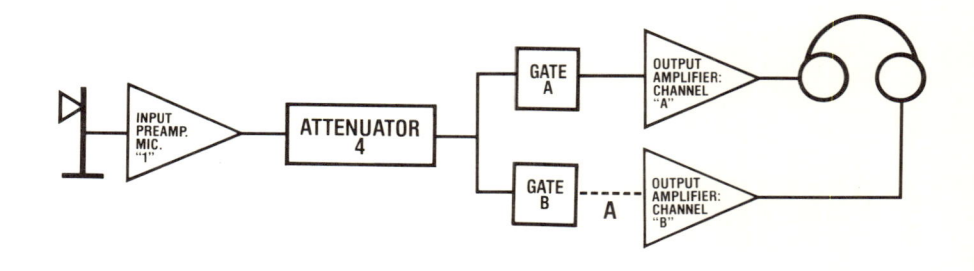

CLOCK SETTINGS			MEMORY ADDRESS		
RANGE SWITCH	PERIOD/ STEP CONTROL	RESPONSE DELAY	MEMORY CHANNEL	00 TO 49	50 TO 99
VARY FROM 10 TO 0.1 MILLISECONDS		SECONDS	GATE "A"	ON	
			GATE "B"		ON
			CLOCK DELAY		
			EXT. SWITCH		

NOTES:

Selected References:

Bocca, E. (1961). Factors influencing binaural interaction of periodically switched signals (messages). *Acta Oto-Lar.*, **53,** 142-144.

Cherry, E.C. (1953). Some experiments on the recognition of speech with one and with two ears. *J. Acoust. Soc. Am.*, **25,** 975-979.

Cherry, E.C. and Taylor, W.K. (1954). Some further experiments upon the recognition of speech, with one and with two ears. *J. Acoust. Soc. Am.*, **26,** 554-559.

Huggins, A.W.F. (1964). Distortion of the temporal pattern of speech: interruption and alternation. *J. Acoust. Soc. Am.*, **36,** 1055-1064.

Huggins, A.W.F. (1972). Perception of temporally-segmented speech. In A. Rigault (Ed.) *Proceedings of the 7th international congress of phonetic sciences.* pp. 531-535. The Hague: Mouton.

Huggins, A.W.F. (1974). On perceptual integration of dichotically alternated pulse trains. *J. Acoust. Soc. Am.*, **56,** 939-943.

Miller, G.A. and Licklider, J.C.R. (1950). The intelligibility of interrupted speech. *J. Acoust. Soc. Am.*, **22,** 167-176.

Schubert, E.D. and Parker, C.D. (1955). Addition to Cherry's findings on switching speech between the two ears. *J. Acoust. Soc. Am.*, **27,** 792-794(L).

Speaks, C. (1976). Comment on "Interaural alternation, information load, and speech intelligibility" [J. Acoust. Soc. Am., **57,** 1219-1220 (1975)]. *J. Acoust. Soc. Am.*, **60,** 272-274.

Speaks, C. and Trooien, T.T. (1974). Interaural alternation and speech intelligibility. *J. Acoust. Soc. Am.*, **56,** 640-644.

Wingfield, A. and Wheale, J.L. (1975). Interaural alternation, information load, and speech intelligibility. *J. Acoust. Soc. Am.*, **57,** 1219-1220.

EXPERIMENT VIII-6: SYMMETRICAL PEAK CLIPPING OF SPEECH AND PURE TONES

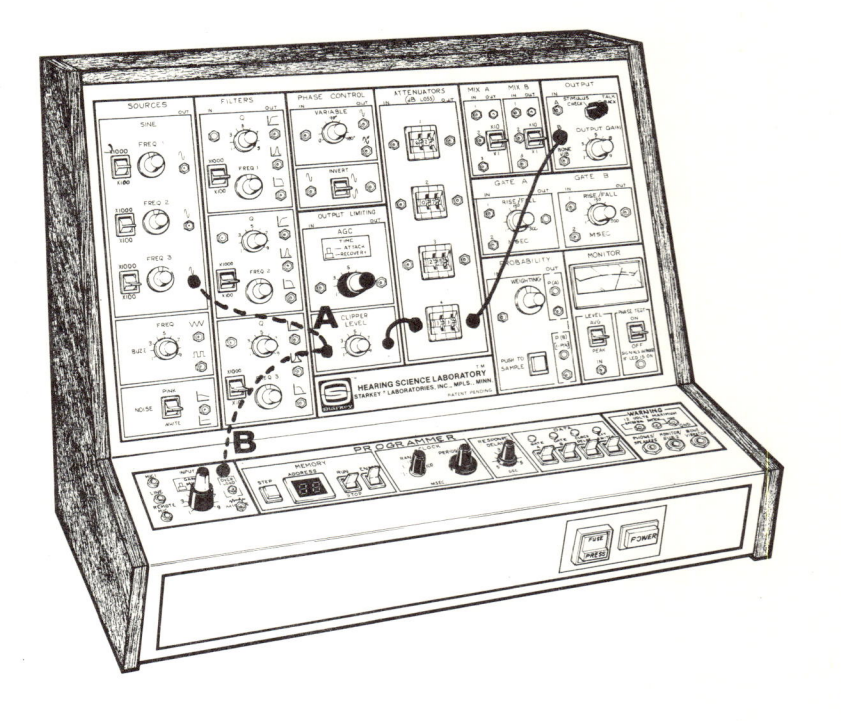

Purpose:
To explore the effects of peak clipping upon the quality and intelligibility of speech signals.

Background Principle:
Individuals who suffer from cochlear pathology may require that sounds be substantially increased in magnitude from normal listening levels in order for detection to occur. These same listeners, however, often exhibit a marked intolerance for stimuli that exceed a particular intensity level. One means of preventing amplified sound from causing listener discomfort is to limit the maximum sound pressure level output of a hearing aid through the use of peak clipping circuitry. See the section on Output Limitation and Figure I-48 in Part I of this text for more details of the peak clipping process. The process of peak clipping distorts the speech waveform and its perceived quality but has surprisingly little effect upon speech intelligibility for normal hearing subjects. This appears to be true, even at extreme clipping levels where the waveform resembles the characteristics of a square wave, because the peaks and valleys of the signal have been clipped in a symmetrical fashion.

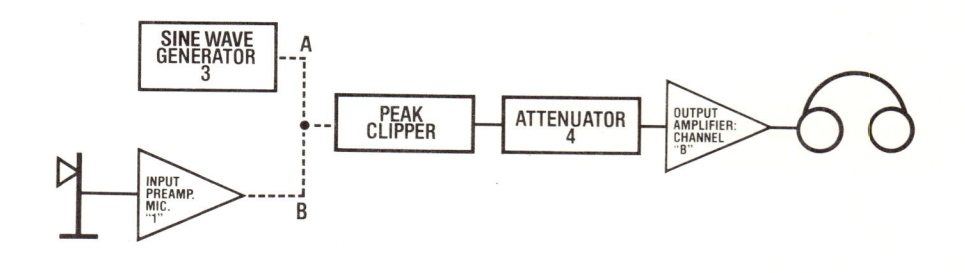

Procedure:
Any desired signal such as speech or pure tones may be used to demonstrate the effects of peak clipping. Connect dashed circuit wire "A" for pure tones or "B" for speech as shown in the wiring guide and block diagram. The test stimulus is passed through the Peak Clipper module, an Attenuator, an Output Amplifier channel, and one headphone. If available, an oscilloscope may be used to monitor the waveform distortions that are created by the clipping process.

Exercises:
(1) Gradually lower the level at which peak clipping occurs for a 500 Hz pure tone and note the change in its perceived quality. This may be achieved by rotating the Clipper Level Control Knob in a counterclockwise direction. Record the relative dial setting at which the distortion first becomes noticeable. Repeat this task for a tone of 4000 Hz. Can you account for any differences between your two results?

(2) Determine the speech discrimination performances of a listener under conditions both of severe and no peak clipping. Repeat this task for different kinds of test stimuli (e.g., spondee or NU6 words, complete sentences, etc.). Are some stimuli less vulnerable to the effects of peak clipping?

NOTES:

Selected References:

Licklider, J.C.R. (1946). Effects of amplitude distortion upon the intelligibility of speech. *J. Acoust. Soc. Am.*, **18**, 429-434.

Licklider, J.C.R., Bindra, D., and Pollack, I. (1948). The intelligibility of rectangular speech waves. *Am. J. Psychol.*, **61**, 1-20.

Licklider, J.C.R. and Pollack, I. (1948). Effects of differentiation, integration, and infinite peak clipping upon the intelligibility of speech. *J. Acoust. Soc. Am.*, **20**, 42-51.

Martin, D. (1950). Uniform speech-peak clipping in a uniform signal-as-noise spectrum ratio. *J. Acoust. Soc. Am.*, **32**, 614-621.

Miller, G.A. and Mitchell, S. (1947). Effects of distortion on the intelligibility of speech at high altitudes. *J. Acoust. Soc. Am.*, **19**, 120-125.

Pollack, I. (1952). On the effects of frequency and amplitude distortion on the intelligibility of speech in noise. *J. Acoust. Soc. Am.*, **24**, 538-540.

Pollack, I. and Pickett, J.M. (1959). Intelligibility of peak-clipped speech at high noise levels. *J. Acoust. Soc. Am.*, **31**, 14-16.

Thomas, I.B. (1968). The influence of first and second formants on the intelligibility of clipped speech. *J. Audio Eng. Soc.*, **16**, 182-185.

Thomas, I.B. and Niederjohn, R.J. (1968). Enhancement of speech intelligibility at high noise levels by filtering and clipping. *J. Audio Eng. Soc.*, **16**, 412-415.

Thomas, I.B. and Niederjohn, R.J. (1970). The intelligibility of filtered/clipped speech in noise. *J. Audio Eng. Soc.*, **18**, 299-303.

Wathen-Dunn, W. and Lipke, D.W. (1958). On the power gained by clipping speech in the audio band. *J. Acoust. Soc. Am.*, **30**, 36-40.

Young, L. L., Jr., Goodman, J. T., and Carhart, R. (1978). The intelligibility of whitened and peak clipped speech. *J. Amer. Audiol. Soc.*, **3**, 167-171.

EXPERIMENT VIII-7: MINIMIZING PEAK CLIPPING DISTORTION

Purpose:
To reduce the unnatural distortion created by peak clipping.

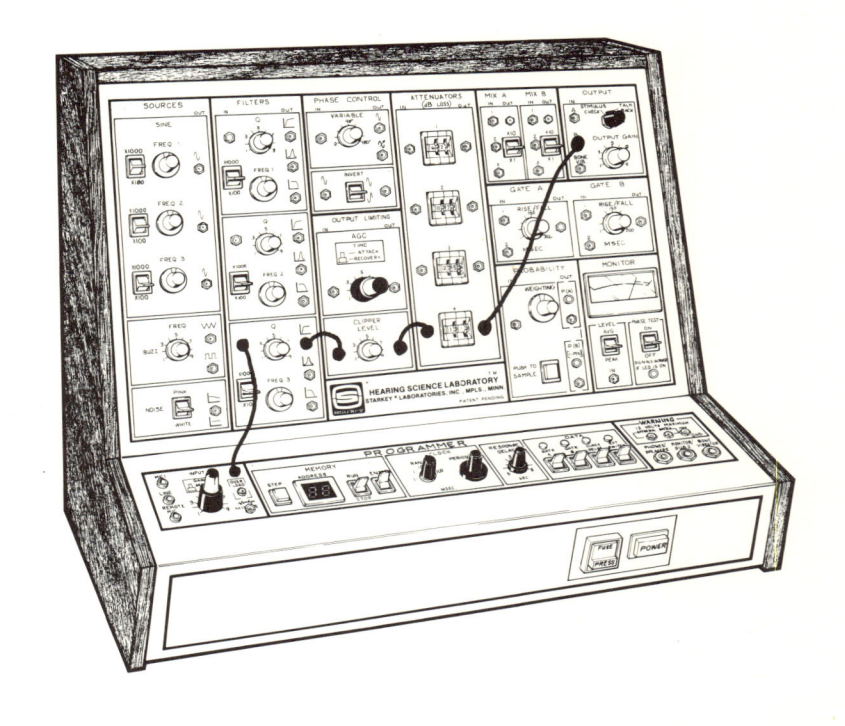

Background Principle:
The hearing impaired individual with poor high frequency acuity may find peak clipped, amplified speech to be harsh and unpleasant sounding. This situation arises from the fact that low frequency vowel sounds may contain 1000 times the energy of the higher frequency speech consonants and are, consequently, the first to reach the peak clipping "ceiling" of a hearing aid. Such low frequency, clipped stimuli generate a series of harmonics (i.e., whole numbered multiples of the waveform fundamental frequency) that lie within the audible range of the listener and contribute to the distortion of speech quality. This problem is not as severe for higher frequency clipped waves since their harmonic components usually lie outside the range which the hearing aid can reproduce or the impaired listener can detect. One way to minimize this distortion is to amplify the high frequency speech components more than their low frequency counterparts, thereby permitting all of the signals to reach the peak clipping level together. This so called "high-tone emphasis" (i.e., high pass filtering) is a common performance feature in most hearing aids because many hearing impairments involve a loss of high frequency acuity and, therefore, require amplification for high frequency sounds.

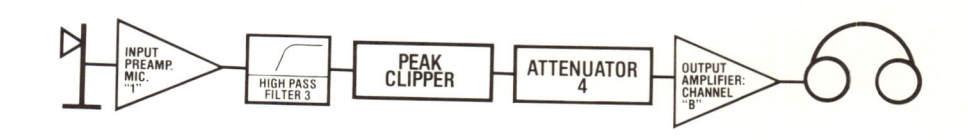

Procedure:
Live speech signals from a microphone are sent to the Mic 1 Preamplifier Input and then to a High Pass Filter and the adjustable Peak Clipper. The Clipper output is then delivered to an Attenuator, one Output Amplifier channel, and headphone (or loudspeaker).

Exercises:
(1) Set the Peak Clipper Level Control for a high degree of peak clipping (i.e., almost fully counterclockwise) and the Filter Frequency Control to an initial value near 100 Hz. Note what effect increasing the Filter cutoff frequency has upon the perceived distortion of live speech stimuli delivered to the microphone. The filter selectivity (Q) control should be left fully counterclockwise.

(2) Repeat exercise #1 with two high pass filters connected in cascade (see Figure I-30). Be sure to adjust the Frequency cutoffs of both Filters to the same settings. Contrast the peak clipping distortion obtained with this steeper filter to that obtained from the single Filter used in exercise #1. Can you explain the differences?

NOTES:

Selected References:

Miller, G.A. and Mitchell, S. (1947). Effects of distortion on the intelligibility of speech at high altitudes. *J. Acoust. Soc. Am.*, **19,** 120-125.

Thomas, I.B. (1968). The influence of first and second formants on the intelligibility of clipped speech. *J. Audio Eng. Soc.*, **16,** 182-185.

Thomas, I.B. and Niederjohn, R.J. (1968). Enhancement of speech intelligibility at high noise levels by filtering and clipping. *J. Audio Eng. Soc.*, **16,** 412-415.

Thomas, I.B. and Niederhohn, R.J. (1970). The intelligibility of filtered-clipped speech in noise. *J. Audio Eng. Soc.*, **18,** 299-303.

Thomas, I.B. and Ravindran, A. (1974). Intelligibility enhancement of already noisy speech signals. *J. Audio Eng. Soc.*, **22,** 234-236.

Thomas, I.B. and Sparks, D.W. (1971). Discrimination of filtered/clipped speech by hearing-impaired subjects. *J. Acoust. Soc. Am.*, **49,** 1881-1887.

Villchur, E. (1973). Signal processing to improve speech intelligibility in perceptive deafness. *J. Acoust. Soc. Am.*, **53,** 1646-1657.

EXPERIMENT VIII-8: ASYMMETRIC PEAK CLIPPING

Purpose:
To compare and contrast symmetrical and asymmetrical peak clipping.

Background Principle:
In Laboratory Experiment VIII-6, we noted that clipping the peaks of a sine wave introduced the odd numbered harmonics to the fundamental frequency of the signal. If, however, we distort the waveform asymmetrically, as in the examples shown in Figures "A" and "B", both the odd and even numbered harmonics appear in the signal, and the second harmonic, or octave, of the fundamental will become quite audible. Some hearing aids will produce asymmetric peak clipping when their amplifiers are "driven" to saturation. Questions remain as to precisely what effect this form of clipping has on speech quality and intelligibility.

Procedure:
We can produce asymmetrically clipped waveforms by combining our test signal with a voltage from a *direct current (D.C.)* source such as a common battery. Unlike *alternating current (A.C.)* signals which fluctuate around some reference voltage value, a battery provides a constant voltage above or below some reference point. An A.C. signal that is mixed with a D.C. voltage will be shifted, or *biased*, above or below its original voltage reference point, causing only one side of the waveform to reach the level at which clipping can take place (see Figures "C", "D" & "E"). A common nine volt transistor radio battery will provide the D.C. bias for the present demon-

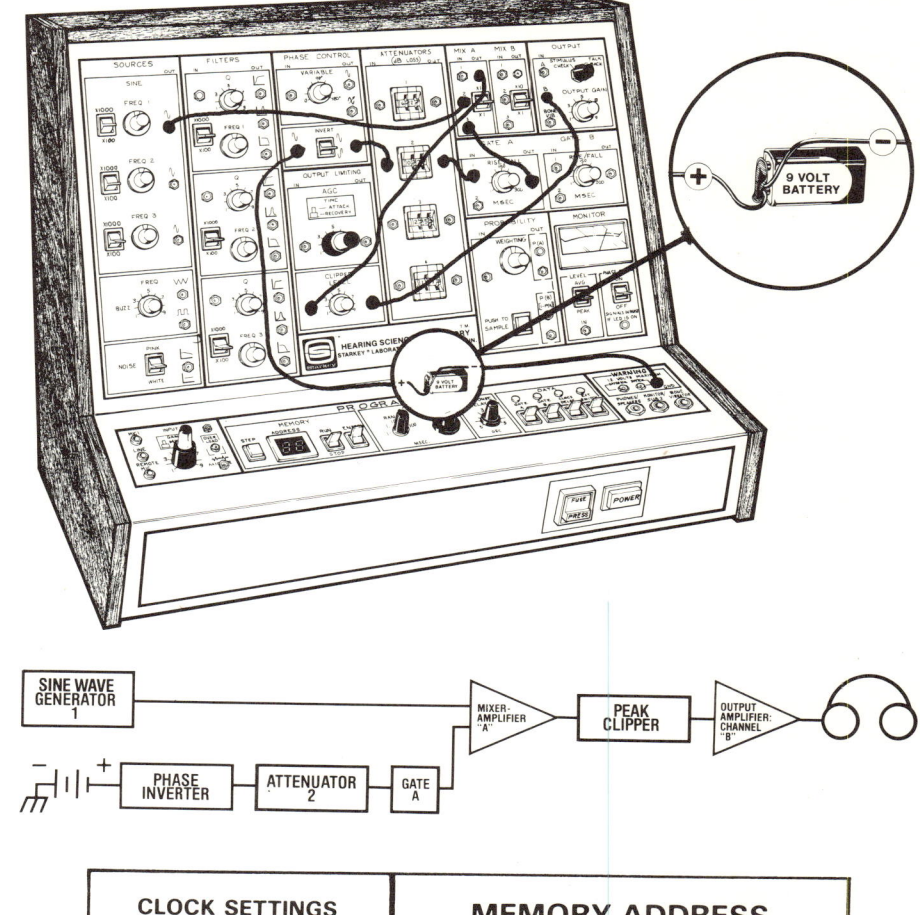

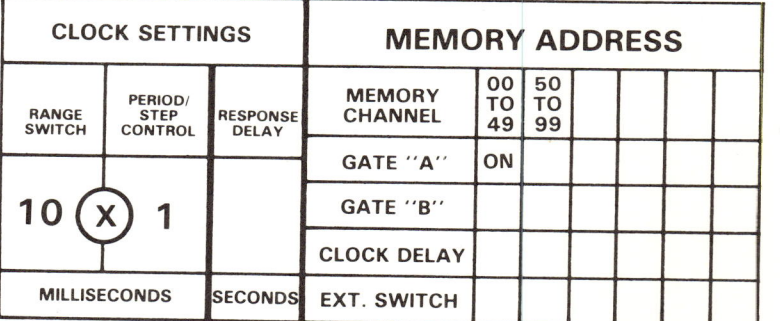

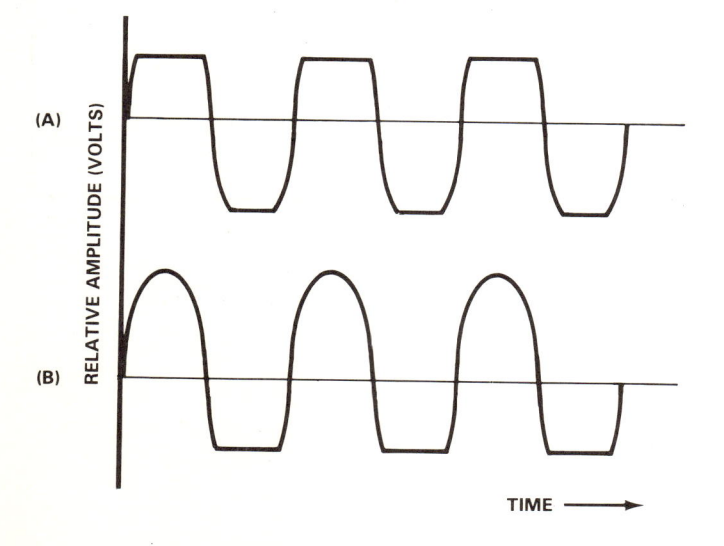

FIGURE (A & B) Examples of asymetrically peak-clipped sinusoids.
(C) The dashed lines indicate the levels at which clipping will occur for this signal.
(D) Effect of applying a "positive bias" to the signal.
(E) Effect of applying a "negative bias" to the signal.

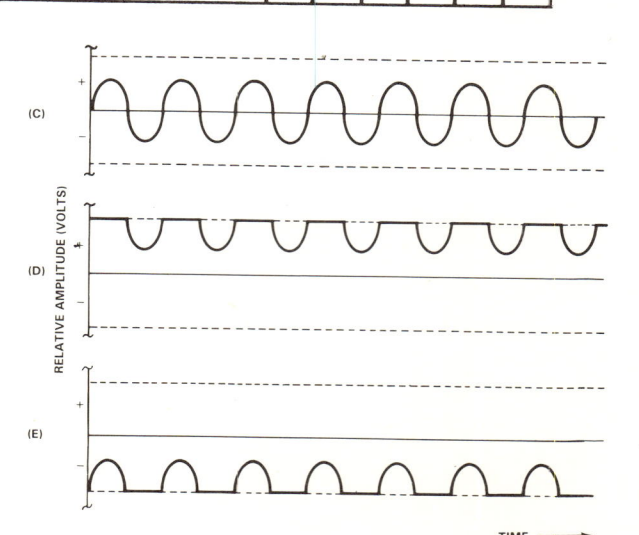

stration (see front panel wiring guide). The battery's negative terminal should be connected to the Ground Jack on the Hearing Science Laboratory, while the positive side should be connected to the Input Jack of the Phase Inverter Module. When the Phase Inverter Switch position is changed, a positive D.C. bias would be inverted in polarity to become a negative D.C. bias. The amount of waveform shift that is introduced can be varied by routing the output of the Phase Inverter through an Attenuator (set the Attenuator to an initial value of 15 dB). The D.C. bias can be added to the test signal on an alternating basis by passing it through Electronic Gate "A" which has been programmed to switch on and off every half-second. The output of the Gate is combined with a sinusoid (or any other desired test signal) in Mixer-Amplifier "A". The Mixer output is sent to the adjustable Peak Clipper and finally to an Output Amplifier and headphone. A symmetrically peak clipped wave is produced when Gate "A" (and the D.C. bias it passes) is switched off, and an asymmetrically clipped wave will be produced each time Gate "A" is switched on.

Exercises:

(1) Select a variety of pure tone frequencies below 1000 Hz and note the differences in sound quality between symmetric and asymmetric clipped waves. Vary the Peak Clipper Level and Attenuator #2 settings to produce the desired waveforms and sound qualities for the signals. Both waveforms may be monitored on an oscilloscope by attaching the scope probe to the output of the Peak Clipper. Can you hear the octave jump in pitch when the symmetrically clipped wave changes to an asymmetric signal? Repeat this task with frequencies above 5000 Hz. Can you still hear the change in pitch? Account for what you do or do not hear.

(2) Send live speech signals through the Mixer Input and note if there is any perceived difference between asymmetric and symmetrically clipped speech.

(3) Repeat exercises #1 and #2 with the Phase Inverter Switch set to the opposite position and note if reversing the D.C. shift polarity results in any audible difference in the effect of clipping.

NOTES:

Selected References:

Licklider, J.C.R. and Miller, G.A. (1951). The perception of speech. In S.S. Stevens (Ed.) *Handbook of experimental psychology.* pp. 1058-1063. Wiley and Sons, Inc., New York.

Preis, D. (1977). Impulse testing and peak clipping. *J. Audio Eng. Soc.*, 25, 2-14.

EXPERIMENT VIII-9: "CENTER CLIPPING" OF SPEECH (CROSSOVER DISTORTION)

Purpose:
To note the effects of zero-crossover distortion on speech quality and intelligibility.

Background Principle:
When a long passage of connected discourse is recorded, and the energies contained at different frequencies of the speech spectrum are analyzed and summated over all time, we find that most of the power is concentrated in the low frequencies. This distribution of speech energy as a function of frequency is called the *long time average speech spectrum* and is shown in Figure "A". It is important to note that while such lower frequency speech sounds as the *vowels* contain substantially greater energy than the higher frequency *consonants,* it is the consonants which contribute most to the information-bearing aspects of speech. Indeed, frequencies below 500 Hz contain about 60% of the power in speech but contribute only 5% to speech intelligibility! In Laboratory Experiment VIII-6, we noted that symmetrical peak clipping did not seriously affect speech intelligibility. A dramatic loss in intelligibility would occur, however, if we distort the low level, "center," portion of the waveform containing high frequency speech information instead of clipping the relatively low frequency — high level

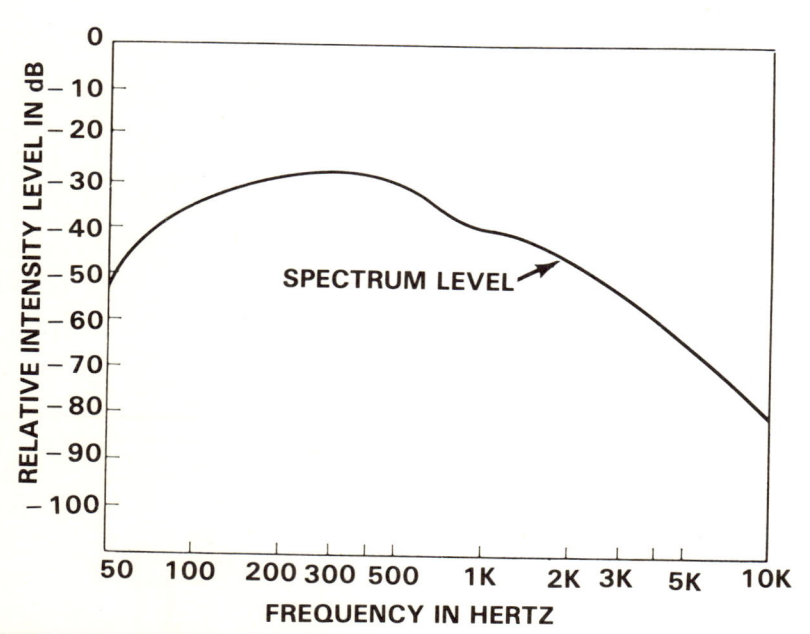

FIGURE A: The long time average spectrum of speech reveals that relatively little speech energy is concentrated in the consonantal frequencies above 500 Hz. (From *The Speech Chain* by P.B. Denes and E.N. Pinson. © 1963 by Bell Telephone Laboratories, Inc. Reproduced by permission of Doubleday & Company, Inc.)

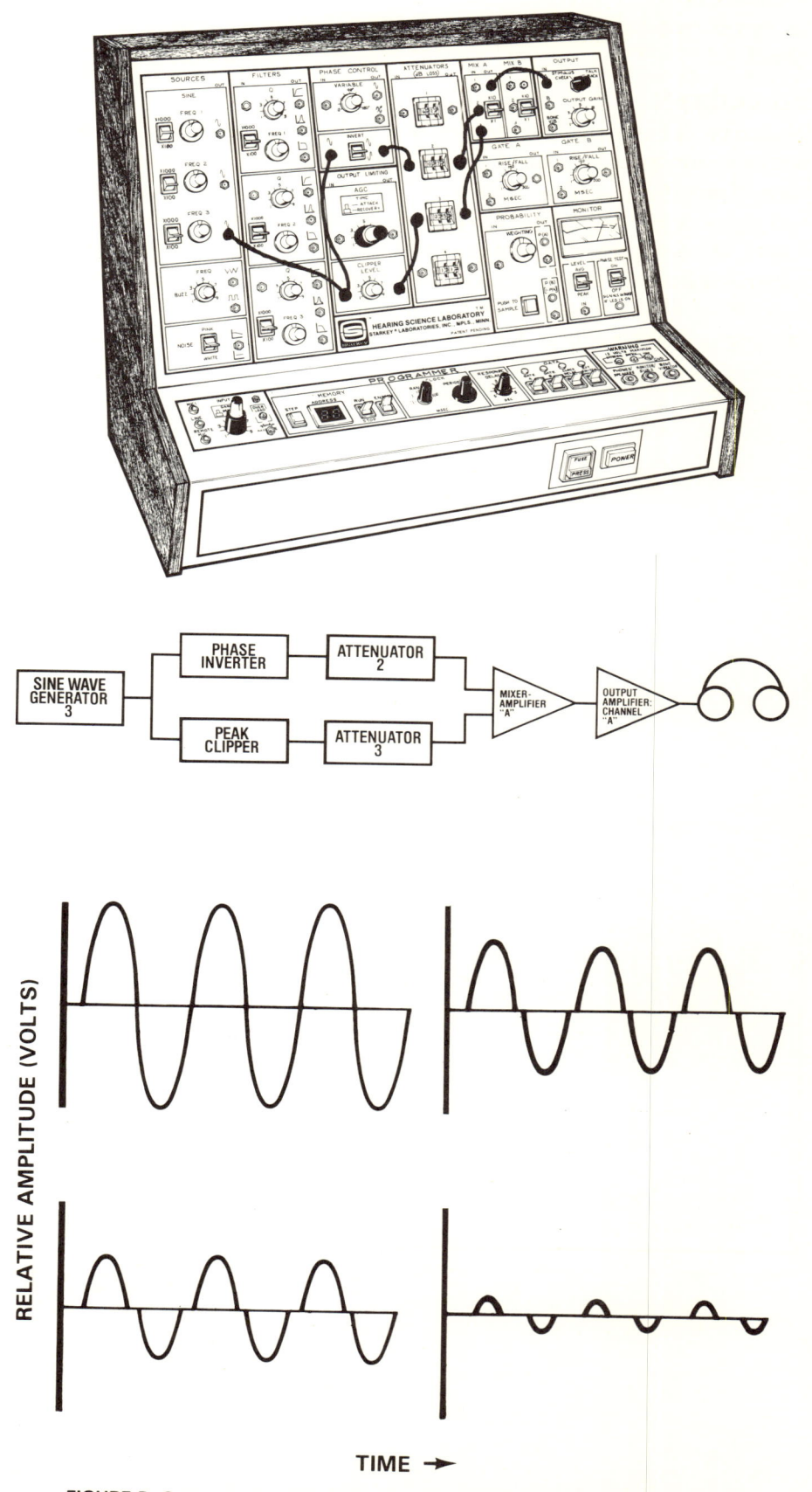

FIGURE B: Crossover distortion clips the central portion of the waveform.

sounds. Clipping a waveform each time it crosses its zero reference level is known as *crossover distortion* and is shown in Figure "B" for a sinusoidal signal.

Procedure:

We can produce crossover distortion by mixing a signal, such as a sinusoid, with a symmetrically peak clipped and inverted version of itself. The inversion process effectively "subtracts" the peak clipped wave from the original signal, yielding a center clipped stimulus similar to the one shown in Figure "B". The same pure tone signal is first routed to both the Phase Inverter and Peak Clipper modules. The outputs from these devices are sent to separate Attenuators and then combined within a Mixer-Amplifier before being delivered to an Output Amplifier channel and headphone (or loudspeaker). Be sure to set the Phase Inverting Switch to the lower, "inverting," position.

Exercises:

(1) Observe the center-clipped waveforms on an oscilloscope. Note what effect varying the Clipper Level Control has upon audible sound quality and waveform shape of the distorted signal. Try this demonstration on a variety of pure tone frequencies and sound levels.

(2) Disconnect the pure tone signal wire from the Peak Clipper. Use a microphone to send live-voice signals to the Mic. 1 Input Jack and connect the output of the Preamplifier to the Peak Clipper module. Vary the Clipper Level Control and note its effect upon speech quality.

NOTES:

Selected References:

Licklider, J.C.R. (1946). Effects of amplitude distortion upon the intelligibility of speech. *J. Acoust. Soc. Am.*, **18**, 429-434.

Licklider, J.C.R. and Miller, G.A. (1951). The perception of speech. In S.S. Stevens (Ed.) *Handbook of experimental psychology.* pp. 1058-1063. Wiley and Sons, Inc. New York.

EXPERIMENT VIII-10: INTELLIGIBILITY OF DICHOTICALLY FILTERED SPEECH

Purpose:
To note the effects of dichotically presented filtered speech upon intelligibility.

Background Principle:
Speech that is passed through a band pass filter will remain fairly intelligible so long as the bandwidth does not shrink below certain limits. The telephone, for example, provides good speech intelligibility by passing frequencies roughly between 300-3000 Hz. Now in this experiment, our binaural hearing mechanism and brain will work together to assist in the discrimination of filtered speech. This effect can be demonstrated by filtering speech into two narrow band signals that are, taken separately, insufficient for complete intelligibility. By delivering these stimuli *dichotically* (i.e., a different speech band to each ear), however, the listener's articulation score improves noticeably. Some studies have even indicated that the intelligibility of speech for the hearing impaired may be augmented by sending only low frequency information to one ear and high frequency components to the other, thereby reducing the masking effect of the high intensity low frequencies upon high frequency stimulus information.

Procedure:
The speech signals from a microphone are passed through the Input Preamplifier and then to the inputs of two Filters. The Band Pass Output from each Filter is sent through a separate Attenuator, Electronic Gate, Output Amplifier channel, and headphone. With the Programmer Clock stopped, one can manually switch either or both of the filtered speech signals on and off by following the suggested programming instructions.

Exercises:
(1) Adjust both Attenuators to identical settings, providing speech levels near the subject's threshold. Rotate the selectivity "Q"-control to position 7 for Filter #2. This narrow band filter will handle the relatively low frequency speech components. Set Filter #3 "Q"-control fully clockwise for the high frequencies. Obtain and contrast the percentage of correctly identified NU6 words a subject achieves for each of the following filter band pass center frequency conditions:

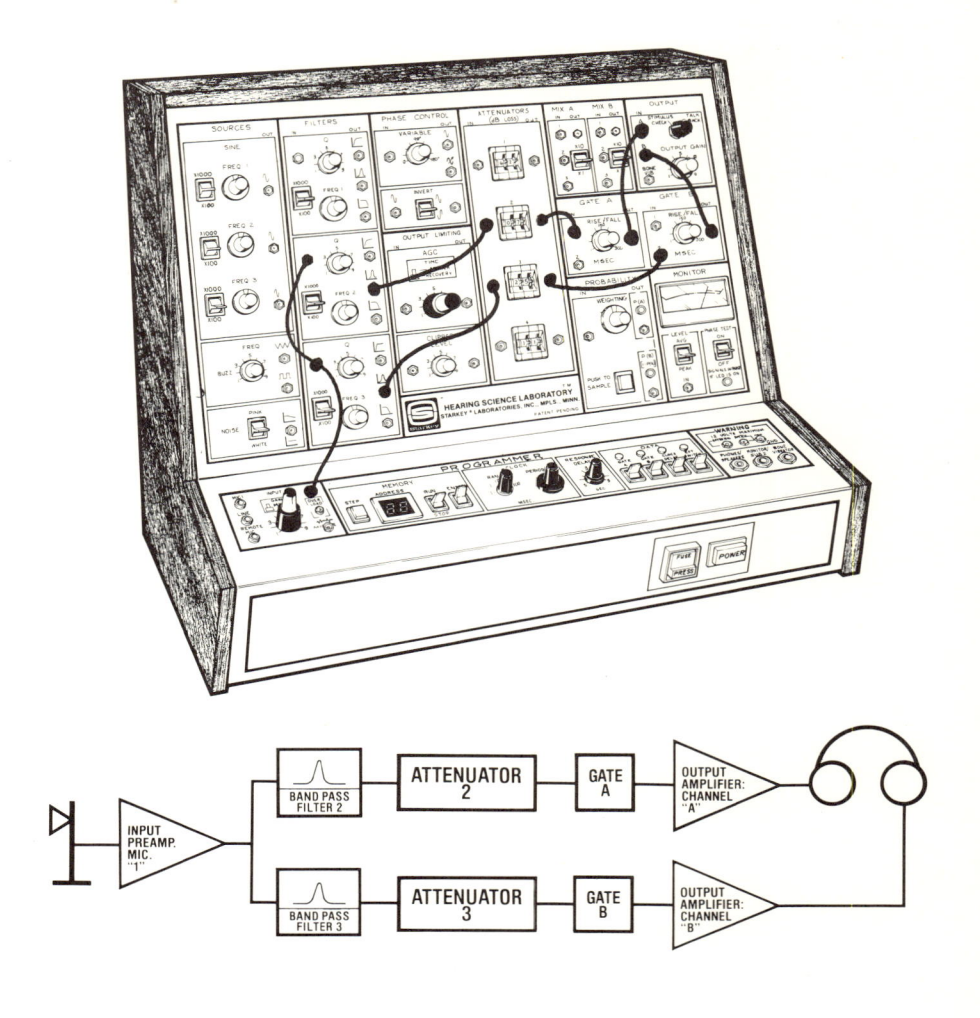

CLOCK STOPPED	BAND PASS TEST CONDITION		
CHANNEL	LOW FREQUENCY	HIGH FREQUENCY	HIGH & LOW FREQUENCY
A	ON		ON
B		ON	ON

	Filter Center Frequency Combinations	
	I	**II**
Low Frequency Band Pass:	350 Hz	650 Hz
High Frequency Band Pass:	1500 Hz	2500 Hz

Next, combine the low and high band pass conditions and note the effect upon intelligibility of the speech.

(2) Repeat exercise #1, using low frequency band pass levels that are about 20 dB and 40 dB above threshold, respectively. Does the subject's articulation score improve for these conditions? Compare your results with those obtained by Franklin (1970) and try to account for any observed differences.

NOTES:

Selected References:

Bocca, E. (1955). Binaural hearing: another approach. *Laryngoscope*, **65,** 1164-1175.

Broadbent, D.E. (1955). A note on binaural fusion. *Q. J. Exp. Psychol.*, **7,** 46-47.

Broadbent, D.E. and Gregory, M. (1964). Accuracy of recognition for speech presented to the right and left ears. *Q. J. Exp. Psychol.*, **16,** 359-360.

Broadbent, D.E. and Ladefoged, P. (1957). On the fusion of sounds reaching different sense organs. *J. Acoust. Soc. Am.*, **29,** 708-710.

Cutting, J.E. (1976). Auditory and linguistic processes in speech perception: inferences from six fusions in dichotic listening. *Psychol. Rev.*, **83,** 114-140.

Franklin, B. (1970). The effect on consonant discrimination of combining a low frequency passband in one ear and a high frequency passband in the other ear. *J. Aud. Res.*, **9,** 365-378.

Franklin, B. (1975). The effect of combining low and high frequency passbands on consonant recognition in the hearing-impaired. *J. Speech Hear. Res.*, **18,** 719-727.

Hayashi, R., Ohta, F., and Morimoto, M. (1966). Binaural fusion test; a diagnostic approach to the central auditory disorders. *Int. Audiol.*, **5,** 133-135.

Huizing, H.C. and Taselaar, M. (1961). Experiments on binaural hearing. *Acta Oto-Lar.*, **53,** 151-154.

Linden, A. (1964). Distorted speech and binaural speech resynthesis tests. *Acta Oto-Lar.*, **58,** 32-48.

Lowe, S.S., Cullen, J.K., Berlin, C.I., Thompson, C.L., and Willet, M.E. (1970). Perception of simultaneous dichotic and monotic monosyllables. *J. Speech Hear. Res.*, **13,** 812-822.

Palva, A. (1965). Filtered speech audiometry, I: Basic studies with Finnish speech toward the creation of a method for the diagnosis of central auditory disorders. *Acta Oto-Lar. Suppl.*, **210.**

Pollack, I. (1948). Effects of high pass and low pass filtering on the intelligibility of speech in noise. *J. Acoust. Soc. Am.*, **20,** 259-266.

Rand, T.C. (1974). Dichotic release from masking for speech. *J. Acoust. Soc. Am.*, **55,** 678-680.

Rosenthal, R.D., Lang, J.K., and Levitt, H. (1975). Speech recognition with low frequency energy. *J. Acoust. Soc. Am.*, **57,** 949-955.

Weiss, M.S. and House, A.S. (1973). Perception of dichotically presented vowels. *J. Acoust. Soc. Am.*, **53,** 51-58.

Willeford, J. (1978). Sentence tests of central auditory function. in J. Katz (Ed.) *Handbook of clinical audiology.* (2nd ed.), chapter 22. Williams & Williams Co., Baltimore.

EXPERIMENT VIII-11: THE INTELLIGIBILITY OF INTERRUPTED SPEECH

Purpose:
To examine the effects of interruption rate and duty cycle upon the discrimination of speech sounds.

Background Principle:
The intelligibility of speech that is periodically switched on and off has been found to vary in a complex fashion with the rate of interruption and the so-called *duty cycle,* or on-time of the signal. The difference between these two variables is portrayed in the figures shown below. Notice in Figure "A" that while the on-time of the signal (per cycle) increases from 10 to 75%, the total period for one complete cycle remains the same. In Figure "B", the same duty cycles shown in Figure "A" are maintained, but the interruption rate for the signal (i.e., its frequency of occurrence) has been doubled. Speech remains quite intelligible at duty cycles greater than roughly 50% for very high interruption rates, even though the actual on-time of the stimulus is small. Some recent findings, however, indicate that the aging process may reduce the ability to process this type of temporal information and, therefore, diminish one's speech intelligibility scores.

Procedure:
The speech signal from a microphone enters the Input Preamplifier module, an Attenuator, and both Electronic Gates. Each Gate can be programmed to have a different on-time, such as those shown in the suggested programming instructions. By connecting either dashed circuit wire "A" or "B", one can easily contrast 50% or 75% speech duty cycles, respectively. The interruption rate of the speech may be altered without disturbing the duty cycle by varying the Period/Step Control of the Programmer Clock.

Exercises:
(1) Determine the discrimination scores for a subject under each of the following arbitrarily selected listening conditions:

Experimental Variables		Programming Suggestions	
Duty Cycle	Interruption Rate	Individual Memory Address Duration	Number of Addresses Programmed To Turn Gate "On"
10%	1 per second	10 milliseconds	10 out of 100
50%	10 per second	10 milliseconds	5 out of every 10
70%	100 per second	1 millisecond	7 out of every 10

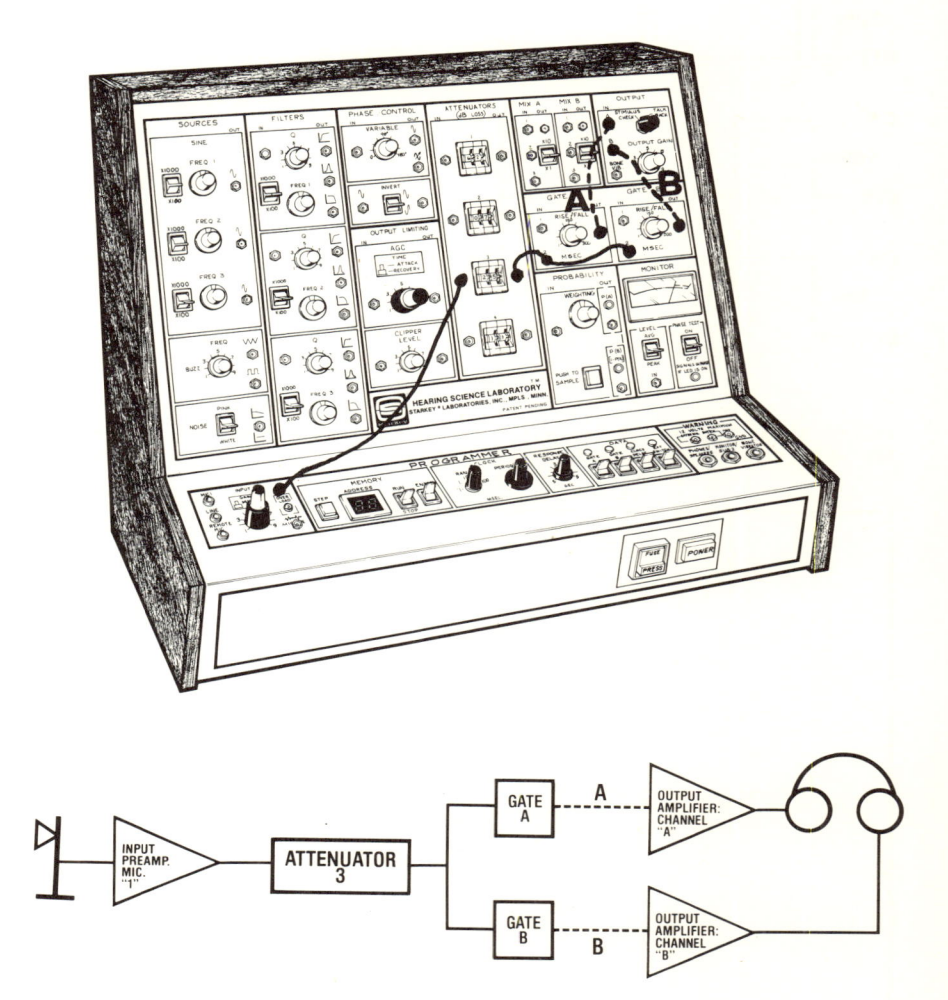

(2) Program the identical interruption rates and duty cycles for both Electronic Gates. Select the same test conditions used in exercise #1. This time, however, send the output from each Gate to a separate ear. Does this binaural listening condition assist in the discrimination of the speech sounds?

SPEECH PERCEPTION

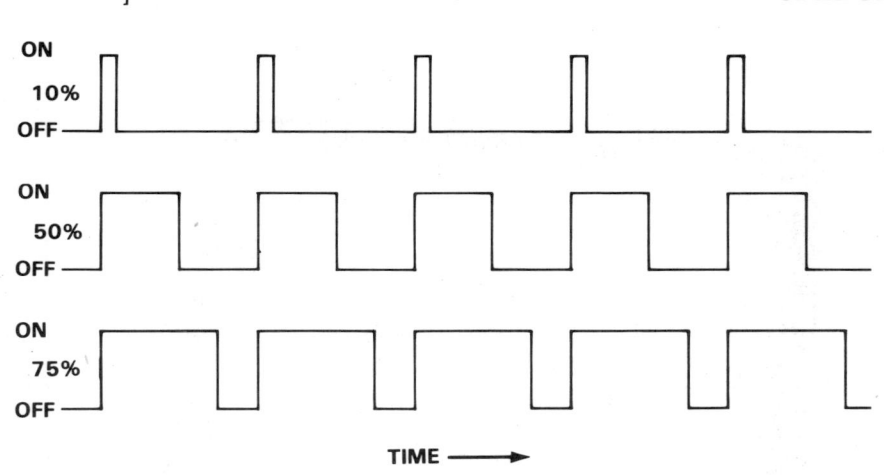

FIGURE A: The duty cycle or "on-time" for these stimuli varies from 10% to 75% while the overall period per cycle (and hence the frequency) for each remains the same.

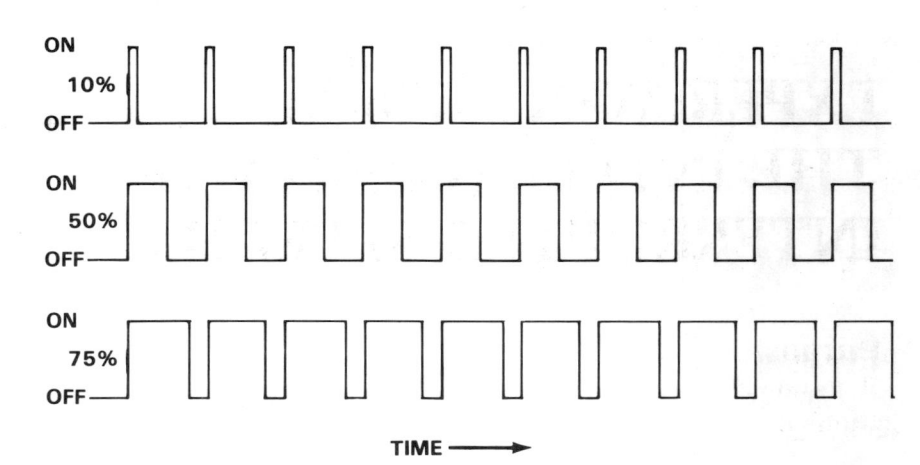

FIGURE B: The duty cycles for these stimuli are identical to their counterparts in Figure "A" but note that the repetition rate (i.e., frequency) for each has been doubled.

NOTES:

Selected References:

Bergman, M. (1971). Hearing and aging. *Audiology,* **10,** 164-171.

Cherry, E.C. and Taylor, W.K. (1954). Some further experiments upon the recognition of speech with one and with two ears. *J. Acoust. Soc. Am.,* **26,** 554-559.

Hopkinson, N.T. (1967). Combined effects of interruption and interaural alternation on speech intelligibility. *Lang. Speech,* **10,** 234-243.

Huggins, A.W.F. (1964). Distortion of the temporal pattern of speech: interruption and alternation. *J. Acoust. Soc. Am.,* **36,** 1055-1064.

Licklider, J.C.R. and Miller, G.A. (1951). The perception of speech. In S.S. Stevens (Ed.) *Handbook of experimental psychology.* pp. 1062-1064. Wiley and Sons, Inc., New York.

Miller, G.A. and Licklider, J.C.R. (1950). The intelligibility of interrupted speech. *J. Acoust. Soc. Am.,* **22,** 167-173.

Schubert, E.D. and Parker, C.D. (1955) Addition to Cherry's findings on switching speech between the two ears. *J. Acoust. Soc. Am.,* **27,** 792-794 (L).

EXPERIMENT VIII-12: THE TRANSFER FUNCTIONS FOR INPUT AND OUTPUT COMPRESSION SYSTEMS

Purpose:
To examine the response of two types of compression amplifiers to steady state (i.e., pure tone) signals.

Background Principle:
One common measure of the performance characteristics of an *Automatic Gain Control (AGC)* circuit is obtained by routing different level pure tone signals through the system and graphing the relationship between the output and input amplitudes. The concept of such an "input/output curve," or *transfer function,* was introduced in Part I of this text (see discussion surrounding Figure I-50). Input signals below the AGC threshold level are amplified in a linear fashion, while those which exceeded the threshold limit give rise to a less than linear or "compressed" output amplification. Hearing aid manufacturers and audiological researchers have recently focused their attention on the relative merits of two AGC techniques. The fundamental difference between the two systems lies in the placement of the AGC monitoring circuit that reduces the amplifier gain when it "senses" an excessive input signal level. Figures "A" and "B" show the location of the sensor for these so-called "output and input compression" systems. With *output compression* (Figure "A"), the sensor monitors the final electrical signal levels that are delivered to the hearing aid receiver. Note that with output compression, the AGC sensor will be affected by changes in input signal level as well as hearing aid "tone" and "volume" control settings. These controls vary the hearing aid's frequency response and output level, respectively. For *input compression* (Figure "B"), the sensor only monitors the first stage of amplification in the hearing aid, and the tone and volume control remain independent of the AGC circuit. Because a change of input signal level may actually alter the desired frequency response of a hearing aid when output rather than input compression is used, researchers are comparing the performance of hearing aid wearers with the two types of compression amplification.

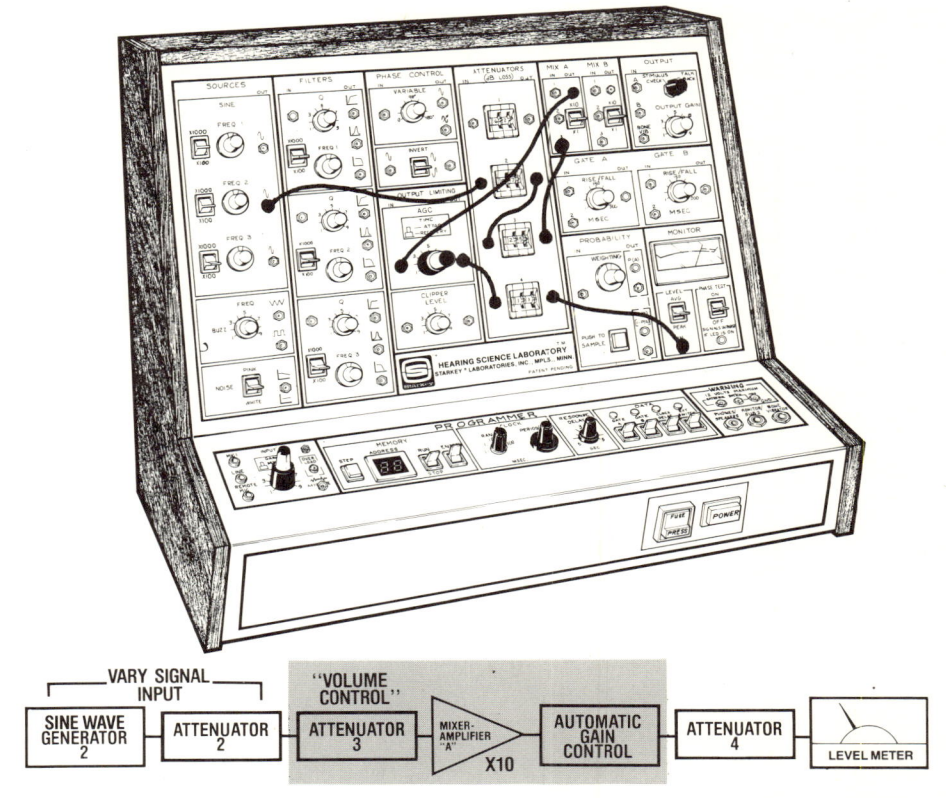

FIGURE A: Output compression system. Note that the AGC sensor follows the "volume control" in the circuit.

Procedure:
Carefully examine the wiring guides and block diagrams for the Input and Output compression configurations. In each case, Attenuator #2 is used to vary the pure tone input signal level, and Attenuator #4 is used to vary the Monitor Meter scale readings. Note that the essential difference between the two types of compression lies with the location of the AGC module within the circuit. For output compression, the AGC is placed after the "volume control" and Mixer-Amplifier (which is set to the X 10 switch position). For input compression, the AGC precedes the "volume control" and Amplifier stage. Attenuator #3 serves in each case as the simulated hearing aid "volume control".

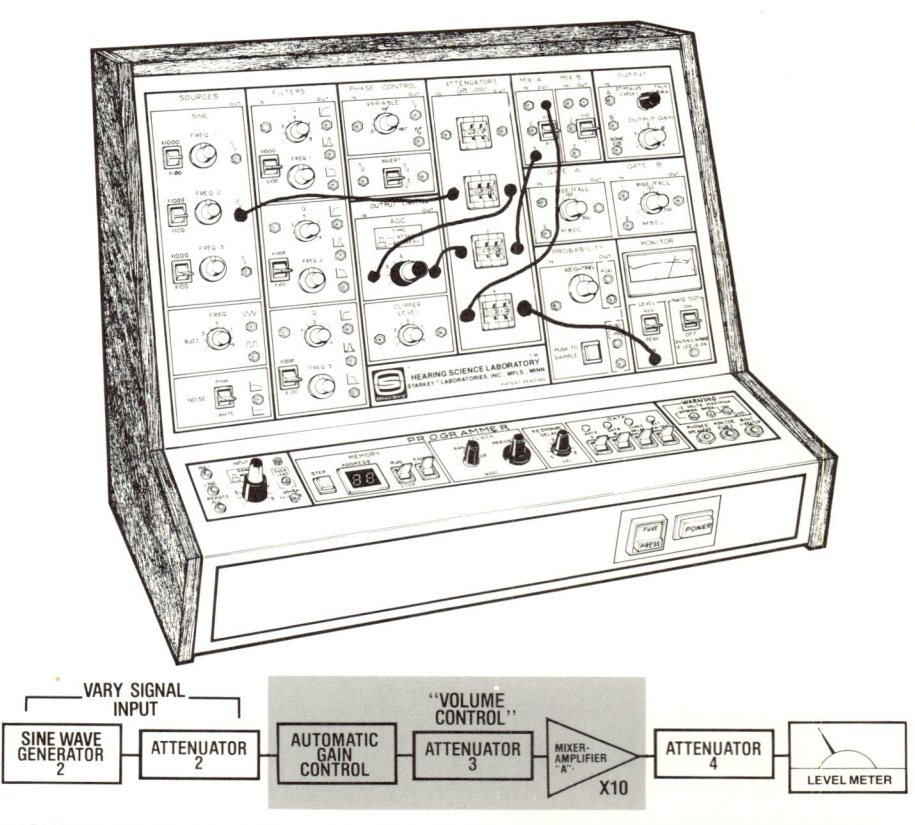

FIGURE B: Input compression system. Note that the AGC sensor precedes the "volume control" in the circuit.

Exercises:

(1) Select a test tone frequency of 1000 Hz. Set the AGC Attack and Recovery Control Knobs to position #3 on the panel scale. Determine the transfer function (i.e., the relationship between the input and output levels of the system) for the output compression circuit (Figure "A") for a "volume control" (Attenuator #3) setting of 20 dB. Begin the experiment with the input Attenuator (i.e., #2) set to 40 dB. Adjust Attenuator #4 until a zero-scale reading is observed on the Monitor Level Meter. Attenuator #4 and Attenuator #2 levels comprise, respectively, the Y-axis and X-axis data values to be plotted on Figure "C." Reduce the input signal Attenuator (i.e., #2) in steps of 2 decibels. Readjust Attenuator #4 for each new input level until the Meter again reads zero. Plot each new data point on Figure "C" and draw a smooth curve to link the points on your transfer function graph.

(2) Repeat exercise #1 for Attenuator #3 ("volume control") settings of 25, 30 and 35 dB, respectively. Note the characteristic shape of the family of curves you obtain.

(3) Rewire the Hearing Science Laboratory to produce an input compression circuit (Figure "B"). Repeat exercises #1 and #2 for this AGC configuration and plot your data on Figure "D." Compare and contrast the families of curves plotted on Figures "C" and "D."

NOTES:

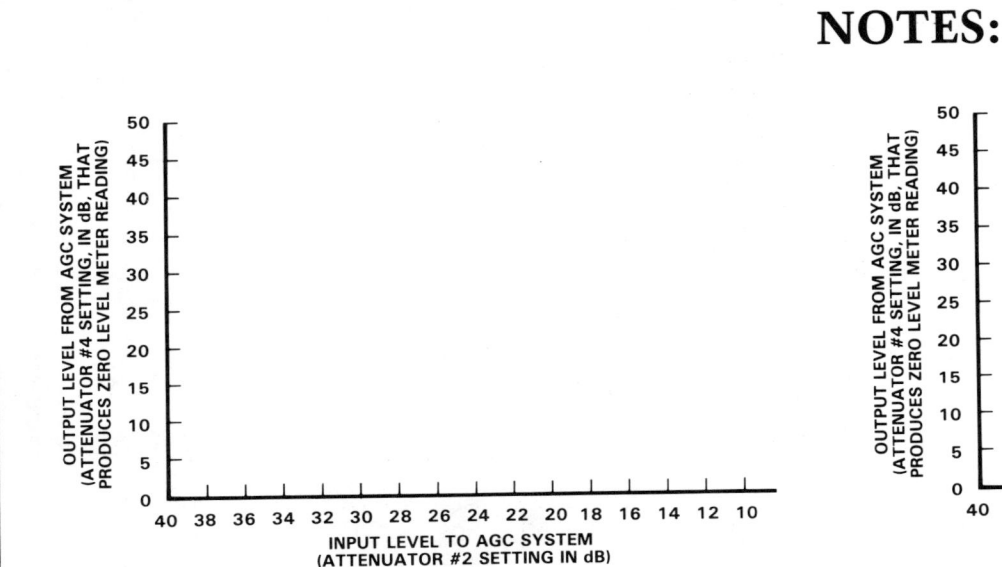

FIGURE C: Data graph for *OUTPUT* compression transfer function.

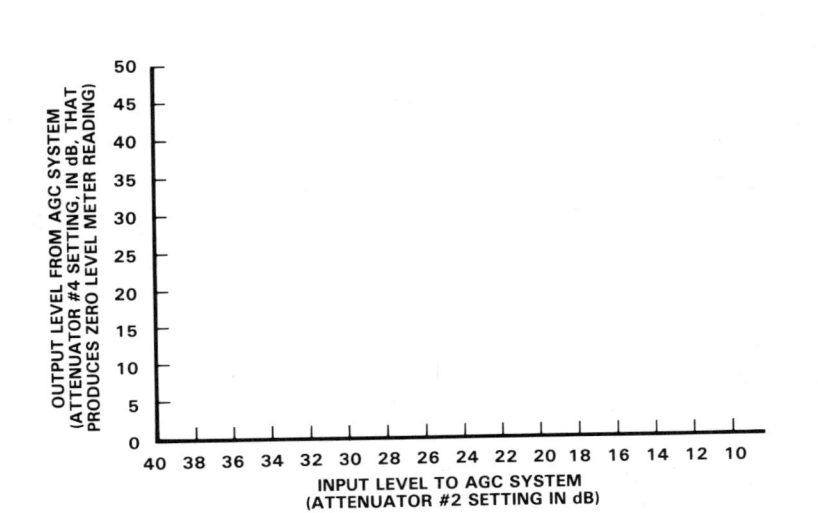

FIGURE D: Data graph for *INPUT* compression transfer function.

Selected References:

Goldberg, H. (1972). Hearing aid compression amplification: varieties. *Natl. Hear. Aid Jour.*, **25**, 9.

Heide, J. (1974). Output limitation. *Hear. Instr.*, **25(8)**, 26-28.

Helle, R.E. (1977). Input and output compression in hearing aids. *Hear. Instr.*, **28**, 12-26.

Hogg, D.C. (1976). Putting compression into perspective. *Hear. Aid Jour.*, **29(7)** 11-36.

Nielsen, T.E. (1972). Information about various methods of output limitation. *Otocongress 2*, Oticon Corp.

EXPERIMENT VIII-13: AGC AND DYNAMIC SIGNALS

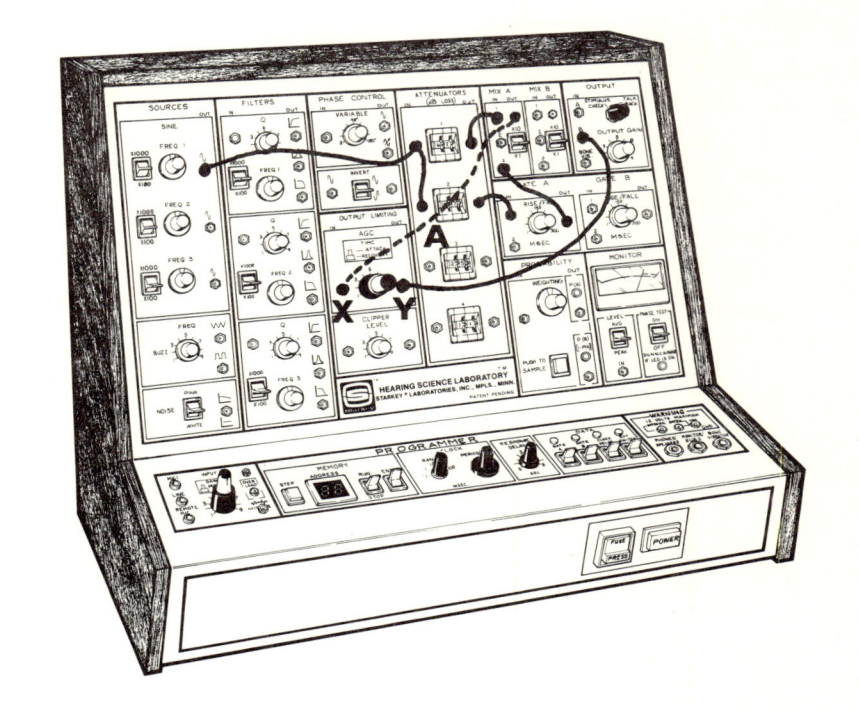

Purpose:
To examine the influence of compression amplification on transient signals.

Background Principle:
It is important to recognize the limitations of testing AGC circuits (as in the preceding experiment) or the hearing capabilities of a listener with steady state signals. The "real-world" sound environment is, after all, filled with ever changing transient sounds like speech, rather than invariant artificial tones. Tests of performance with "dynamic" sounds more closely approximate the conditions under which both the human and hearing aid must operate. A recent *Acoustical Society of America* standard for hearing aid AGC performance testing requires the use of a 2 kHz tone which abruptly alternates between two signal levels 25 dB apart. When such a dynamic stimulus is delivered to an AGC circuit, its output, when viewed on an oscilloscope, will be similar to the waveform shown earlier in Figure I-48. Varying the AGC attack and recovery times may have an effect, not only upon the waveform, but also upon the quality and intelligibility of speech signals passed through the system.

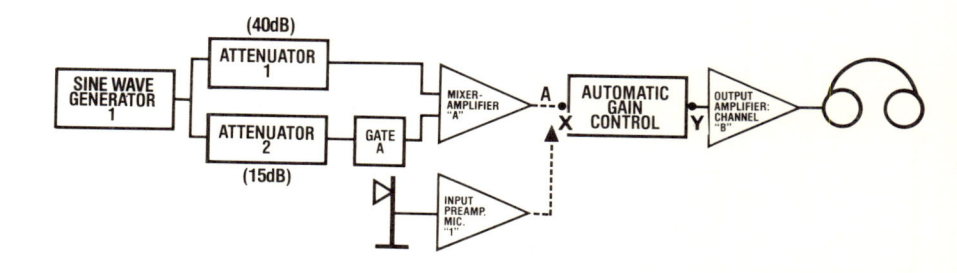

Procedure:
The pure tone signal is sent to two separate Attenuators. The output from Attenuator #1 is sent directly into a Mixer-Amplifier. The output from Attenuator #2 is passed through an Electronic Gate before it is combined with the first signal in the Mixer-Amplifier. Set Attenuator #2 to 15 dB and Attenuator #1 to 40 dB (i.e., 25 dB more attenuation). The suggested programming instructions permit the Gate "A" signal to add its higher intensity to the continuous lower level tone 50% of the time. The Mixer-Amplifier output is sent through the AGC module and finally to one Output Amplifier channel and headphone.

Exercises:
(1) Connect an oscilloscope probe to points labeled "X" and "Y" on the wiring guide and block diagram and note how the AGC module processes the test signal. Vary the Attack and Recovery Time Control Knobs and compare the oscilloscope waveforms you see with those shown in Figure I-48. (Note: for different attack and recovery times, it will be necessary to alter the Programmer Clock rate by adjusting the Period/Step Control in order to obtain the desired waveform pattern on the oscilloscope.)

(2) Disconnect dashed wire "A" from Mixer-Amplifier "A" and route it to the Output Jack of the Input Preamplifier. Use a microphone to send live speech signals to the Preamplifier and listen to the effect which AGC has upon connected discourse for various attack and release times. Note especially the effect of a short attack and long recovery time upon the smooth flow of continuous speech.

NOTES:

Selected References:

Blesser, B.A. (1969). Audio-dynamic range compression for minimum perceived distortion. *IEEE Trans. Audio-Electroacoustics*, **AU-17**, 22-32.

Caraway, B.J. and Carhart, R. (1967). Influence of compressor action on speech intelligibility. *J. Acoust. Soc. Am.*, **41**, 1424-1433.

Edgardh, B.H. (1952). The use of extreme limitation for the dynamic equalization of vowels and consonants in hearing aids. *Acta Oto-Lar.*, **40**, 376-386.

Kretsinger, E.A. and Young, N.B. (1960). The use of fast limiting to improve the intelligibility of speech in noise. *Speech Monogr.*, **27**, 63-69.

Lynn, G. and Carhart, R. (1963). Influence of attack and release in compression amplification. *J. Speech Hear. Dis.*, **28**, 124-140.

Nábělek, I.V. (1973). On transient distortion in hearing aids with volume compression. *IEEE Trans. Audio Electroacoustics*, **AU-21**, 279-285.

Nábělek, I.V. (1975). Amplitude compression in hearing aids. *J. Audio Eng. Soc.*, **23**, 213-216.

Niederjohn, R.J. and Grotelueschen, J.H. (1976). The enhancement of speech intelligibility in high noise levels by high-pass filtering followed by rapid amplitude compression. *IEEE Trans. Acoust. Speech, and Sig. Proc.*, **ASSP24**, 23-28.

Nunley, J. (1973). Automatic volume control instrumentation. *Hear. Instr.*, October.

Punch, J.L., Lawrence, W.F., and Causey, G.D. (1978). Measurement of attack-release times in compression hearing aids. *J. Speech Hear. Res.*, **21**, 338-349.

Schweitzer, H.C. and Causey, G.D. (1977). The relative importance of receiver time in compression hearing aids. *Audiology*, **16**, 61-72.

Trinder, E. (1972). An attempt to correct speech discrimination loss in cochlear deafness by graded instantaneous compression. *Sound*, **6**, 62-67.

Vargo, S. (1972). Compression amplification and hearing aids. *Maico Audiological Library Series*, Vol. 12.

Vargo, S. and Carhart, R. (1972). Amplitude compression on speech intelligibility in quiet with normal and pathological groups. *J. Acoust. Soc. Am.*, **53**, 327(A).

Villchur, E. (1973). Signal processing to improve speech intelligibility in perceptive deafness. *J. Acoust. Soc. Am.*, **53**, 1646-1656.

Wanink, A. (1975). The effect of limitation, compression factor and recovery time on sound production via AGC circuits. *Fenestra*, 12.

Yanick, P. (1973). Improvement in speech discrimination with compression vs. linear amplification. *J. Aud. Res.*, **13**, 333-338.

EXPERIMENT VIII-14: OSCILLOSCOPIC SPEECH DISPLAYS

Purpose:
To demonstrate two novel types of real-time visual displays for speech.

Background Principle:
Special intensive training is needed to assist the severely, or profoundly, hearing impaired child in the acquisition of speech and language. Numerous scientists and educators of the deaf have explored the use of instantaneous visual displays as one tool for providing feedback cues for the speech training of the deaf individual. Modern electronics now makes possible the display and storage of visual patterns produced by normal speech sounds so that the hearing impaired student may compare and match them with his or her own vocalizations. The *oscilloscope* visually displays electrical waveforms on a florescent screen. The typical patterns produced by speech sounds on such a device are, however, too complex for most speech training applications (see Figure "A"). Alternative electronic processing techniques can, however, be used to create simple visual patterns for speech on the oscilloscope. In one procedure (Pronovost, et al., 1968), speech signals are passed through phase-shifting networks that render the speech display in the form of a variety of circular oscilloscopic images (see Figure "B").

Yet another type of oscilloscopic display makes use of patterns named after the French physicist, Jules Antoine Lissajous (1822-1880), who first explored their nature. Lissajous patterns are created when the instantaneous amplitudes of two oscillations are displayed at a 90 degree angle to one another. For two sinusoids having identical frequencies and amplitudes, a circle, elipse, or straight line will be viewed on the oscilloscope, depending upon the phase relationship existing between the two component signals (see Figure "C"). A variety of simple and complex patterns are created when dissimilar signal frequencies are employed (see Figure "D"). Before the advent of more modern frequency measuring devices, Lissajous patterns provided a simple means of determining the frequency of an unknown signal. Specifically, a calibrated reference signal was paired with an unknown frequency sinusoid and adjusted until a circular pattern was obtained. The frequency of the unknown stimulus would then be equal to that of the known reference signal. Splitting a speech signal into two channels and presenting the separated components to the different input terminals of an oscilloscope can produce Lissajous-type images for speech training experiments.

Procedure:

(A) **"Circular" Speech display (After Pronovost, et al., 1968):**
Live microphone signals are routed through the Mic. 1 Preamplifier, the AGC module (which serves to control maximum display size), and the Variable Phase Shifter (adjusted to provide 90° phase shift). The Hear-

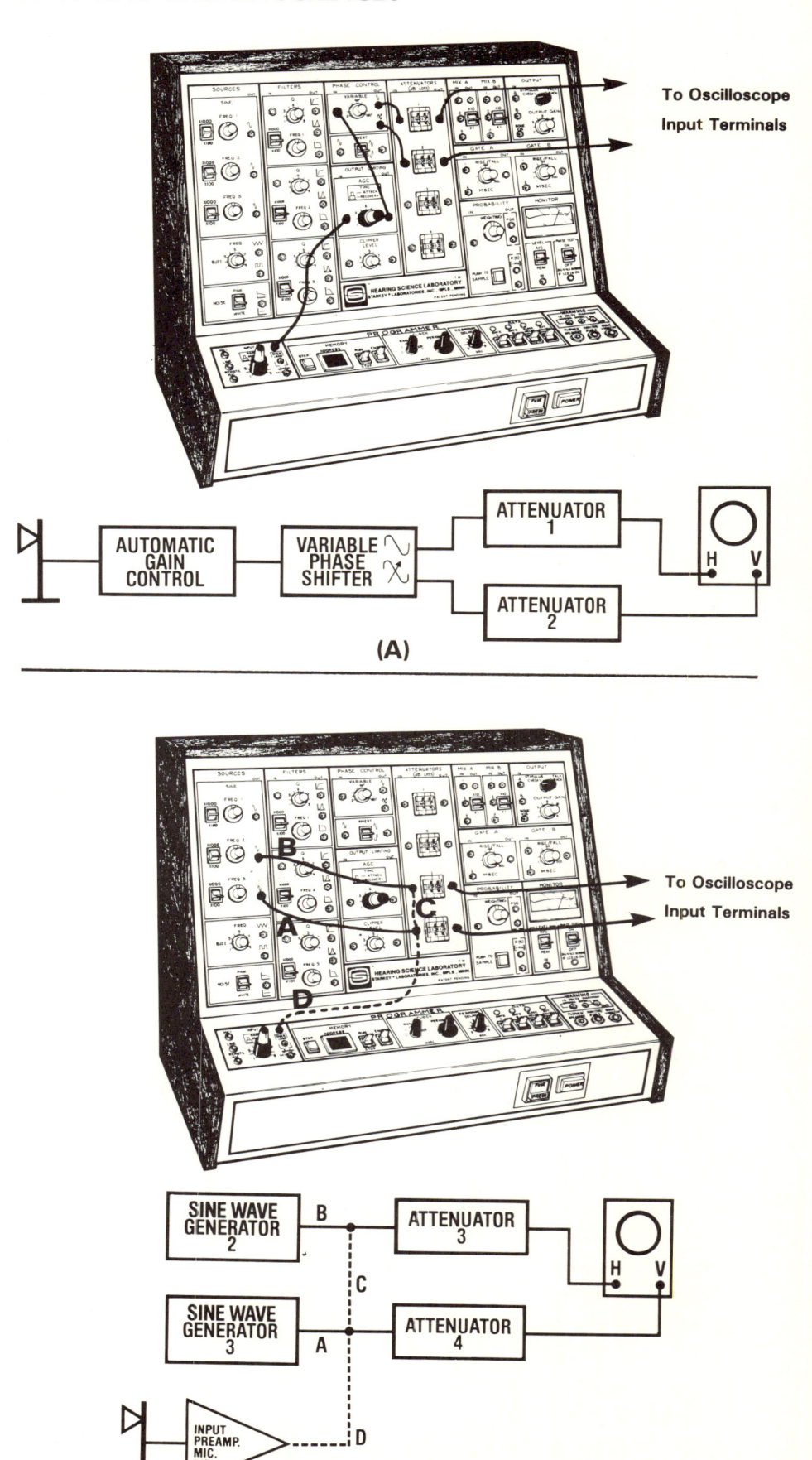

ing Science Laboratory Variable Phase Shifter will provide the same phase shift, in degrees, for frequencies between 100 Hz to 6000 Hz. The two Phase Shifter outputs are passed through separate Attenuators before being sent to the horizontal ("X") and vertical ("Y") input terminals of an oscilloscope. Adjustments of the Preamplifier Gain Control Knob and the Attenuators will alter the size of the oscilloscopic patterns.

(B) **Lissajous-Type Displays:**

(1) **For Tones:** Route two different sinusoids through separate Attenuators before they are sent to the "X" and "Y" input terminals of an oscilloscope. Observe the different patterns produced for various frequency combinations and signal levels.

(2) **For Speech:** Disconnect both pure tone signal wires "A" and "B". Connect dashed circuit wires "C" and "D", which will permit preamplified microphone signals to be routed to the input terminals of the oscilloscope. Adjust the Preamplifier Gain Control Knob and both Attenuators until a satisfactory image size is obtained on the scope.

Exercises:

(1) Examine the various patterns produced by procedures "A" and "B" above for individual speech sounds as well as connected discourse. Contrast the relative pattern complexity for several different classes of speech sounds, including: *fricatives* such as /s/, /z/, /f/, and /v/; *vowels* such as /o/, /e/, and /i/; and *plosives* such as /p/, /b/, /k/, and /g/. Sketch and characterize the basic patterns of each broad class of sounds.

(2) Examine each of the oscilloscopic patterns produced for exercise #1 in terms of its *sensitivity* to slight changes in the speaker's vocalization. Is one type of display more effective at revealing differences between speech sounds?

(3) Use an assortment of other signals to produce graphic displays on the oscilloscope. Note, for example, the visible differences produced by a variety of complex sounds that possess different spectral components (e.g., asymmetric and symmetric clipped sine waves, narrow band noises, synthetic vowels, and series of pulsed signals).

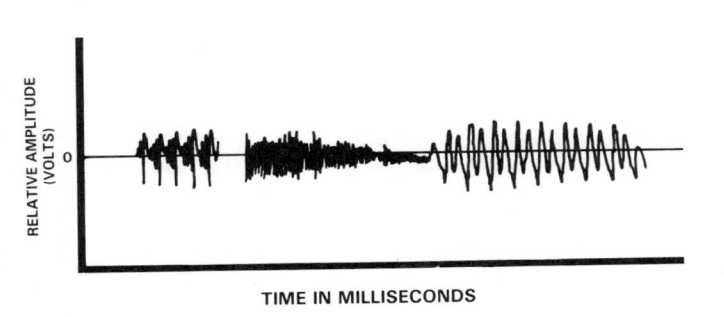

FIGURE A: Typical oscilloscopic display of brief sample of connected discourse.

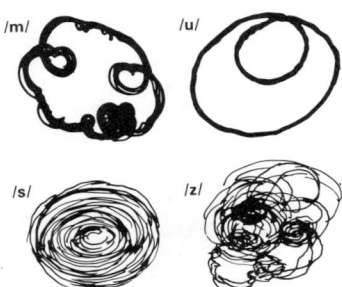

FIGURE B: "Voice Visualizer" patterns. (After Pronovost et al., 1968).

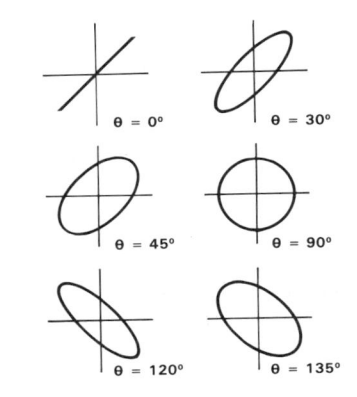

FIGURE C: Lissajous figures for two identical sinusoids which share different phase relationships.

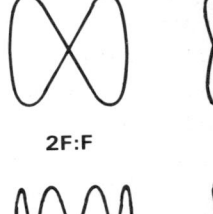

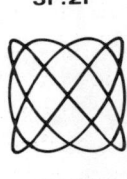

FIGURE D: Lissajous patterns for two sinusoids of differing frequency.

Selected References:

Børrild, K. (1968). Experiences with the design and use of technical aids for the training of deaf and hard of hearing children. *Am. Ann. Deaf,* **113,** 168-177.

Boston, D.W. (1973). Synthetic Facial Communication. *Brit. J. Audiol.,* **7,** 95-101.

House, A.S., Goldstein, D.F., and Hughes, G.W. (1968). Perception of visual transforms of visual stimuli: learning simple syllables. *Am. Ann. Deaf,* **113,** 215-221.

Kringlebotn, M. (1968). Experiments with some vibratactile and visual aids for the deaf. *Am. Ann. Deaf,* **113,** 311-317.

Phillips, N., Remillard, W., Pronovost, W., and Bass, S. (1968). Teaching of intonation to the deaf by visual pattern matching. *Am. Ann. Deaf,* **113,** 239-246.

Pickett, J.M. (Ed.) (1968). Proceedings of the conference on speech-analyzing aids for the deaf. *Am. Ann. Deaf,* **113,** 116-330.

Pickett, J.M. and Constam, A.A. (1968). Visual speech trainer with simplified indication of vowel spectrum. *Am. Ann. Deaf,* **113,** 253-258.

Pickett, J.M. (1971). Speech science research and speech communication for the deaf. In L.E. Conner (Ed.) *Speech for the deaf child: knowledge and use.* Alexander Graham Bell Association for the Deaf, Washington, D.C.

Potter, R.K., Kopp, G.A., and Kopp, H.G. (1966). *Visible Speech.* Dover Publications, Inc., New York.

Pronovost, W., Yenkin, L., Anderson, D.C., and Lerner, R. (1968). The voice visualizer. *Am. Ann. Deaf,* **113,** 230-238.

Risberg, A. (1968). Visual aids for speech correction. *Am. Ann. Deaf,* **113,** 178-194.

Stark, R., Cullen, J., and Chase, R. (1968) Preliminary work with the new Bell Telephone visible speech translator. *Am. Ann. Deaf,* **113,** 205-214.

Stark, R. (1971) The use of real-time visual displays of speech in the training of a profoundly deaf, non-speaking child: a case report. *J. Speech Hear. Dis.,* **36,** 397-409.

Upton, H. (1968). Wearable eyeglass speechreading aid. *Am. Ann. Deaf,* **113,** 222-229.

Appendix

EXPERIMENT   :

Purpose:

Background Principle:

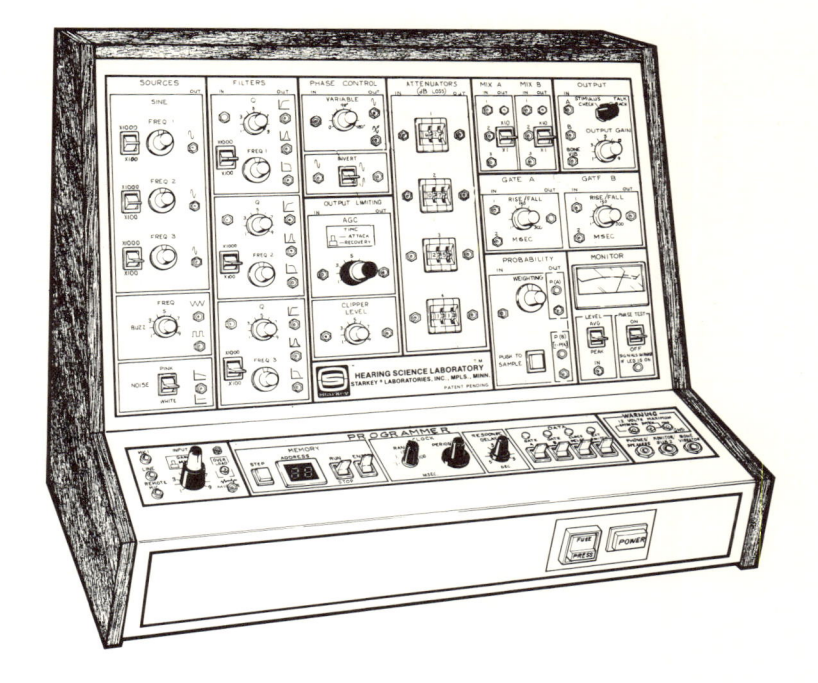

Exercises:

Procedure:

	CLOCK SETTINGS			MEMORY ADDRESS
RANGE SWITCH	PERIOD/ STEP CONTROL	RESPONSE DELAY	MEMORY CHANNEL	
			GATE "A"	
	Ⓧ		GATE "B"	
			CLOCK DELAY	
MILLISECONDS		SECONDS	EXT. SWITCH	

Block Diagram:

NOTES:

Selected References:

180

EXPERIMENTING IN THE HEARING AND SPEECH SCIENCES

EXPERIMENT   :

Purpose:

Background Principle:

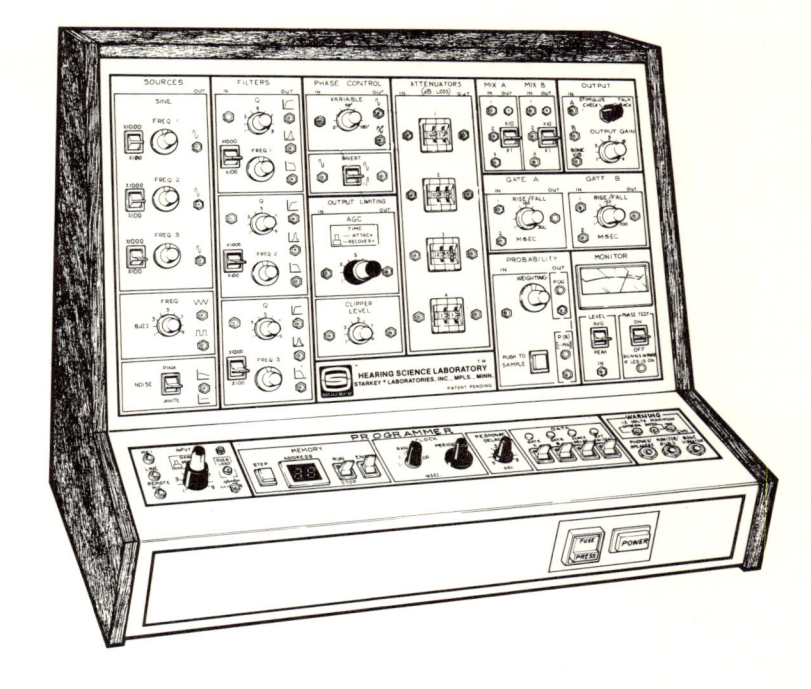

Exercises:

Procedure:

APPENDIX

CLOCK SETTINGS			MEMORY ADDRESS
RANGE SWITCH	PERIOD/ STEP CONTROL	RESPONSE DELAY	MEMORY CHANNEL
ⓧ			GATE "A"
^			GATE "B"
^			CLOCK DELAY
MILLISECONDS	SECONDS		EXT. SWITCH

Block Diagram:

NOTES:

Selected References:

EXPERIMENT   :

Purpose:

Background Principle:

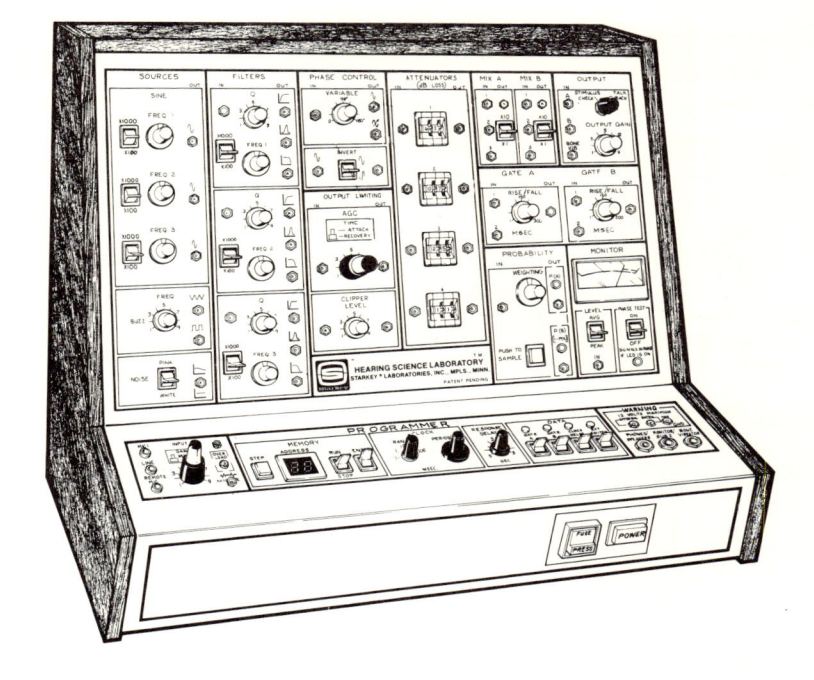

Exercises:

Procedure:

APPENDIX

CLOCK SETTINGS			MEMORY ADDRESS																						
RANGE SWITCH	PERIOD/ STEP CONTROL	RESPONSE DELAY	MEMORY CHANNEL																					
			GATE "A"																					
	⊗		GATE "B"																					
			CLOCK DELAY																					
MILLISECONDS		SECONDS	EXT. SWITCH																					

Block Diagram:

NOTES:

Selected References:

184

EXPERIMENT   :

Purpose:

Background Principle:

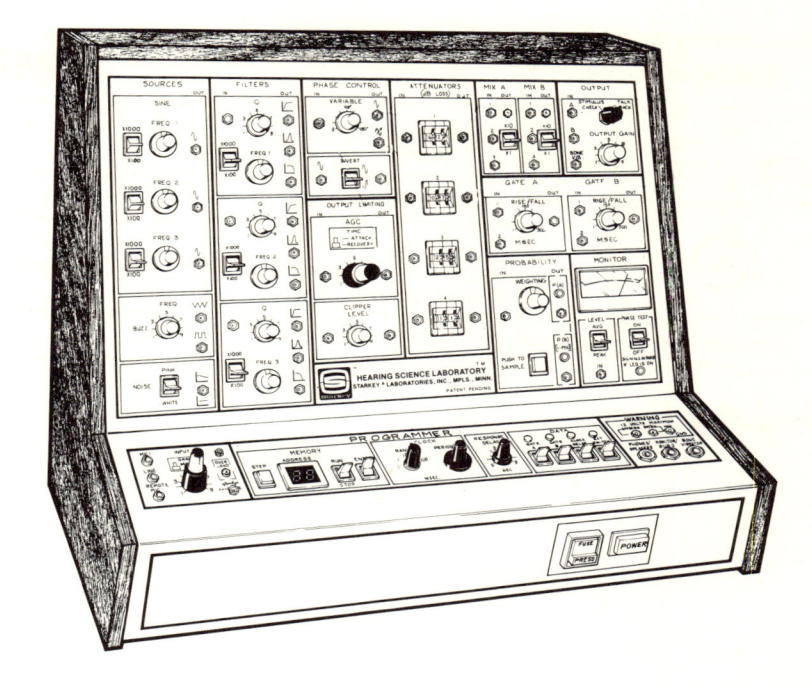

Exercises:

Procedure:

APPENDIX

CLOCK SETTINGS ||| MEMORY ADDRESS																							
RANGE SWITCH	PERIOD/ STEP CONTROL	RESPONSE DELAY	MEMORY CHANNEL																				
⊗			GATE "A"																				
			GATE "B"																				
			CLOCK DELAY																				
MILLISECONDS		SECONDS	EXT. SWITCH																				

Block Diagram:

NOTES:

Selected References:

EXPERIMENT   :

Purpose:

Background Principle:

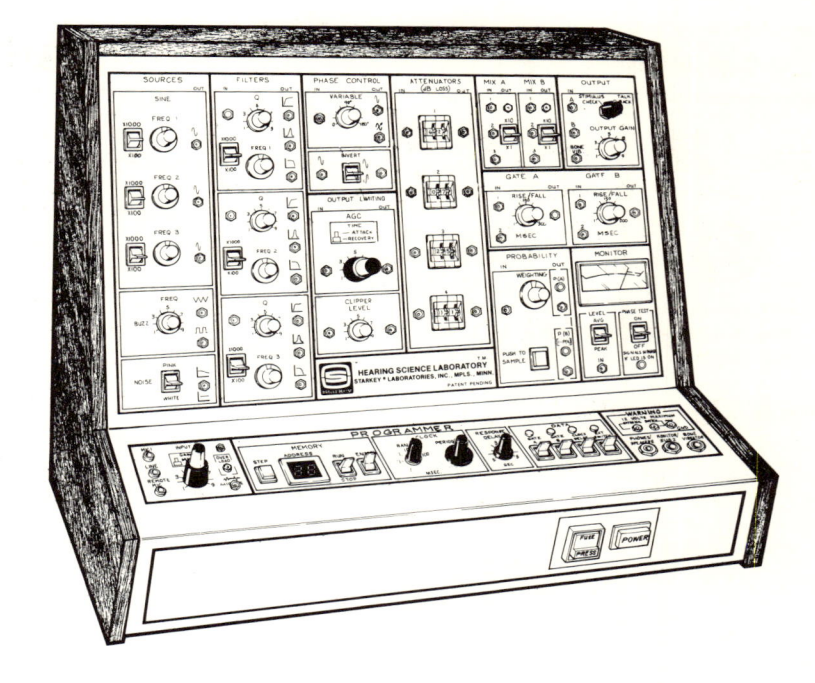

Exercises:

Procedure:

APPENDIX

CLOCK SETTINGS ||| MEMORY ADDRESS																								
RANGE SWITCH	PERIOD/ STEP CONTROL	RESPONSE DELAY	MEMORY CHANNEL																						
⊗			GATE "A"																						
^^^			GATE "B"																						
^^^			CLOCK DELAY																						
MILLISECONDS	^^^	SECONDS	EXT. SWITCH																						

Block Diagram:

NOTES:

Selected References:

188 EXPERIMENTING IN THE HEARING AND SPEECH SCIENCES

EXPERIMENT   :

Purpose:

Background Principle:

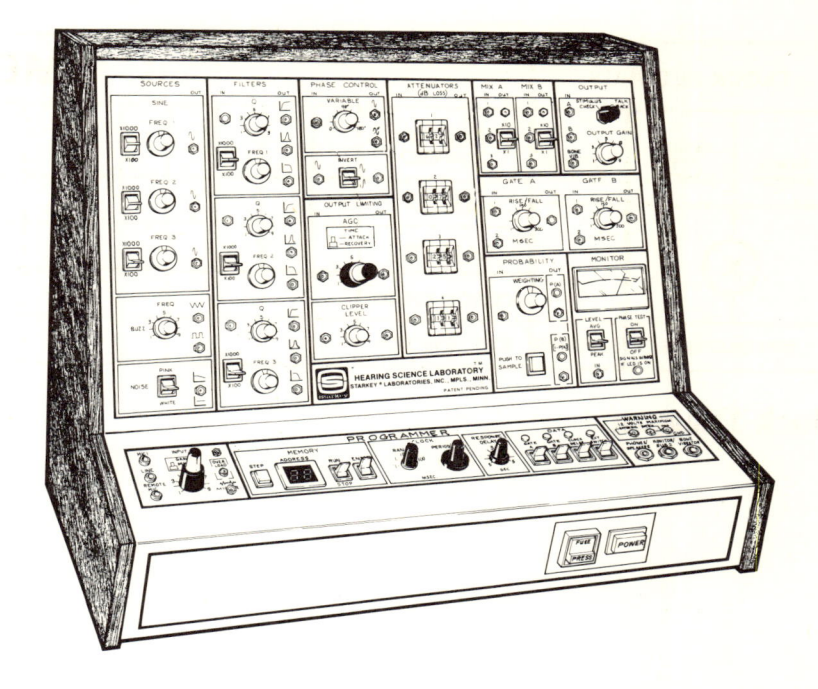

Exercises:

Procedure:

APPENDIX

CLOCK SETTINGS			MEMORY ADDRESS																						
RANGE SWITCH	PERIOD/ STEP CONTROL	RESPONSE DELAY	MEMORY CHANNEL																					
			GATE "A"																					
⊗			GATE "B"																					
			CLOCK DELAY																					
MILLISECONDS		SECONDS	EXT. SWITCH																					

Block Diagram:

NOTES:

Selected References:

Index

A. C. voltmeter, 37
AGC threshold, 25
Absorption, 144
Acoustical Society of America, 172
Adaptive procedures, 48
Air conduction, 24, 54, 56, 144
Alternate binaural loudness balance (ABLB), 70
Alternating current (AC), 162
Ambient air pressure, 4
American National Standards Institute (ANSI), 52
Amplification, 22
Amplitude, 4, 36
Amplitude spectrum, 13
Antilog, 115
Aperiodic signals, 13
Arithmetic graph rulings, 6
Articulation gain function, 152
Articulators, 150
Attack time, 26
Attenuation, 9, 10
Audiogram, 52
Audiology, 3
Audiometric threshold, 48
Automatic gain control (AGC), 25, 170-174
Average voltage values, 11, 36

Backward masking, 120
Band pass filter, 15
Band reject filter, 15
Bandwidth of a band pass filter, 16
Base number, 7
Beats, 80, 138
Beat frequency, 80
Bel, 7
Bell, A. G., 7
Best beats, 80
Bias, 162
Binaural beats, 138
Binaural fusion, 130, 156
Binaural hearing, 128-144
Bone conduction, 24, 54, 56
Bone conduction vibrator, 23, 24

Cancellation, 12, 30
Canonical signals, 98
Cascade connection, 17
Center frequency, 16
Central masking, 118
Coefficient, 7

Combination tone, 84
Comparison stimulus, 66
Complex sound, 32
Compression, 4, 170
Conductive hearing loss, 53
Consonance, 82
Consonants, 164
Continuity effect, 122
Continuous spectrum, 14
Contralateralization, 144
Correlated signals, 9
Critical bandwidth, 114
Critical ratio, 114
Crossover distortion, 165
Cutoff frequency, 15
Cycle, 4
Cycles per second, 4

Decibels (dB), 6-10
Decibels gain, 9
Decibels hearing level (dB HL), 52
Decibels intensity level (dB IL), 8
Decibels per octave (dB/oct), 16
Decibels sensation level (dB SL), 112
Decibels sound pressure level (dB SPL), 8
Detection index (d'), 47
Dichotic signals, 142, 166
Difference limen (DL), 60
Differential sensitivity, 90
Direct current (DC), 162
Discrimination score, 152
Dissonance, 82
Distortion, 24, 36, 84, 160, 164
Duty cycle, 102, 168
Dynamic range, 6

Echo suppression, 136
Electrolarynx, 150
Electronic switch, 18, 19
Envelope of waveform, 19
Equal loudness contours, 64
Equivalent duration of a signal, 99
Esophageal speech, 150
Exploring tone, 84
Exponents, 7
External auditory meatus, 54

Fall-time, 19
Feedback, 38
Filtering, 15

Filtered speech, 154, 166
Flutter fusion, 102
Formants, 148
Forward masking, 120
Fourier, J.B., 12, 32, 78
Free sound field, 134
Frequency, 4
Frequency domain, 13
Full-on amplitude, 19
Fundamental frequency, 13, 86, 148

Geometric mean, 16
Geometric scale, 6

Harmonics, 13, 160, 162
Headphones, 23
Hearing levels (dB HL), 52
Hearing threshold levels (dB HTL), 52
Hertz (Hz), 4
High pass filter, 15, 160
High tone emphasis, 160

Impedance, 16
In-phase, 5
In-series, 12
Initial stimulus value, 48
Input compression, 170
Input-output graph, 26
Instantaneous amplitude, 36
Integration of sound energy, 100
Intensity, 6, 59-74
Interaural attenuation, 144
Interference, 30
Interrupted speech, 168
Intervals (musical), 82
Inverse relationship, 4

Just noticeable difference (JND), 60, 62, 90, 142, 108

Lateralization, 54, 130-134
Law of superposition, 30
Light-emitting diode, 6
Line spectrum, 13-14
Linear function, 25, 68, 116
Linear ruled graph paper, 6
Lissajous, J. A., 174
Localization, 134-135
Log-log coordinates, 69
Logarithms, 7
Long-term spectrum of noise, 14

Long time average speech spectrum, 164
Loudness level, 64-65
Loudness recruitment, 70-73
Loudspeakers, 23
Low pass filter, 15
Lower AGC limit, 25

Masking level differences, 140, 141
Masking phenomena, 112-124, 140
Mastoid process of the temporal bone, 56
Maximum power output, 24
Mels, 88
Method of compensation, 144
Method of fractionation, 66
Method of limits, 48
Method of magnitude estimation, 68
Method of multiple stimuli, 66
Micropascals, 6
Missing fundamental, 86
Modulus, 68
Monophonic, 135

NU6 Lists, 152
Narrow bandwidth filter, 16
Numerosity, 106

Observation interval, 44
Occlusion effect, 54
Octave, 14, 162
Offset of signal, 17
Ogive curve, 42
Ohm, G. S., 78
Oscillate, 3
Oscilloscope, 32, 174
Onset of signal, 17
Ossicular-chain, 54
Out-of-phase, 5
Output compression, 170
Overshoot, 26

PB max, 152
Parallel connection, 15
Passband of a band pass filter, 16
Peak amplitude, 4, 36
Peak clipping, 24, 158-164
Peak-to-peak amplitude, 4, 36
Pedestal experiment, 62
Period of a wave, 4
Performance intensity function, 152
Phantom sound image, 134
Phase, 5, 6, 92, 142
Phase spectrum, 13
Phon line, 64

Phonation, 13
Phonetically balanced (PB) words, 152
Physical acoustics, 3
Pink noise, 15
Pitch, 74-92
Positive feedback, 38
Power, 6, 8, 36
Power amplifiers, 23
Power function, 69
Power of a number, 7
Precedence effect, 136
Pressure, 6, 8
Probability, 46
Probe tone, 84
Propagation of sound, 4
Psychoacoustics, 3
Psychometric function, 42
Psychophysical power law, 69
Pulsation threshold, 122
Pure tone audiometer, 52
Pure tones, 4, 98

Quality factor of a filter, 16

Rarefaction, 4
Ratio estimation, 66, 67
Ratio production, 66
Receiver operating characteristic (ROC), 46
Recovery time, 26
Recruitment, 70-72
Reference level, 7
Reinforcement, 11, 30
Release time, 26
Release from masking, 124, 140
Resonance, 16
Response time of a filter, 16
Rise-fall time, 18
Roll-off rate, 16
Root-mean-square (RMS) amplitude, 36

Saturation output level, 24
Scientific notation, 6
Selectivity of a filter, 16
Series conection, 15
Short increment sensitivity index (SISI), 62
Signal to noise ratio, 153
Simple harmonic motion, 3
Sine waves, 4
Sone scale, 66-68
Sound level meter, 9
Sound medium, 3
Spectrum, 13, 32
Spectrum level, 114

Speech perception, 148-174
Speech reception threshold (SRT), 152
Spondee words, 152
Square waves, 13
Standard stimulus, 66
Steady-state signal, 26
Stereophonic effect, 134
Stop band of a notch filter, 16
Switched speech, 156
Synthetic vowels, 148

Temporal integration, 100
Threshold of audibility, 41-56
Threshold of speech intelligibility, 152
Threshold shift, 112, 124
Time domain, 13
Tonality, 96-98
Transduction, 22
Transfer function, 170
Transformed up-down strategy, 50
Transient signal, 26, 98
Triangle wave, 13
True RMS meter, 37
Two interval forced choice (2IFC) technique, 50
Two-tone suppression, 124
Tympanic membrane, 54

Undershoot, 26
Unity gain, 10
Up-down technique, 49
Upward spread of masking, 112

Voltage, 9
Vowels, 164

Watts per square centimeter (W/cm^2), 6
Waveform graph, 4, 13
Weber, E. H., 60
Weber fraction, 60, 90
White noise, 14, 116
Wide band filter, 16
Work, 36

Yes-no procedure, 44

Zero reference point, 9